CULTURES OF CHILD HEALTH IN BRITAIN AND THE NETHERLANDS IN THE TWENTIETH CENTURY

THE WELLCOME SERIES IN THE HISTORY OF MEDICINE

Forthcoming Titles:

Dental Practice in Europe at the End of the Eighteenth Century
Edited by Christine Hillam

The Cape Doctor in the Nineteenth Century:
A Social History
Edited by Harriet Deacon, Howard Phillips
and Elizabeth Van Heyningen

War, Medicine and Britain, 1600-1815
Edited by Geoff Hudson and Roy Porter

Sex and Seclusion, Class and Custody
Perspectives on Gender and Class in the
History of British and Irish Psychiatry
Edited by Anne Digby and Jonathan Andrews

The Wellcome Series in the History of Medicine series editors are
V. Nutton, C. J. Lawrence and M. Neve.
Please send all queries regarding the series to Michael Laycock,
The Wellcome Trust Centre for the History of Medicine at UCL,
24 Eversholt Street, London NW1 1AD, UK.

CULTURES OF CHILD HEALTH IN BRITAIN AND THE NETHERLANDS IN THE TWENTIETH CENTURY

Edited by Marijke Gijswijt-Hofstra and Hilary Marland

Amsterdam – New York, NY 2003

First published in 2003
by Editions Rodopi B. V., Amsterdam – New York, NY 2003.

Gijswijt-Hofstra, Marijke and Marland, Hilary © 2003

Design and Typesetting by Michael Laycock,
The Wellcome Trust Centre for the History of Medicine at UCL.
Printed and bound in The Netherlands by Editions Rodopi B. V.,
Amsterdam – New York, NY 2003.

British Library Cataloguing in Publication Data
A catalogue record for this book is available from the British
Library
ISBN 90-420-1044-4 (Paper)
ISBN 90-420-1054-1 (Bound)

'Cultures of Childhealth in Britain and the Netherlands in the
Twenthieth Century' –
Amsterdam – New York, NY:
Rodopi. – ill.
(Clio Medica 71 / ISSN 0045-7183;
The Wellcome Series in the History of Medicine)

Front cover:
Image from a 1904 postscard of children photographed in a studio, with
the legend 'Croydon, Raw Material' underneath.
Courtesy, the *Wellcome Library,* London.

© Editions Rodopi B. V., Amsterdam – New York, NY 2003
Printed in The Netherlands

All titles in the Clio Medica series (from 1999 onwards) are available to
download from the CatchWord website: http://www.ingenta.com

Contents

Acknowledgements

This volume is based on papers presented at the Anglo-Dutch Workshop 'Child Health and National Fitness in the Twentieth Century', held at the University of Warwick, 9-11 July 1999. We would like to acknowledge the Wellcome Trust, the Research and Development Services Office at the University of Warwick, the Huizinga Instituut and the Gebiedsbestuur Geesteswetenschappen of the Nederlandse Organisatie voor Wetenschappelijk Onderzoek for their extremely generous funding of the conference. We would also like to warmly thank the Humanities Research Centre at Warwick for their financial support and particularly for the assistance of the Humanities Research Secretary, Sue Dibben, who contributed enormously to the smooth running of the Workshop.

The articles presented here owe a great deal to the comments of the participants at the Workshop, and their continued response with ideas and feedback subsequently; they have contributed much to the overall structure and content of the book. We are also indebted to the three referees who read through the chapters at an earlier stage and provided helpful feedback. Roy Porter and the other series editors at the Wellcome Trust Centre for the History of Medicine in London smoothed the process of taking the book through to production and offered encouragement throughout. Angela McShane Jones has been of inestimable help in the final stages in assisting with the correction of English.

Notes on Contributors

Nelleke Bakker is Associate Professor of the History of Education at the University of Groningen, the Netherlands. Her PhD on the history of child-rearing literature in the Netherlands (1845-1925) was published in 1995. She has published on a broad variety of themes from the history of Dutch education in edited volumes and journals, including *Paedagogica Historica, History of Education Quarterly* and the *Journal of Social History.*

Gemma Blok studied history at the University of Amsterdam. From 1995 to 1998 she worked at the Trimbos Instituut, the Netherlands Institute of Mental Health and Addiction in Utrecht, where she did research into the history of Dutch psychiatry. Together with Dr Joost Vijselaar, she has published several books on the history of psychiatric hospitals in the Netherlands. She is currently working on her PhD thesis on 'Antipsychiatry in the Netherlands', at the University of Amsterdam.

Roger Cooter was Professor of History and Director of the Wellcome Unit for the History of Medicine at the University of East Anglia, Norwich. He is the author of *The Cultural Meaning of Popular Science* (Cambridge University Press, 1984), *Surgery and Society in Peace and War* (Manchester University Press, 1993), and the editor of volumes on the history of alternative medicine, child health, the social relations of accidents, and war in connection with medicine and modernity. He recently co-edited with John Pickstone, *Medicine in the Twentieth Century* (Harwood International, 2000). Current work includes studies of the politics of rural medicine, food science, medical members of parliament, and a history of the practice and concept of medicalisation.

Marijke Gijswijt-Hofstra is Professor of Social and Cultural History at the University of Amsterdam. She has published on the granting of asylum in the Dutch Republic, deviance and tolerance, witchcraft and cultures of misfortune in the sixteenth to twentieth centuries, the reception of homoeopathy in the Netherlands, and on women and alternative health care in the Netherlands in the twentieth century. She has recently edited, with Godelieve van Heteren and Tilli Tansey, *Biography of Remedies: Drugs, Medicines and Contraceptives in Dutch and Anglo-American Healing Cultures* (Rodopi, 2002), and, with Roy Porter, *Cultures of Neurasthenia from Beard to the First World War* (Rodopi, 2001). She is currently working on the history of psychiatry and mental health care in the Netherlands in the twentieth century.

Lyubov Gurjeva is a Research Associate at the Centre for the History of Science, Technology and Medicine at the University of Manchester, where she is working on a project entitled 'From the Patient's Point of View: Health and Healing in Russia, 1945-2000' (funded by the Wellcome Trust). She was educated at Moscow State University, the University of Amsterdam and the University of Cambridge. Her thesis was entitled 'Everyday Bourgeois Science: The Scientific Management of Children in Britain, 1880-1914' (University of Cambridge, 1998), and she has published various articles on the subject of the creation of expertise and transmission of knowledge on childhood in Britain around 1900.

Ido de Haan is a researcher in the Department of History at the University of Amsterdam. He has published books and articles on political philosophy and Dutch political history, on collective memory and the persecution of the Jews. He is now working on a project on institutional and cultural reconstruction after large-scale violence in France and the Netherlands.

Bernard Harris is Senior Lecturer in Social Policy in the Department of Sociology and Social Policy at the University of Southampton. He is author of *The Health of the Schoolchild: A History of the School Medical Service in England and Wales* (Open University Press, 1995), and he is currently completing a book on the history of welfare provision in Britain between 1800 and 1945.

Harry Hendrick is an Associate Professor in the Institute of History at the University of Southern Denmark. His principal publications are *Images of Youth: Age, Class and the Male Youth*

Problem, 1880-1920 (Clarendon Press, 1990), *Child Welfare. England, 1872-1989* (Routledge, 1994), *Children, Childhood and English Society, 1880-1990* (Cambridge University Press, 1997). He is currently working on a study, *Children and Grown Ups since the Eighteenth Century* for London Books.

Mark Jackson is Reader in the History of Medicine in the Department of History at the University of Exeter. After qualifying in medicine in 1985, he pursued doctoral research in the social history of infanticide. More recently, he has been researching not only the history of feeble-mindedness in Britain but also the history of allergic diseases, such as asthma and hay fever, in the modern world. His publications include *New-Born Child Murder: Women, Illegitimacy and the Courts in Eighteenth-Century England* (Manchester University Press, 1996), *The Borderland of Imbecility: Medicine, Society and the Fabrication of the Feeble Mind in Late Victorian and Edwardian Britain* (Manchester University Press, 2000), as well as several edited volumes and numerous articles.

Hilary Marland is Reader in History and Director of the Centre for the History of Medicine at the University of Warwick. She is former editor of *Social History of Medicine*, and has published on midwifery and childbirth in the Netherlands, nineteenth-century medical practice, women and medicine, and infant and maternal welfare. She is currently working on puerperal insanity in nineteenth-century Britain and preparing a monograph study, *Dangerous Motherhood: Insanity and Childbirth in the Nineteenth Century.*

Hugo Röling is Associate Professor in the History of Education at the University of Amsterdam. He has published mainly on the history of childhood and the family and on the history of sex education in the Netherlands. His next book will be a history of childhood based on nineteenth- and twentieth-century memories of youth in the Netherlands and Belgium.

Deborah Thom is a Fellow of Robinson College Cambridge and lectures on twentieth-century British history in the Faculties of History and Social and Political Sciences and the Department of History and Philosophy of Science. She has published on the history of women's employment, war, child psychology and education. Her book *Nice Girls and Rude Girls: Women Workers and the First World War* was published by I.B. Tauris in 1998.

John Welshman was educated at the Universities of Oxford and York and his main area of interest is the history of health care and social policy. He is author of numerous articles in this field, and of *Municipal Medicine: Public Health in Twentieth-Century Britain* (Peter Lang, 2000). He is currently based in the Institute for Health Research at Lancaster University, where he is Lecturer in Public Health.

Ido Weijers teaches the history of education at the University of Utrecht. He wrote his dissertation *Terug naar het behouden huis. Romanschrijvers en wetenschappers in de jaren vijftig* (Back to the Safe House. Novelists and Scientists in the 1950s) in 1991. He has written extensively on the history of mental retardation and on the history and theory of juvenile justice. His latest books are *Schuld en schaamte. Een pedagogisch perspectief op het jeugdstrafrecht* (2000) (Guilt and Shame. A Pedagogical Perspective on Juvenile Criminal Justice) and *De creatie van het mondige kind. Geschiedenis van pedagogiek en jeugdzorg* (2001) (The Creation of the Mature Child. A History of Pedagogics and Child Welfare). He is currently working on the history of Dutch psychiatry in the twentieth century.

1

Introduction:
Cultures of Child Health in Britain and the Netherlands in the Twentieth Century

Hilary Marland and Marijke Gijswijt-Hofstra

The twentieth century was pronounced by politicians and reformers in various national settings as the 'century of the child'. Late nineteenth-century reforms regulating children's employment and education set the scene for a redefinition of the child as being less a unit of labour and more an object of care.[1] The narrow vision of the child as a worker pure and simple developed into a wider-ranging concept of citizenship to encompass the child as a pupil and a responsibility of the state, who could be entitled to care and assistance. The child's contribution to the national good would no longer be measured in current physical toil but in terms of future citizenship and ability to contribute to the needs of the state as part of the future labour force. These shifts in ideas were put into effect through a range of educational and social welfare initiatives during the early twentieth century. Initially, such action was framed very much in the language of national efficiency and national fitness, but the requirements of the state subsequently became enmeshed with the needs of children as individuals. The movement to give children a 'proper childhood' became well established early in the twentieth century,[2] as childhood was recognised as a distinct phase of life, children having special needs and rights, which added up to more than a concern with national good. Yet, it could be argued at the same time that children were in many ways still regarded as citizens in the making, requiring care, guidance, and sometimes compulsion to enable them to contribute to the general welfare of the nation.

It was under the heading of 'child health and national fitness' that a group of British and Dutch academics met together at the University of Warwick in July 1999. However, as the essays in this volume show, the dominance of national efficiency as a theme was challenged, particularly within a comparative framework. The articles contained in this volume are based on the pre-circulated

7

papers presented at the workshop, mediated by the contributions of the invited commentators and participants.[3] Many themes emerged from the discussions, with the papers engaging with child health and welfare in its broadest sense: infant welfare, school medicine, sport and physical education, mental hygiene and health, child psychology, corporal punishment, sex education, and children's experiences of institutional care. The workshop also reflected on Roger Cooter's landmark collection of essays, *In the Name of the Child*, published in 1992. The papers spoke to and developed a number of the themes covered in Cooter's volume, allowing for reflection about how historical research on the child as a subject of educational, welfare and health policies has moved on in the intervening decade. Appropriately, Roger Cooter has contributed the final chapter to this volume.

Through our selection of the title *Cultures of Child Health* we could well be accused of misrepresentation, for there is little in the chapters to follow on illness, curative medicine, paediatrics, the child as patient, or images of the sick child.[4] The contents of the book reflect the fact that the history of the sick child has not advanced far,[5] and certainly warrants more work, while the child as an object of welfare has attracted more attention by historians particularly over the last decade.[6] What we have set out to achieve are ways of understanding child health provision in Britain and the Netherlands in its broadest sense, linked to welfare and the creation of new preventative medical services, with education, with the care of those deemed mentally deficient and the psychologisation of society.

How can we define 'the child' in terms of age and how can we map changing definitions over time? The boundaries between infant and child (and pre-school child) and between childhood and adolescence, that starts to emerge as a category early in the twentieth century, and even more so after the Second World War, are difficult to pin down. According to the historian John Gillis, the category 'adolescents' came into usage at the end of the nineteenth century in England, while in the Netherlands this group started to be distinguished by the 1920s.[7] In the Netherlands, distinctions were also drawn by the late-nineteenth century between the child and 'youth' (*jeugd*) in regulating care and provision, categories not replicated in Britain in quite the same way, 'juvenile' coming to have a stronger association with delinquency. For the purposes of this volume we have broadly accepted 'the child' as being school-aged, between the ages of 4 and 14, and most of the essays focus on this age group, while also exploring the boundaries between these categories in the two countries.

As indicated, the purpose of much action in connection with the health and welfare of the child in the twentieth century was predicated on the idea of the child as citizen in the making. As there was a shift in thinking about the child as an actual worker to a future worker, so too did child health concerns tend to shift from the immediate to the future. This in part was due to a dramatic fall in death rates, particularly the infant mortality rate, across Western Europe.[8] Once epidemic disease was in decline, and once infant mortality rates began to drop after 1900, attention moved from issues of preventing deaths to longer-term health issues. This included, as many of the essays show, the invocation of proper child-rearing practices, the education of families and mothers, and safeguarding the child's ability to obtain an education and then participate in the workforce. As a result, the topic of child health in the twentieth century has in many ways far stronger links with notions of 'fitness' and 'welfare' than with illness *per se*. The early twentieth century saw emphasis shift from addressing infection, disease and death, to concerns about the quality of populations and anxieties about the feeble or mentally defective child. The eugenics movement highlighted these concerns around the period of the First World War and into the 1930s, although its impact in practical terms was limited in both Britain and the Netherlands.[9] Prior to governments expressing the will to ensure better health for all children, it was the infant who first symbolised fears of national decline - falling populations and enfeebled populations - particularly around the time of the Boer and First World Wars. It was the emaciated and sickly infant that became symbolic of national anxieties about populations in decline, qualitatively and quantitatively, and re-enforced fears about falling middle-class fertility.[10] Yet, at the same time, the infant was held up as the nation's hope, expressed emblematically through the 'infant soldier', 'bringing up the reinforcements'.[11] Services, however, for infant and then older children, were to be largely about prevention or damage limitation rather than removing the root causes of poverty.

Agents involved in improving physical and mental welfare - doctors, social workers, psychiatrists, and so on - would make further shift in the mid-twentieth century, to emphasise the importance of the individual child's development and achievement, from children with special problems to all children. Childhood at the same time became more socially homogeneous and reconstructed in largely psycho-medical terms.[12]

Background

By the turn of the twentieth century the child's move in Britain and the Netherlands from the factory and workshop[13] to school and home was underway.[14] The working-class child was turned slowly 'from a component of the labour force into a subject of education'.[15] In 'a progressive lengthening of childhood as a stage in life',[16] in the 1840s the age of 8 became established as the minimum for half-time employment in textile mills in England, and by the 1860s this had been extended to many other industries. During the 1870s the minimum age was raised to 10, while certain tasks were recognised as being unsuitable for children. The number of children employed as 'half-timers' tumbled in the 1880s, although the Education Act of 1902 permitted 12-14 year old children to combine work with school attendance, a provision which remained in force until the Fisher Act of 1918. The regulation of child labour commenced later in the Netherlands, but when it was introduced in 1874 with the Kinderwetje (Children's Law) of Sam van Houten, it went much further, forbidding the employment of children below the age of 12 in factories. Further restrictions followed in the Arbeidswet (Labour Law) of 1889, extending control over children aged between 12 and 16, banning night work and Sunday employment, and introducing a maximum 11 hour day with proper breaks.

Early in the twentieth century, the child became the focus of attention in other areas of law and policy-making. In England and Wales Forster's 1870 Education Act saw the introduction of legislation giving school boards the power to make primary education compulsory in their districts; this was made compulsory across the whole country in 1880. A series of acts was also passed during the last quarter of the nineteenth century seeking to prevent child cruelty, neglect and exploitation.[17] Concern about child protection in the Netherlands culminated in a cluster of Kinderwetten (Children's Acts) in 1901, which came into force in 1905. These dealt with the punishment of juvenile offenders, the protection of neglected children, provision for criminal youths, the regulation of parental authority over their children and proper conditions of guardianship. Compulsory schooling for children aged between 6 and 12 was introduced in 1900. In both countries issues relating to child welfare, health and education came to the forefront of national debate. A number of social surveys of the late nineteenth and early twentieth centuries (including those of state committees investigating the mental and physical condition of working children in the Netherlands, and of Charles Booth in London and Seebohm Rowntree in York), provided detailed evidence on the status of children and their conditions of work and life.

In Britain where 'childhood became inextricably implicated in the most critical public issues of the time',[18] the condition and status of the child was closely bound up with concerns of national efficiency and citizenship, and the early twentieth century saw a proliferation of services and experts dealing with child health and welfare. Mothers were urged not to abdicate their responsibilities by choosing paid employment over motherhood, and great concern was also expressed about family limitation and abortion. In the Netherlands, Catholics and Orthodox Calvinists encouraged families to have large numbers of children and both prohibited birth control, but in general there was less concern about family limitation.[19] In the Netherlands fewer women worked in factories or were confronted by the lure of paid work. Nor did the War years provide a major stimulus to female employment, as the Netherlands remained neutral in World War I and was occupied in World War II.[20] Fertility rates remained high in the Netherlands compared with other European nations, with an exceptional baby boom after World War II.

Despite the very different demographic experiences of the two countries, the needs of the child were addressed through a similar gamut of new or expanded services, dealing principally with infant welfare and the health of the school child. Infants were the first to receive state and voluntary attention, with local government bodies, charities and denominational organisations setting up clinics to weigh and inspect babies, and to advise and school mothers on feeding and hygiene. In the Netherlands, these would mainly be organised through *Kruisverenigingen* (Cross Societies), private organisations, first neutral and then also Catholic and Protestant, which after the 1870s dealt with disease prevention, district nursing, health education, tuberculosis, and infant welfare. In 1908 the *Nederlandsche Bond voor Moederschapszorg en Kinderhygiene* (Dutch Society for Maternal Care and Child Hygiene) was set up, and *consultatiebureaus*, infant welfare centres, were further stimulated by the *Gezondheidswet* (Health Act) of 1919, which established a separate inspectorate for child health, and by the introduction of government subsidies in 1927; by 1929 there were a total of 246 *bureaus* across the country.[21] In England and Wales the first infant milk depots were set up after 1902, and voluntary infant welfare clinics from 1907 onwards, government grants were introduced in 1912 for medical treatment and in 1913 for medical inspection.[22]

11

Infant welfare centres proliferated in the 1920s and 1930s to reach a total of 3,145 in 1937, [23] advice literature was produced in reams, and teams of health visitors monitored the condition of the infant at home, some 5,350 by 1937. Notification of births was first introduced in 1907 giving local authorities the power to insist on notification of birth in their areas and the Notification of Births (Extension) Act made this compulsory throughout the whole country in 1915. This was long after a system of notifying the Dutch municipal authorities of births, marriages and deaths had been established when in 1810 the Kingdom of Holland was incorporated into the French Empire.

By the 1920s attention was turning in many European countries to the welfare of mothers prompted by persistently high maternal death rates. This rate had levelled off at a much lower plateau in the Netherlands, due largely to its well-trained domiciliary midwife services.[24] The provision of material aid took a poor second-place to advice and education, though some countries established maternity benefits in an attempt to deflect falling birth rates and to give financial incentives to mothers giving birth and raising children in poverty.[25] The British National Insurance Act of 1911 included cash maternity benefits for insured women and the wives of insured men, and the Maternity and Child Welfare Act of 1918 encouraged the further development of local maternity clinics and services. Family allowances were introduced in most European countries in the 1930s and 1940s: in the Netherlands in 1941 for labourers, and later to all families with children in 1963, in Britain in 1945.[26]

From the end of the nineteenth century, the Dutch Cross Societies tackled general child health and school medicine as well as infant welfare, and from 1901 the medical inspection of school children was instituted under the auspices of the public health authorities. In England and Wales school medical inspection was introduced on a national basis in 1907.[27] In both countries the focus on improving the child's physical status, particularly that of the urban child, led to the establishment of summer camps, open-air schools and tuberculosis sanatoria.[28] Sport came to fulfil a social function, but also to place emphasis on fitness of body and mind, preparedness to work and to fight.

Clinics for nervous and mental illness, care for mentally defective children and child psychiatry clinics were also set up by the Cross societies, or by other private organisations or indeed by local or provincial authorities in the Netherlands, and by the private and voluntary sectors and later local authorities in Britain.[29] *Medisch*

Opvoedkundige Bureaus (Medical-Pedagogical Bureaus) were established from 1928, and, by the end of the 1930s, seven MOBs had been set up in the Western, urbanised provinces of the Netherlands. Concern with mental hygiene developed in the early twentieth century with efforts to redefine and refine definitions of the 'feeble-minded', and base classification on educability, ability to work and proximity to citizenship.[30] In the 1940s and 1950s a new wave of advice books appeared, with Benjamin Spock and John Bowlby becoming pre-eminent and widely available in both countries, offering guidance on socialisation and the mental and emotional wellbeing of children. At this point it could be argued that a new phase was entered, as the potential for problems was seen as not resting with the individual child but with the family unit. So too was emphasis in terms of health and welfare needs focused increasingly on the normal child, rather than the physiologically or mentally handicapped child.

Themes:
Cultures of child care

One of the more striking aspects of this volume is the varied engagement with the subject of child health on the part of English and Dutch scholars, which may be an accurate representation of the differing concerns historically in connection with child health and welfare issues. While the English, perhaps living up to national typologies, have worked around the topics of physical health, physical education and sport, and role of beating as punishment, particularly focusing on the period before the Second World War, Dutch research has placed much more emphasis on the 'psychologisation' of the child, particularly in the post-Second World War period.

Issues around definitions and the use of different frameworks were also encountered during the course of the workshop. In particular, the concepts of national efficiency and pillarization (*verzuiling*) were challenged as setting too narrow an agenda, and their value to the historian as models and analytical tools was also questioned. Yet, we were also interested to see how persistent these models were throughout the twentieth century. At the turn of the twenty-first century the concept of national efficiency does not seem to have withered away altogether. This is demonstrated by the current debates in Britain about under-achievers, boys who fail to meet their potential in schools geared as they are increasingly to 'national' curricula, as compared with the ambition to impose a minimum level of education at the beginning of the century. Concern with obesity amongst children has replaced anxieties about under-nourishment and feebleness, while the drug estate youth has substituted the street Arab and juvenile delinquent as an object of public anxiety. The *bête noire* at the close of the twentieth century was no longer the mother who 'claimed to know all about childbearing and childrearing because she had "born 12 and buried 8"',[31] but the single, welfare mother, a burden to the state and society because of her moral ineptitude and inability to work to support her family. Writing in his typical strain in *The Sunday Times* of 13 February 2000, the American right-wing academic, Charles Murray, expressed grave concern about the growth of a British 'underclass'. Based on three indicators - dropout from the labour force amongst young males, violent crime, and births to unmarried women - Murray predicted 'the growth of a class of violent, unsocialised people who, if they become sufficiently numerous, will fundamentally degrade the life of society'.[32] Current debates in the Netherlands focus rather more on questions of ethnicity, with media discussions referring to an unfolding 'multicultural drama' and the formation of an 'ethnic underclass'. With reference to children in particular, the press in recent years has printed numerous articles expressing concern about schools dominated by one ethnic group and the effect of this upon levels of education.

Differences of approach as well as topic between Britain and the Netherlands became evident during the course of the workshop. Questions of national fitness and efficiency have, if not dominated, then at least played a very large role, in directing the focus of research into child health and welfare in Britain. This has been demonstrated particularly in work on the health and wellbeing of infants and school children, and more recent studies focusing on mental hygiene and fitness. In the Netherlands, industrialisation took off much later, with the 1890s initiating a period of economic growth and modernisation. The country largely missed out on the worst horrors of industrialisation and child labour, which may explain in part at least why legislation regulating labour was introduced later than in England. Involvement in the First World War was confined to aiding refugees, and, though concern with the health and strength of future generations was expressed in the Netherlands, it was offset by a constantly rising population. Under German occupation in the Second World War, the Netherlands was not confronted with the problems of mass recruitment and concerns about the physical and mental fitness of the forces. A law introducing compulsory health insurance was passed under German occupation in 1941 (the *Ziekenfondswet*),[33] reducing regional differences and ensuring health care for the poor. Yet the country was very concerned about its children, particularly following the deprivations of the '*hongerwinter*' of 1944-45. After the war there was much anxiety about the moral degeneration of young people, juvenile delinquency, and child neglect; Jewish foster children, children whose parents had been interned and those returning from the Dutch East Indies were singled out for particular attention.[34] More than in Britain, there was a sense of a generation of children who had missed out on childhood, and who were physically and mentally scarred by the war, and 'spiritually uprooted'.

The link between child health and national fitness turned out to be a troublesome one, a concept which could be said to have been over-used by historians as an explanatory model, and often with little subtlety (see the discussions in the essays of Harris and Welshman). It is argued that ideas concerning national efficiency had a role to play in policy decisions for much of the twentieth century in assessing the future development of the child. But it is also clear that we need to see these ideas as being subject to enormous change during the twentieth century, as different aspects of child health were prioritised, and as relations changed between the state, community, family and children. Several of the papers offer more nuanced ways forward in dealing with the concepts of national fitness and citizenship. It has been pointed out that we must also be careful to make distinctions between theory and rhetoric and practice and implementation. National fitness does not emerge as *the* dominant theme of this book, but it figures in the chapters in many important ways. It would be better to frame the book as being focused on different ways in which children or the idea of the child have been configured in different welfare or health related debates, and how this interacted with changing ideas on fitness and citizenship in both national settings.

While ideas of national fitness have played a key role in focusing historical research in Britain, Dutch scholarship in many areas of health and welfare has been shaped by the concept of 'pillarization'. Though this arrangement has been described as rapidly breaking down since the 1970s, the provision of and the rationale behind the establishment and organisation of services was linked up until then to 'pillars', determined by belief systems, religion and world-view rather than social-economic condition and class. Dutch society has been 'pillarized' since the last quarter of the nineteenth century, broken into the pillars of, for example, Roman Catholic, Orthodox Calvinist, Social Democrat and Liberal, and the much smaller Jewish pillar. Public life was organised along the lines of different pillars 'living apart together', and covered numerous aspects of social and cultural life: health and welfare, schools, youth organisations, infant welfare services, sports facilities, clubs, housing associations, health institutions, even the media and the universities. Other 'neutral' bodies also carried out activities in the fields of health and welfare, set up by law and supported by public monies, including a system of medical inspection and the expanding public health machinery, which employed its own doctors and sanitary inspectors.[35]

The state accommodated and supported the system of pillarization. State subsidies were allocated to the pillars, according to the principle of proportionality, and the presence of this intermediate layer of ideologically-based private organisations, distributing money for educational, medical, social, and cultural purposes, became a salient feature of the Dutch welfare state in the twentieth century. Pillarization saw the development of a cradle-to-grave pluralistic organisation of society, which provided a strong sense of identity and social cohesion, which has been said to override considerations of class, national or regional forms of solidarity and in some cases even kinship.[36] Pillarization complicates ideas of national fitness, as the promotion of national fitness was seen in part at least as being the task of different pillars, as well as the state. Pillarization also seems to have mitigated against the emergence of a large voluntary sector, in contrast to Britain where voluntarism balanced out state involvement in many areas of health and welfare (although the balance between state, local provision and the voluntary sector varied considerably from region to region and town to town).[37] Only after the Second World War and the setting up of the National Health Service in 1948, which extended free medical treatment to women and children, did the role of the voluntary sector diminish in Britain.[38]

National efficiency and pillarization have been key in shaping research and research questions in Britain and the Netherlands respectively, and perhaps have acted as a limitation on other ways of thinking about social processes and change. As De Haan argues in his chapter, however, liberal thinking greatly influenced law and regulation before and also during the period of pillarization. There was great consensus between the liberal and confessional groups too on areas concerning the morals and welfare of children. Many organisations continued to work throughout the period of pillarization without a strong denominational colouring. Pillarization also modified ideas of national efficiency, citizenship, and the rights and duties of individuals *vis à vis* the state in the Netherlands, but certainly did not do away with these ideas altogether.

Ido de Haan's article offers a comprehensive introduction to the topic of national fitness and citizenship. He takes on board issues of child labour and health, physical and mental embodiment, the role of the child as client, and the shifts in concerns reflecting the changing political and social environment in the Netherlands from the late nineteenth century through to the years after the Second World War, through phases defined as 'liberal citizenship', 'citizenship within ideological bounds', and 'citizenship as self-development'. De Haan's paper takes citizenship as its core theme, describing conceptions that shaped policy decisions, of the child as incomplete, undeveloped, irresponsible and weak, needing projection and care, not as a right, but in order to become a complete 'rights-bearing' citizen. He also traces the debates about the form of support children needed to become good citizens, and on the kind of citizen that they were supposed to develop into. The evolving story is one of the mental and bodily status of children as it pertains to nation and state building, and interrelated change in the concepts of human development and citizenship.

Several of the contributions further develop the notion of citizenship, examining different ways in which concepts of health, citizenship and class can be approached and linked. They point to the strong links between educatability and health, either in terms of ideas of regeneration through education or the necessity of a healthy physique to facilitate learning (Welshman, Harris, Jackson, Röling). John Welshman examines sport and physical education to test his supposition that the 'movement for national efficiency was a key influence on the development of child health and welfare in Britain' during the period 1900-1940. Focusing on changes in emphasis during periods of 'imagined' crisis in the 1900s and 1930s, he stresses, referring to Searle's influential work,[39] that national efficiency is not a homogeneous political label, but a complex series of beliefs, assumptions and demands. Tracing the ideological background to health policy, particularly through the work and writings of George Newman, Chief Medical Officer to the Board of Education (1907-35) and to the Ministry of Health (1919-35), he points to the complexities of the debate on child health in terms of class, region, gender and localism, the gap between rhetoric and action which resulted from these complexities, and the mediation of the voluntary approach and local initiatives. Physical education was intended to address problems of weakness, and to counter the debilitating effects of urban life, bringing the classes together and training for work and the military. It was presented as being preventive, remedial and curative.

Bernard Harris approaches the links between health and citizenship through his analysis of the origins of the school medical service as a feature of educational legislation rather than a medical service which happened to be located in school. Divorcing the discussion from its usual partners, as part of an evolving series of health provisions for children, he moves the focus from the interests of the state in promoting the education and health requirements of the next generation to the question of the desire to serve the child's own interests. The language of children's rights made itself felt in connection with reforms introducing school meals and school medical inspection, but, Harris argues, it is hard to believe that these services would have been introduced in the early years of the twentieth century without the spur of national efficiency.

The contributions to the book demonstrate the need to think hard about the use of references to themes such as 'citizenship' and 'rights' as catch-all terms; they need to be used rigorously, specifically and carefully, also paying attention to the issues of region, localism, class and gender indicated by Welshman. They have different meanings in different periods, and different implications for health and welfare provision. They need to be understood in terms of civil society and community, and, as Lyubov Gurjeva points out in her account, in terms of family values. Ideas of being a valued family member might not differ significantly from being a good citizen.

Links between family and experts, child health and wellbeing, and consumerism and commercialism - the commerce of health - have been explored in connection with the infant welfare movement and child-rearing advice.[40] With her focus on the middle-class family, Gurjeva interprets domestic child care as an element of the (re)production of the middle classes and consumerism in relation to the production and circulation of goods outside the home. Taking as her case studies, artificial feeding and anthropometric measurement, Gurjeva focuses on the relationship between parents and medical and scientific experts.[41] She also situates domestic child-care practices firmly in the arena of contemporary practices of production and consumption, the mass production of consumer goods, advertising, publishing, and shopping. Rhetoric on national good and efficiency, and the well-being of the child, is seen, following Gurjeva's account, as being influenced and mediated by middle-class interpretations of childhood and their understanding of the (consumer) needs of middle-class children.

Nelleke Bakker's focus on advice to parents locates much of the debate in the Netherlands to issues of morality rather than child health. As in Britain, printed child-rearing advice proliferated around 1900, and mapped increasing sensitivity to the quality of the child's treatment and environment, at least among the middle classes. Yet attention shifted from issues of physical wellbeing and from infants, toward the mental hygiene of the child and moral education, splintered along denominational lines in terms of interpretation and support. Around 1930 a second shift began to emerge, as the 'notion of the autonomous individual' took hold and the moral concept of child-rearing was replaced by a medical approach. It was no longer the moral authority of the parents over the child that mattered most, but rather the interaction between parents and children. Child psychiatrists and psychologists claimed authority to tell parents how to raise their children, at the same time making them responsible for their emotional stability. The emphasis on individualism perhaps reinforced the formation of a more direct link between child, family and nation-citizenship.

Gurjeva and Bakker address issues connected to the production of normal, largely middle-class children. Some children, partly by virtue of their class origins and environment, had less chance of reaching a healthy adulthood and a state of responsible citizenship.[42] Class appears to have played a less pronounced role in the Netherlands, with its very small aristocracy and late and less drastic industrialisation, while pillarization, particularly along religious lines, also had a mitigating impact on class differences. However, poverty, bound in both Britain and the Netherlands to particular regions, both rural and urban, as well as to the growth of towns, was a decisive factor in influencing children's environment and access to services. Distinctions - increasingly subtle - were also drawn in both nations between the healthy and unhealthy, and normal and physically or mentally handicapped child during this period. In Britain this was represented by the increasingly subtle breakdown of the categories of idiot through to feeble-minded, on the 'borderland of imbecility', and efforts to educate the mentally deficient, encapsulated in the Mental Deficiency Act of 1913 and subsequent legislation.[43] In 1920 provision was first made in the Netherlands, in the revised law on primary education, for special education, and in 1923 the government established special schools for mental defectives and imbeciles and boarding schools for mentally handicapped children (also for the deaf, dumb and blind).[44]

As part of the process of reconceptualising the child during the early twentieth century, came the possibility of regenerating the seemingly hopeless. Mark Jackson, focusing on the Edwardian period, explores the concept of the 'borderland' of mental degeneration and feeble-minded children. This definition of borderland had positive as well as negative aspects, placing the feeble-minded in a murky half-way house between educationally and socially normal children and the pathologically hopeless. Jackson also sees these children as positioned – like other children – in a borderland between childhood and adulthood, but these children were less likely to make this transition becoming trapped as 'grown-up children' in a 'psychiatric no-man's land'. The response of government and the medical profession was to place faith in the medico-pedagogical approach, and the idea of educating to develop body and mind. Yet the failures of 'developmentalism' reflected concern about racial degeneration, and bolstered panic about the physical decline of the race. The poorly developed child became equated with the poorly developed nation. Jackson is talking for the most part about institutionalized children, children outside the normal bounds of family, by reason of their handicap or because the family unit had broken down. Just as many of the feeble-minded would never reach adult maturity and full citizenship, becoming locked in a state of 'permanent childhood', so too were the problems of children in institutions redefined in terms of their potential and difficulties in achieving citizenship.

Ido Weijers identifies the absence in the series of children's acts passed in 1901 of ideas and processes geared specifically to protecting and improving children, particularly children in institutions. Weijers focuses on a key figure in Dutch child protection, D.Q.R. Mulock Houwer, who, influenced by a range of authorities representing ideas of self-government, personalism and the psychoanalytical approach, developed his notion of 'education for responsibility'. Institutions were to be turned around from being asocial environments to function as little societies where 'pupils' would 'learn citizenship'. The stress was on tolerance, moral education, and self-government, and on the child's needs and rights. Mulock Houwer's highly influential approach encapsulated the notion of the individual development of the child, with the aim of the child being enabled to reach his or her full potential - as did the work of Mary Dendy outlined by Mark Jackson, albeit with a rather different end in view.

Jackson and Weijers, and to a certain extent Thom, focus on children in various forms of educational institutions. Several of the essays also develop the role of the family in mediating child health and welfare, and as recipients of specific advice on education and upbringing which changed over the course of the twentieth century. Gurjeva's middle-class families adopted a robust stance towards the advice being proffered, integrating it into their own social ambitions, consumerism and views of child health and development. Bakker, taking a longer chronological time span, monitors shifting responses, with at some points the family apparently co-towing to the expert, medicalised view. The shifting emphasis on the family is addressed in different ways in other essays. The reconceptualising of the 'problem' child or child with potential problems as being positioned in the 'problem family' is clearly an issue of great significance in talking about both health and mental wellbeing.[45]

At the beginning of the twentieth century, parents were supposed to act as a form of bridge between the state and child, for example, carrying out the advice of infant welfare reformers concerning the care and feeding of infants, or in ensuring the child was fit and able to attend school. In the second half of the twentieth century this was still valid, but the state, local government bodies and medical and educational experts also mediated increasingly and more directly between the family and child.

One specific form of interaction and debate centred around corporal punishment, explored by Deborah Thom through the extensive discourse which developed in Imperial Britain on beating young offenders. The parental relationship could be fundamentally altered by state intervention, and Thom explores the way in which, state, civil society and the family interacted. She asks why beating remained so important in dealing with delinquency in the face of general acceptance among professionals of the uselessness of physical punishment and the acceptance of psychological approaches to criminal or anti-social behaviour.

The articles map a gradual shift in emphasis during the twentieth century from concerns with physical fitness and physical good health to issues related increasingly to the mental wellbeing and mental hygiene of the child, first the abnormal child, then increasingly the normal. This was in part a response to the fact that physical health and wellbeing did improve over this period and the problems were seen in part as having been dealt with, however a misguided view that may appear on reflection to be. By early in the twentieth century infant and child mortality had been significantly reduced, some of the major killer diseases of childhood were in decline, due to improved living conditions, better disease management and the smallpox vaccination campaign,[46] and children were in general more robust and healthy. The problems of 'defective' children were monitored and attempts made to deal with them from early in the century. By the 1930s advice books for parents written by child psychiatrists and psychologists were addressing the mental health of 'normal children'. This group of experts was highly influential in mediating between the parents and child, as shown in the articles of Gurjeva and Bakker. This period also saw the emergence of childhood gurus, Bowlby and Spock being particularly noteworthy, but also individuals like Dendy and Mulock Houwer, who became highly influential in shaping pedagogical approaches. Holding up the dangers of the dysfunctional family, they were able to superimpose on ideas of how to raise healthy children notions of how to protect and improve their moral, mental and emotional welfare.

Harry Hendrick uses the origins of the National Association for the Welfare of Children in Hospital (NAWCH) to trace the growing post-1945 interest in children's emotional wellbeing with respect to mental health. The emphasis, he argues, during the inter-war period, within psychoanalytic and child guidance circles, was on individual analysis, 'troubled' children and childrearing. Hendrick engages primarily with the campaign to achieve unrestricted visiting of hospitalised young children by their families, which led to the founding of the NAWCH in 1961. This organisation was inspired by John Bowlby and his colleagues and the 'Tavistock Programme', the Platt Report on the Welfare of Children in Hospital, and the popular and medical press. The essay also offers explanations for the take off and eventual success of this campaign. Children's emotional contentment was seen increasingly as being crucial for the development of mature and stable adults, and was important in the more general promotion of national and familial health. This concept of mental health was part of a wider concern with 'social citizenship' in a popular democracy.

Hugo Röling's chapter on sex education in the Netherlands also shows how experts dictated different approaches at different periods. At the end of the nineteenth century most experts in educational philosophy favoured a minimum of information on sexual matters for children and adolescents. The little that could be done to prevent premarital pregnancies and venereal diseases had to be left to parents. In the course of the twentieth century sex education became the subject of public debate, and the role of the family was questioned. Yet despite the failings of parents, the resistance of confessional political parties, especially Catholics, to the teaching of sex education in school countered efforts to introduce it into the curriculum. The movement for sexual reform became embodied in the Dutch Society for Sexual Reform (Nederlandse Vereniging voor Seksuele Hervorming, the NVSH) which gained great popularity in the 1960s, collaborating closely with mental health specialists. In a very short time, attitudes were turned around and educational policy changed.

Implicit in a growing awareness of the need for sex education, is the awareness of a separate category of young person, the adolescent or 'youth', which, though dating from much earlier in the century, gained much greater significance in the 1950s. The post-war baby boom resulted in more young people, with more time, money, knowledge and awareness of their distinctive status to create a separate youth culture, which also became a new topic and market for the experts, including sociologists, psychologists and psychiatrists. For some it was growing non-conformism and delinquency which became a cause of anxiety, but others had a more positive view which praised the dynamic quality and free spirit of youth as a force for social renewal and revitalisation. This positive notion had close links with the 'anti-psychiatric' view that presented psychosis as being a potentially positive phase in one's life. The 'romantic view' of the adolescent and psychotic was part of a growing tendency to stress the values of individual autonomy and creativity and the dangers of conformism and traditional values. Gemma Blok explores this dovetailing of ideas on adolescence in anti-psychiatric throught and youth sub-culture, also exploring the case study of Jan van der Lande's unit, Amstelland, founded in 1968, in an 'extreme (and ultimately failed) expression' of important structural and conceptual changes.

The aim of this volume was to take forward work on the history of child health in the twentieth century, framing the health of the child in its broadest sense as being preventive as well as curative, dealing with physical and mental fitness and wellbeing, and the 'abnormal' and 'normal' child. Comparing the Netherlands and Britain has thrust some issues and debates into a sharper focus. It has also highlighted differences in approaches to child health in the twentieth century, as well as approaches in ways of undertaking historical work, forcing reflection on commonplaces, historical tools and methodologies, challenging, for example, the dominant explanatory structures of national fitness and pillarization. In particular, the essays have sought to develop ideas of how state, local government, experts, families and children interacted in formulating discourses and practices of child health. The essays have reinforced the view that we cannot divorce child health from emerging conceptions of welfare, education, mental and physical hygiene, professionalisation, the role of the state, family, sexuality and gender.

Much remains to be done; that too is clear. Some themes included in this volume could be fruitfully developed. The impact of class, poverty and regionality on health differentials and approaches to care and services needs more unpacking than could be achieved here, although several of the essays do develop ideas of middle-class methods of child rearing which sharply contrast with the dealings of experts with poorer families.[47] The relative roles of the state, professionals, family and child in realising the boundaries of care and provision are explored in the contributions to this volume, as is the question of how children were distinguished from each other on lines of gender as well as social class. Gender-related themes have been developed in terms of ideas of the 'sexless child' and parental roles have been discussed in several chapters, but could also be pushed further along the lines of divisions of labour between mothers and fathers, and the creation of divergent rearing and educational advice for girls and boys. The most difficult aspect of all is to find the child in the competing discourses surrounding health, and to develop a child-centred approach. On many issues the silence or absence of sources is frustrating: how did children experience institutions, or beatings, why did they engage in sport, how did they respond to expert advice mediated by their families? Harry Hendrick's essay in particular indicates the kinds of sources that could be drawn upon to achieve a child-centred history, exploring the politics of children's emotions.[48] Other essays in the volume demonstrate how using other sources sympathetically and creatively bring us closer to the child's view. Sources such as diaries, letters, and memoirs need to be drawn on more resolutely, [49] while reports, case notes, advice literature and so on can bring us closer to a reconstruction of the child's sense of illness and health. There is a need to continue to look for the child – define him or her in terms of age, the worlds of work, education and leisure, in relation to state, family, community, neighhourhood, society, school, and other children - and to search out the child's own sense of potential to be ill, feeble, sick, 'abnormal' or fit, well and strong, to become full developed and healthy citizens.

Acknowledgement

We have drawn freely on the ideas of the contributors to this volume in the introduction, and are particularly grateful to Bernard Harris for his comments on an earlier version.

Notes

1. See Roger Cooter, 'Introduction', in *idem* (ed.), *In the Name of the Child: Health and Welfare, 1880-1940* (London and New York: Routledge, 1992), 1–18.

2. Harry Hendrick, *Children, Childhood and English Society 1880-1990* (Cambridge: Cambridge University Press, 1997), 11.

3. With the addition of a further invited contribution by Nelleke Bakker.

4. There is little detailed work on paediatrics in Britain or the Netherlands during this period, but see for children's diseases, e.g. Paul Weindling, 'From Isolation to Therapy: Children's Hospitals and Diphtheria in *Fin de Siècle* Paris, London and Berlin', in Cooter (ed.), *op. cit.*(note 1),124–45; Anne Hardy, 'Rickets and the Rest: Diet and Infectious Children's Diseases, 1850-1914', *Social History of Medicine*, 5 (1992), 389-412; Elizabeth Lomax, 'The Control of Contagious Disease in Nineteenth-Century British Paediatric Hospitals', *Social History of Medicine*, 7 (1994), 383–400; for specific children's hospitals, e.g. Thera Wijsenbeek, *Zieke lieverdjes: 125 jaar kinderzorg in het Emma Kinderziekenhuis* (Amsterdam: Ploegsma, 1990); M.J. van Lieburg, *Het Sophia Kinderziekenhuis 1863-1975* (Vereniging Sophia Kinderziekenhuis, Rotterdam, 1975); P.D. 't Hart, *Het zieke kind in goede handen: 100 jaar gezondheidszorg in het Wilhelmina Kinderziekenhuis* (Zwolle: Catena, 1988); J. Klosky, *Mutual Friends: Charles Dickens and Great Ormond Street Children's Hospital* (London: Weidenfeld & Nicolson, 1989), for a general survey E. Seidler, 'An Historical Survey of Children's Hospitals', in Lindsey Granshaw and Roy Porter (eds), *The Hospital in History* (London: Routledge, 1989), 181–97; and for the US Thomas E. Crone, Jr., *History of American Pediatrics* (Boston: Little Brown, 1979). See also Harry Hendrick's essay in this volume.

5. See Russell Viner and Janet Golden, 'Children's Experience of Illness', in Roger Cooter and John Pickstone (eds), *Medicine in the Twentieth Century* (Amsterdam: Harwood International, 2000), 575–87, and Roger Cooter's essay in this volume.

6. Cf. Cooter's comment in *op. cit.* (note 1), 2, that 'the child as patient or "welfare object" has hardly obtained a toe-hold in historical

studies'. See e.g. Hendrick, *op. cit.* (note 2) and Pamela Horn, *Children's Work and Welfare, 1780-1890* (Cambridge: Cambridge University Press, 1994).

7. J.R. Gillis, *Youth and History: Tradition and Change in European Age Relations, 1770-Present* (New York: Academic Press, 1974). See also De Haan's essay in this volume.

8. Significantly death rates also tumbled rapidly in the Netherlands after 1880, and infant mortality rates, though starting out at a much higher level, were also quicker to decline than in Britain. By the late nineteenth century the Netherlands had one of the highest levels of infant mortality in Europe, but between 1871, when 227 out of every 1,000 live-born children died before their first birthday, and 1920 it declined to 83 per 1,000, one of the lowest rates in Europe. By the years 1931–35 one estimate put the IMR at 45 per 1,000 in the Netherlands, compared with 62 in England and Wales: B.R. Mitchell, *European Historical Statistics 1750-1970* (New York: Columbia University Press, 1975), 40–1, 43; J.H. de Haas, *Kindersterfte in Nederland. Child Mortality in the Netherlands* (Assen: Van Gorcum, 1956), 80–3.

9. See Jan Noordman, *Om de kwaliteit van het nageslacht: Eugenetica in Nederland 1900-1950* (Nijmegen: SUN, 1989); Geoffrey Searle, *Eugenics and Politics in Britain 1900-1914* (Leiden: Noordhoff, 1979) and *idem, The Quest for National Efficiency* (Oxford: Blackwell, 1971).

10. Simon Szreter, *Fertility, Class and Gender in Britain, 1860-1940* (Cambridge: Cambridge University Press, 1996).

11. See Cynthia R. Commacchio, '*Nations are Built of Babies': Saving Ontario's Mothers and Children 1900-1940* (Montreal: McGill-Queen's University Press, 1993), and *idem,* '"The Infant Soldier": Early Child Welfare Efforts in Ontario', and L. Marks, 'Mothers, Babies and Hospitals: "The London" and the Provision of Maternity Care in East London, 1870-1939', in Valerie Fildes, Lara Marks and Hilary Marland (eds), *Women and Children First: International Maternal and Infant Welfare 1870-1945* (London and New York: Routledge, 1992), 97–120, 48–73 and Deborah Dwork, *War is Good for Babies and Other Young Children: A History of the Infant and Child Welfare Movement in England 1898-1918* (London and New York: Tavistock, 1987).

12. Harry Hendrick, 'Constructions and Reconstructions of British Childhood: An Interpretative Study', in A. James and A. Prout (eds), *Constructing and Reconstructing Childhood: Contemporary Issues in the Sociological Study of Childhood* (London: Falmer, 2nd edn, 1997),

34–62.

13. Though not field. See, for example, Pamela Horn, *The Victorian Country Child* (1974, Stroud: Allan Sutton, 1985) and *idem, op. cit.* (note 6).

14. See e.g. Clark Nardinelli, *Child Labor and the Industrial Revolution* (Bloomington, I.N.: Indiana University Press, 1990); Horn, *op. cit.* (note 6), and Henk te Velde, 'Van grondwet tot grondwet. Oefenen met parlement, partij en schaalvergroting, 1848-1917', in Remieg Aerts et al., *Land van kleine gebaren. Een politieke geschiedenis van Nederland 1780-1990* (Nijmegen: SUN, 1999), 99–175.

15. Carolyn Steedman, 'Bodies, Figures and Physiology: Margaret McMillan and the Late Nineteenth-Century Remaking of the Working-Class Childhood', in Cooter (ed.), *op. cit.* (note 1), 19–44.

16. Horn, *op. cit.* (note 6), 69.

17. See George K. Behlmer, *Child Abuse and Moral Reform in England, 1870-1908* (Stanford, C.A.: California University Press, 1982).

18. Hugh Cunningham, *The Children of the Poor: Representations of Childhood since the Seventeenth Century* (Oxford. Blackwell, 1991), 190.

19. Barbara Brookes, *Abortion in England, 1900-1967* (London: Croom Helm, 1988); Jan de Bruin, *Geschiedenis van de abortus in Nederland* (Amsterdam: Van Gennep, 1979); Dirk Damsma, *Familieband. Geschiedenis van het gezin in Nederland* (Utrecht and Antwerpen: Kosmos, 1999).

20. See Hettie A. Pott-Buter, *Facts and Fairy Tales about Female Labor, Family and Fertility. A Seven Country Comparison, 1850-1990* (Amsterdam: Amsterdam University Press, 1993). From 1840 to 1990 the Dutch population increased five times, from 3 to 15 million, compared with a threefold increase in Britain. The Dutch population totalled over 4 million 1879, 5 million in 1899, almost 7 million in 1920, and 16 million in 1999. In Great Britain by 1881 the population was 37 million, in 1901 41 million, and 1991 56 million.

21. Hilary Marland, 'The Medicalization of Motherhood: Doctors and Infant Welfare in the Netherlands, 1901-1930', in Fildes, Marks and Marland (eds), *op. cit.* (note 11), 74–96, esp. 81. For details of infant welfare services in the Netherlands, see R.N.M. Eykel, *Overzicht over het Sociaal Hygiënisch Werk in Nederland op het Gebied van den Dienst der Volksgezondheid* ('s-Gravenhage: Algemeene Landsdrukkerij, 1932); N. Knapper, *Een Kwart Eeuw Zuigelingenzorg in Nederland* (Amsterdam: Scheltema & Holkema, 1935).

22. See, e.g. Elizabeth Peretz, 'The Costs of Modern Motherhood to

27

Low Income Families in Interwar Britain', in Fildes, Marks and
Marland (eds), *op. cit.* (note 11), 257–80.

23. *Ibid.*, 258.

24. See Irvine Loudon's comparative study of maternal mortality, *Death
in Childbirth: An International Study of Maternal Care and Maternal
Mortality 1800-1950* (Oxford: Clarendon, 1992).

25. E.g. France. See the essays in Gisela Bock and Pat Thane (eds),
*Maternity and Gender Policies: Women and the Rise of the European
Welfare States 1880s-1950s* (London and New York: Routledge,
1991), including the essays of Anna Cova and Karen Offen on
France.

26. See introduction to *ibid.*, 4–5.

27. For the school medical service in England and Wales, see e.g.
Bernard Harris, *The Health of the Schoolchild* (Buckingham: Open
University Press, 1995); Harry Hendrick, 'Child Labour, Medical
Capital, and the School Medical Service, c. 1890-1918', in Cooter
(ed.), *op. cit.* (note 1), 45–71.

28. See, e.g., Linda Bryder, '"Wonderlands of Buttercup, Clover and
Daisies": Tuberculosis and the Open-Air School Movement in
Britain, 1907-39', in Cooter (ed.), *op. cit.* (note 1), 72-95; Bryder,
*Below the Magic Mountain: A Social History of Tuberculosis in
Twentieth-Century Britain* (Oxford: Clarendon, 1988);
Wijsenbeek,*op. cit.* (note 4); Eykel, *op. cit.* (note 21); Ernest Hueting
and Agnes Dessing, *Tuberculose. Negentig jaar tuberculosebestrijding in
Nederland* (Zutphen: Walburg Pers, 1993); J.M. Fuchs and W.J.
Simons, *Ter wille van het kind. Vijfenzeventig jaar Centraal
Genootschap voor Kinderherstellingsoorden 1901-1976* (Naarden:
A.J.G. Strengholt, 1977).

29. Cathy Urwin and Elaine Sharland, 'From Bodies to Minds in
Childcare Literature: Advice to Parents in Inter-War Britain' and
Deborah Thom, 'Wishes, Anxieties, Play, and Gestures: Child
Guidance in Inter-War England', in Cooter (ed.), *op. cit.* (note 1),
174-99, 200-19; Tom van der Grinten, *De vorming van de ambulante
geestelijke gezondheidszorg. Een historisch beleidsonderzoek* (Baarn:
Ambo, 1987); Leonie de Goei, 'Psychiatry and Society: The Dutch
Mental Hygiene Movement 1924-1960', in Marijke Gijswijt-Hofstra
and Roy Porter (eds), *Cultures of Psychiatry and Mental Health Care
in Postwar Britain and the Netherlands* (Amsterdam and Atlanta,
G.A.: Rodopi, 1998), 61-78.

30. Mathew Thomson, *The Problem of Mental Deficiency* (Oxford:
Clarendon, 1998); *idem*, 'Sterilization, Segregation and Community
Care: Ideology and Solutions to the Problem of Mental Deficiency

in Inter-War Europe', *History of Psychiatry*, 3 (1992), 473-98; Mark Jackson, ' Images of Deviance: Visual Representations of Mental Defectives in Early Twentieth-Century Medical Texts', *British Journal for the History of Science*, 28 (1995), 319-37; Inge Mans, *Zin der zotheid . Vijf eeuwen cultuurgeschiedenis van zotten, onnozelen en zwakzinnigen* (Amsterdam: Bert Bakker, 1998); Ido Weijers, 'Christianization of the Soul: Religious Traditions in the Care of People with Learning Disabilities in the Netherlands in the Nineteenth Century', *Social History of Medicine*, 12 (1999), 351-69.

31. Jane Lewis, *The Politics of Motherhood* (London: Croom Helm, 1980),13.

32. *Sunday Times,* 13 February 2000, 'News Review', 1-2.

33. Henk van der Velden, *Financiële toegankelijkheid tot gezondheidszorg in Nederland, 1850-1941* (Amsterdam: Stichting beheer IISG, 1993).

34. De Goei, *op. cit.* (note 29), 65.

35. J.C.H. Blom and C.J. Misset (eds), *'Broeders sluit U aan'. Aspecten van verzuiling in zeven Hollandse gemeenten* ('s-Gravenhage: De Bataafsche Leeuw, 1985).

36. A. Lijphart, *The Politics of Accommodation: Pluralism and Democracy in the Netherlands* (Berkeley: University of California Press, 1968); J. Sturm, L. Groenendijk, B. Kruithof and J. Rens, 'Educational Pluralism - A Historical Study of So-Called "Pillarization" in the Netherlands, Including a Comparison with Some Developments in South African Education', *Comparative Education,* 34 (1998), 281-97.

37. See, e.g., in the field of maternity provision, Jane Lewis, 'Mothers and Maternity Policies in the Twentieth Century' and Elizabeth Peretz, 'A Maternity Service for England and Wales: Local Authority Maternity Care in the Inter-War Period in Oxfordshire and Tottenham', in Jo Garcia, Robert Kilpatrick and Martin Richards (eds), *The Politics of Maternity Care: Services for Childbearing Women in Twentieth-Century Britain* (Oxford: Clarendon, 1990), 15-29, 30-46.

38. Charles Webster, *The Health Services since the War: Volume 1: Problems of Health Care the National Health Service before 1957* (London: HMSO, 1988).

39. Searle, *op. cit.* (note 9).

40. E.g. Peretz, *op. cit.* (note 22); Hilary Marland, 'Childbirth and Maternity', in Cooter and Pickstone (eds), *op. cit.* (note 5), 559–74.

41. Cf. Rima Apple's work on the United States: Rima D. Apple, *Mothers and Medicine: A Social History of Infant Feeding 1890-1950*

(Madison, W.I.: University of Wisconsin Press, 1987); *idem*, 'Constructing Mothers: Scientific Motherhood in the Nineteenth and Twentieth Centuries', in Rima D. Apple and Janet Golden (eds), *Mothers and Motherhood: Readings in American History* (Columbus, Ohio: Ohio State University Press, 1997), 90–110.

42. Jacques Donzelot's work indicates that child policy is also about the regulation of working-class life. He also argues that the relationship between families and the state has been centred on mothers, in the fields of infant welfare, child health, education and development: Jacques Donzelot, *The Policing of Families: Welfare versus the State* (New York: Pantheon, 1979).

43. Thomson, *op. cit.* (note 30).

44. Mans, *op. cit.* (note 30), 245.

45. John Welshman, '"In Search of the "Problem Family": Public Health and Social Work in England and Wales 1940-1970', *Social History of Medicine*, 9 (1996), 447–65; Jane Lewis and John Welshman, 'The Issue of Never-Married Motherhood in Britain, 1920-70', *Social History of Medicine* 10 (1997), 401–18; Pat Starkey, 'The Medical Officer of Health, the Social Worker, and the Problem Family, 1943 to 1968: The Case of Family Service Units', *Social History of Medicine*, 11 (1998), 421–41.

46. For the complexities of this decline, see Anne Hardy, *The Epidemic Streets: Infectious Disease and the Rise of Preventive Medicine 1856-1900* (Oxford: Clarendon, 1993).

47. Nick Spencer, *Poverty and Child Health* (Abingdon, Oxon.: Radcliffe Medical Press, 1996), esp. chapter 4 on the historical relationship.

48. See also Harry Hendrick, 'The Child as a Social Actor in Historical Sources: Problems of Identification and Interpretation', in Pia Christensen and Allison James (eds), *Research with Children: Perspectives and Practices* (London and New York: Falmer Press, 2000), 36–61; Viner and Golden, *op. cit.* (note 5).

49. Rudolf Dekker, has explored the world of the child through letters and diaries for the seventeenth century: *Uit de schaduw in 't grote licht. Kinderen in egodocumenten van de Gouden Eeuw tot de Romantiek* (Amsterdam: Wereldbibliotheek, 1995), also showing the great potential for this form of research for the modern period. See also John Burnett (ed.), *Destiny Obscure: Autobiographies of Childhood, Education and Family from the 1820s to the 1920s* (London: Allen Lane, 1982), Anna Davin, *Growing up Poor: Home, School and Street in London 1870-1914* (London: River Oram Press, 1996), and Carolyn Steedman, *The Tidy House: Little Girls Writing* (London: Virago, 1987).

2

Vigorous, Pure and Vulnerable:
Child Health and Citizenship in the Netherlands
Since the End of the Nineteenth Century

Ido de Haan

Politics has never been child's play. Like the mentally disturbed, criminals, foreigners and, for most of our history, women, children tended to be considered as mere denizens. Their fate, if poor, generally depended on charity, not on rights, and they lacked the privileges of citizenship including the ability to make to personal judgments in public affairs.

Even if children were denied the rights of citizenship, however, modern Western states developed a considerable political interest in the lives of children. After the seventeenth century, political authorities began to view the population not only as a threat, but also as an asset. Developing the productivity of the nation enhanced the power of political authorities, and, at the same time, strengthened the bargaining position of the population. Children were understood to be the future of the nation. The care of a healthy and loyal, resilient and responsible citizenry was considered to be a *sine qua non* of national wealth and international prominence.[1]

Since the eighteenth century, the debate on how to turn children into good and useful citizens has turned on two issues. There has been debate about the support children needed in order to become good citizens, as well as about the kind of citizen they were supposed to become. In both dimensions dominant conceptions have altered over time, and the history of the mental and bodily state of children as it pertains to nation and state building is a story of shifting and interrelated change in concepts of human development and citizenship.

In this article, I want to outline three phases of this development in the Netherlands. All three are defined by successive dominant conceptions of citizenship and human development. The first is the phase defined by the transformation of citizenship in the liberal state around the turn of the century; the second phase concerns the rejuvenation of citizenship in the consociational state of the Interbellum. The final phase is that of the post-war welfare state, when citizenship became increasingly embedded in a system of social rights and institutions of social care.

One of the noteworthy aspects of the developments I will sketch is the change, not just in the conception of the major threats to the health of the nation's stock of new citizens, but of the relationship between their physical and mental health. There seems to be a cycle in which the transformation of children into citizens was initially understood to be a mental issue; since the turn of the century, attention shifted to physical aspects. After 1945, the focus was once again on mental aspects, be it that they were related to physical aspects in a different way.

Finally, changes in the conceptions of citizenship are also related to shifting notions of childhood and gender. For much of the period under discussion, child health concerns were actually directed at juveniles. Even though infant health care was an important issue, especially at the end of the nineteenth century, the greatest debates evolved around the health of youngsters. Moreover, all of these debates were gendered: while in the earlier period, the implied subject of debate often turned out to be male, in the later phases, the health of young females was the centre of attention.

The demise of liberal citizenship, 1870–1900

At the end of the nineteenth century there was a growing awareness in the Netherlands that the bodily health of children mattered to the nation. A law to restrict child labour was promulgated in 1874, and expanded at the end of the following decade. In the first year of the new century, a whole series of laws was issued, all concerned with juvenile care and discipline. There was also growing attention to physical education, which eventually resulted in the adoption of obligatory physical education as part of the education act of 1920.

The growing emphasis on the physical well-being of children implied a major shift in the dominant perspective on the development of children into citizens. During most of the nineteenth century, it was the mind, not the body that was the object of struggle between contesting groups. The liberal elite of the Netherlands, which dominated the political arena for most of the second half of the century, held a restrictive view on the *pays légal*, and accepted the exclusion of most of the inhabitants except for a small group of independent tax payers. However, if not in practice, they recognised the gradual extension of citizenship in principle, even though they assumed that a fully extended citizenship still had a long way to go. The main road to citizenship was through public education based on a fusion of Christianity and humanism, civilising the poor and backward inhabitants, in order to prepare youth for an independent and productive existence.[2]

Their main opponents were orthodox Protestants and sections of the Catholic elite, who feared that liberal Christianity overriding denominational distinctions would lead to a lack of true piety, and, consequently, a loss of morality and order. They opposed both the religious neutrality of the public school and the economic utilitarianism of the liberal conception of poor relief. However, they did not propose an alternative to this liberal conception of public and juvenile health, with the exception of vaccination against smallpox, which was required for admission to primary education between 1823 and 1857, and again after 1872. Orthodox Protestants objected particularly to the intrusion of the human body by the state and the attack on parental authority which obligatory vaccination implied.[3]

This, however, was the exception to the rule that the mind, not the body, was what mattered most. Yet slowly this conviction began to erode. Ever since the end of the eighteenth century there had been some attention placed on the bodily state of children. Physical exercise and fresh air was recommended in advisory books for parents.[4] But it was only in the 1850s that the child's bodily health was focused on in a more systematic way. An important protagonist of this development was the 'hygienist' movement. In the wake of the liberal era from 1848 onwards, Dutch physicians, general practitioners and health inspectors to the local and provincial boards, established in 1818, began to follow the French and British examples of the 1820s and 1830s of formulating a more activist health policy. Among their most important concerns were the living conditions of the poor, and their influence on the health of children. Applying new statistical methods, they argued that the mortality rates of children in the poorest sections of society were much higher than in the richer neighbourhoods, and that this was best explained by bad living conditions: damp houses, an absence of fresh air, a lack of adequate sewerage, and so on. Nutrition also was considered to be an important factor. With regard to small children, neglect of breast-feeding was pointed to as an essential factor in explaining mortality rates.[5]

Up until the end of the century, the impact of hygienist ideas was limited. Its main promotors were a section of the liberal middle classes, who met in the local departments of the Society for the Common Good, the *Maatschappij tot Nut van 't Algemeen.* Through publishing reports and handbooks on education and child care, this Society focused particularly on instructing lower-class women. Yet, as a result of their style and organisation, the bourgeois social reformers probably reached only members of their own class.[6] Moreover, juvenile care was part of the poor relief system dominated by Christian charity and denominational interests. This blocked the way for state intervention and the national regulation of child care. On a local level, however, and on the initiative of private foundations, innovations in child care were instituted.

Between 1850 and the 1870s, the number of institutions for the relief of orphans, unruly or criminal children quadrupled from 11 to 41, most of them founded by denominational private organisations. There were only three state institutions, *Rijksopvoedingsgestichten,* where convicted children were held until their eighteenth year.[7] Private initiatives also formed the basis of the first hospitals specialising in child care. In Amsterdam, the first children's hospital opened in 1865, following a fund-raising campaign by the local elite, led by N.G. Pierson, a progressive liberal banker and later Minister of Finance in the government that introduced a series of child legislation in 1901. Following foreign examples, such as Charles West's children's hospital in Brighton, private organisations also founded holiday resorts for children in the Netherlands.[8] At the end of the century, plans were made for the organisation of infant welfare services. The first *consultatiebureau* opened in 1901 to advise young mothers and to distribute fresh milk to children who were not being breast-fed.[9] In all of these cases, innovations in child care were initiated by private organisations, sometimes even by a cooperation of liberals and orthodox Protestants.[10] Yet, while infant welfare was not centralised and regulated by the state until 1932, other aspects of juvenile care became the object of state intervention by the turn of the century.

The first area to be regulated by government was child labour. Again, hygienists played a leading role in this. They observed a close connection between health and social issues. Bad working conditions were a threat to parents and children alike, both because parental care deteriorated when parents had to work too hard, especially when mothers were unable to breast-feed their children, and working children themselves succumbed under such harsh conditions. In the course of the 1860s, leading hygienists such as S.Sr. Coronel, published alarming reports in the journal *Schat der Gezondheid*

(Treasure of Health, established in 1858) on children who worked in some cases ten to twelve hours a day. Under pressure from Coronel and the Dutch Medical Society, a state committee was appointed in 1863 to investigate the mental and physical condition of working children.[11] The report of this committee was ambiguous in its findings and oriented towards a strict *laissez-faire* ideology in its rejection of all state intervention. Child labour was considered an economic fact of life, given the low wages of the parents. A ban on child labour would automatically lead to a search for alternative sources of income, perhaps in even worse circumstances than the current workplaces. The report also followed the standard liberal creed in its most radical recommendation, that is, that compulsory primary education was 'the most reasonable and effective legal means to ensure and promote the physical and mental development of children'.[12]

Notwithstanding the modest outcome of these first attempts to improve the living and health conditions of children, the official report was the first of a series of reports and petitions, which eventually resulted in the so-called *Kinderwetje* of S. van Houten of 1874. This law restricted the labour participation of children under the age of twelve, without, however, providing a means of control and sanction. At least part of the reason for the law's inadequacy was that very few people favoured direct state intervention in economic relations. The ban on child labour was considered as a threat to the 'normal' determination of wages for adult workers. The initiator of the law, S. van Houten, actually held the position that in the long term education, not state intervention, was the solution to degrading social conditions.[13] However, proposals for mandatory primary education were opposed by religious groups.[14]

In the last decade of the nineteenth century, the climate for further government intervention gradually improved. In 1889 the law of 1874 was expanded and strengthened through the introduction of sanctions against contravention.[15] In the following years, progressive liberals began to plead for a new set of laws in reaction to what was called in an influential report of the *Maatschappij tot Nut van 't Algemeen* of 1896, 'the question of the care for the neglected child'. It focused mainly on the unruly and criminal behaviour of children, and, although it recommended, among other things, revision of the penal law, its main interest concerned the protection of both the child and society. Following the *Nieuwe Richting*, a re-orientation in the debate on penal law, the line dividing penalising the criminal child and civilising the unruly child began to blur. In a remarkably short and effective episode of law-making, these recommendations were passed into law in 1901, combining a revision of both the penal and the civil code, thereby limiting the authority of parents and expanding the means of disciplining the child. Finally, in 1901, a law instituting obligatory primary education was passed, as it were to round off the legal incorporation of the citizens-to-be.[16] This remarkable episode seems to confirm the dominance of the liberal conception of citizenship. Legal measures determined the limits of civil society, disciplining the unruly and criminal child, and instituting a stringent norm of child health development.

However, in the traditional historiography, this episode is presented as the rise of consociational democracy, or pillarization (*verzuiling*), followed by a subsequent demise of liberalism in the Netherlands. *Verzuiling* indicates the development of networks of organisations, based around the same world-view, and coordinated by political parties. And indeed, Protestant 'anti-revolutionaries', Roman Catholics and Social Democrats attracted growing electoral support through their promises to advance the interests of their section of the nation. Liberal groups, claiming to represent the nation as a whole, withered away. Child care also came to be organised on a denominational basis. Child protection agencies, juvenile homes, hospitals and schools were divided along denominational lines and served the needs of their own constituencies.[17]

Yet, there are a number of caveats against the idea of a clear transition from a liberal to a pillarized society. To begin with, the moral foundations of the pillars, especially those of the Protestants and Catholics, were substantially the same, even though they aimed to be exclusive. All of the pillarized organisations emphasised obedience to paternal and political authority, sexual restraint, productivity and parsimony. Moreover, many of the special care organisations worked on the basis of professional standards with little denominational colouring. They also shared information on improvements in treatment and supervision at meetings of overarching national boards and state committees, such as the *Staatscommissie tot onderzoek naar de ontwikkeling der jeugdige personen van 13–18 jaar*, established in 1915 (see below). Furthermore, many of the improvements, such as the development of the clinics for infant care, were pursued by, often locally based, non-denominational professionals. And their clientele in the local community, especially in bigger cities, were also not denominationally divided.[18]

Nevertheless, the liberal, rationalist conception of citizenship, and with it the conception of child development, was on the wane. This had less to do, however, with the formation of societal pillars, and more to do with changes within the liberal perspective, which Dutch liberalism shared with liberal movements in other countries.[19] The new penal doctrine, codified in the laws of 1901, was based on a pedagogical concept, aiming not to punish the unruly child for immoral behaviour, but to re-educate the child as a means of protecting society and improving the child's character. It rejected moral responsibility as the central concept of the law, and put public order and social improvement in its place.[20] This also implied a shift in the concept of education. Beginning in the 1870s, both in the family and in formal education, intellectual development began to lose its dominance.[21] Character building, responsibility and resilience became more central concerns. This was first of all a consequence of denominational resistance to the religious neutrality of the public school. The school's deficient contribution to the formation of character had to be compensated, not only by private denominational schools, but also by a more vigorous education within the family. Earlier notions of a caring education in the family, in which the mother was central, were thus replaced by a more fatherly authority, stimulating strength and robustness.[22]

This change in perspective started long before the development of a pillarized society, and it was primarily the work of liberals, both conservative and progressive. As the conservative liberal W.H. de Beaufort argued in 1880, the liberal conception of the school mistakenly neglected physical education and manual dexterity: 'Brain-work stands in a certain sense at a higher level than manual labour, yet both are necessary for conservation and progress.'[23] Also more progressive liberals began to argue for a shift in focus in public education, arguing for a greater emphasis on the preparation for manual labour, and also for gymnastics as an obligatory element in the school programme.[24]

The latter element in particular received increasing public attention. One of the greatest promotors of gymnastics was 'the Dr. Spock of the nineteenth century', the hygienist G.A.N. Allebé.[25] He lamented the 'deplorable one-sidedness', as the 'consecutive generations grew richer in knowledge, yet physically weaker than their predecessors and this weakness had negative repercussions on the freshness, originality and on the productiveness of the spirit'.[26] He participated in the establishment of a society of instructors of gymnastics in 1862, which pleaded for the introduction of gymnastics as an obligatory part of the curriculum of primary education. The main argument was that it was 'in the national interest to have solid, vigorous, well-built manual labourers, rather than to have the poor relief and the hospitals suffer the consequences of a weakened population, which forms the majority of the nation', as stated in the journal, *Volksheil, weekblad voor turnbelangen* (People's health, weekly for the interests of gymnastics, founded in 1873).[27]

In the 1890s these appeals began to receive more enthusiastic support. On the one hand, progressive liberals were looking for more practical issues in the reform of the curriculum to bypass the unsolvable questions of 'who is allowed to found and administer schools and whether different groups of the population will receive financial support'.[28] On the other hand, conservative liberals, who felt marginalised by the rise of the new liberalism and of the Protestant and socialist mass parties, turned to a nationalistic and in some cases even militaristic discourse, stressing the importance of vigour and manly virtue.

Initially, gymnastics was not advocated for male youngsters only. In 1857, Allebé acknowledged that the value of gymnastics for boys was obvious, but for girls it was less evident. There were dark sides to physical exercise for girls, who would get accustomed to bad habits like 'climbing and jumping'. But it was undeniable 'that the general health condition, as a result of physical exercise, would improve', and this was 'especially with respect to the female sex – an essential, a primary, perhaps the most primal need of our century'. Allebé scorned contemporary education, which 'created ladies [*dames*] – against her will mostly weakish, very often infirm ladies – it does not create true *women*'. Moreover, the cognitive learning abilities, 'for both sexes equally', depended on regular distraction through physical exercise. Even if a wrongly applied gymnastics could turn girls into 'Amazones of the nineteenth century', this was not an argument against gymnastics as such, provided that it did not intervene in the 'softer female characteristics'.[29]

At the end of the century, when the argument for gymnastics became closely connected to a growing enthusiasm for military virtues, attention to physical exercise became more exclusively focused on boys. For example, J.T.T.C. van Dam van Isselt, colonel of the infantry, lamented that 'we lack the moving, creative force, a higher leading, a resilience of will and character', and quoted approvingly from *Das Volk in Waffen* of a certain Von der Goltz, who announced the day of a *Völkerentscheidungskampf*. However, Van

Dam called for an improvement of the resilience of the people and popular education, 'not to militarise our children, but to make them strong, independent, freedom-loving and liberal [in the sense of ready to make a sacrifice] men, adequately trained for the hard struggle of life'. He praised the Anglo-Saxon race for taking such good care of its public education: 'As a result of physical exercise, the Englishman has become modest and sober. The fat-bellied, over-eaten, purple-colored congestive race from the times of George III has completely disappeared. John Bull is replaced by the Christian gentleman of Arnold.'[30]

In the Netherlands, however, Van Dam van Isselt observed a strong resistance to stressing military virtues, and pleaded in vain for a military popular education. The reason for this failure was not so much an inborn pacifism of the Dutch nation. The nationalist campaign at the end of the century and the enthusiasm for the struggle of the South-African Boers made clear that military zeal was also common in the Netherlands.[31] Other reasons explain why the campaign for physical education was also less successful in the twentieth century. One barrier was the internal contradiction in the argument advocating gymnastics. On the one hand, it was meant to teach military discipline, molding the child's character by disciplining the body. On the other hand, instructors of gymnastics, but also others concerned with the physical state of the youth, stressed the importance of natural development. As one handbook on school hygiene argued, 'There shall be no military discipline in the school, but a discipline, which leaves ample room for a free movement of mind and body alike'.[32] Another reason for the relative lack of success of the gymnastics movement in the Netherlands was its anti-clericalism. It often justified its cause by referring to the 'spirituality of Christianity' as a result of which 'physical education was neglected'.[33] Instead it exalted the hellenistic virtues. 'Poor Leiden, Nordic Athens, blessed memory', exclaimed the secretary of the gymnastics society in 1893, when the city council of Leiden banned gymnastics in primary schools.[34]

Even though the Netherlands remained neutral during the First World War, it is very likely that the threat of war, and also the mobilisation of a substantial part of the male population, reinforced the call for better physical education. In 1917, a government committee recommended that gymnastics should be part of the obligatory curriculum of primary education, arguing that it was 'an eminent interest of the State, that the nation in its struggle for existence as a whole has at its disposal both the maximum of physical as well as the maximum of intellectual and moral force'.[35] Eventually, the new law on primary education of 1920 mentioned gymnastics as one of the standard elements of the curriculum, although schools still had ample opportunity to exempt themselves from this obligation.

After 1900, the liberal conception of citizenship, stressing intellectual capacities as a precondition for recognition as a citizen, was replaced by a much more embodied and less intellectual formulation. In a sense, this depended on a reversal of the hierarchy of body and soul. According to the earlier conception, the soul commanded the body, and poverty and illness had to be overcome by working on the mind and the beliefs of the pupil. Now body and soul worked jointly. Character had as much to do with mental responsibility as with physical resilience, while to some enthusiastic promoters of gymnastics, it was self-evident that physical exercise 'serves to create courage, self-reliance and determinacy in action'.[36]

At the same time, care of the body was also disconnected from the larger concerns of the development of a vigorous character.[37] Part of the hygienist movement put all of its efforts behind the development of juvenile care: consultation bureaus for the infant child and its mother, hospitals for children, and, after the promulgation of the laws of 1901, a series of custody boards, councils for the protection of minors and the 'medical-pedagogical bureaus' to assist the 'difficult child'. This development led to another strand of citizenship, which viewed the child as a client of social and medical help and intervention. Given the fact that most of these institutions were not first and foremost founded in the interest of the child, but for the good of public order, it is clear that this did not create full-blown civic entitlements. Yet it was a first step in the development of a special status for children, which at the same time granted them some rights of citizenship, and created a separate societal domain of juvenile care and development.

Rejuvenating citizenship, 1900–1950

The laws of 1901 created not only a separate domain of juvenile care, but also contributed to the formation of childhood and in particular adolescence as a separate social category and phase in the life of both the individual and society. In the first decade of the twentieth century, the youth became a pivotal concern of the state and private organisations. For instance, in 1915 a state committee was set up to investigate the development of children aged between 13 and 18; the committee prepared reports that were discussed at a major conference in 1919. The participants were aware of a growing interest in childhood. In the final report they argued that this was the result of new insights into the psychology of adulthood, recent socio-economic changes and the ethical and pedagogical issue that they had put on the agenda. The war had reinforced these tendencies. From this official point of view, the motive behind promoting special attention to childhood and adolescence was that the child's 'accumulated energy which does not find a normal outlet, in combination with other factors, will easily lead to criminality'.[38] A more important aspect was the belief that developments since the 1870s had undermined the moral standing of both the family and school. The latter was too intellectual, while the former was often considered deficient. This led to the notion that the education of children needed a 'third' educational environment, as the influential pedagogue C.P. Gunning had described it.[39] Moreover, youngsters experienced increasing opportunities to participate in this environment after the new labour laws of 1911 and 1919 created more leisure time for them.[40]

As John Gillis among others has argued, the development of a separate sphere of adolescence at the end of the nineteenth century in England, and one or two decades later in the Netherlands, was not the result of a simple generational shift, but the consequence of a more fundamental change in the perspective on children.[41] Adolescence, but also childhood in general, came to be seen as a societal category, the meaning of which was not just a preparation for adult citizenship, but an alternative conception of what it meant to be a citizen. This alternative lay in the energy and resilience of the youthful body. As one of the early representatives of the socialist youth movement stated:

> We are the Youth. We differ in thoughts and deeds from our surroundings. We have the feeling to be a modern man, and this feeling burns inside us, and the flames of our enthusiasm burst out. We want to set the world on fire ... we will subvert the stuffiness, repress the conventional in our free enjoyment of the truth, trample the rut with our swift feet.[42]

There was a strong tension between the discovery of the youth as a separate societal category and a new object of care and discipline, and the expectation that the future lay with the young and contained the promise of a better world. The diverging evaluation of youngsters as potential criminals versus potential redeemers was translated at an institutional level as the distinction between disciplinary youth care and a utopian youth movement. The discovery of youth thus made it an object of political struggle, of organisation, counter-organisation and self-organisation.

To begin with, the laws of 1901 had reinforced the position of denominational organisations for child care, if not relative to non-denominational organisations, at least in absolute numbers, as a result of growing state subsidies.[43] Child care had always been an important part of the poor relief system and dominated by denominational organisations, and it remained in denominational hands as it became a more or less independent branch of social work. It appears that one of the main reasons for the quick acceptance of the laws of 1901 was that a compromise was struck between denominational interests and the state. Just as the solution of the struggle against the public school was found in an administratively independent, yet state-financed private school system, child care also largely remained in private hands, even when the state accepted financial responsibility.[44] As a result, the extended network of denominational child care organisations inherited the clerical control and the concomitant proselitising objectives of denominational administrators. Child care and (religious) discipline were thus closely intertwined.

Roman Catholic and Protestant leaders of child care organisations were suspicious about the development of an independent youth movement. They abhorred the lack of adult leadership, rejected the stress on sports and play, and considered camping out and walks in the woods to be a threat to virtue and piety.[45] The development of a Roman Catholic scouting organisation was barred by a ban on a national federation by the Dutch bishops in 1920. Yet at the end of the 1920s, the climate began to change. The development of Catholic scouting organisations was permitted, provided that a priest kept a close eye on the boys camping in the woods.[46] The main reason that the clergy changed its mind was that it wanted to tap into the strong current of idealism that the independent youth movement generated. Yet in the process, it kept a keen eye on its own interests, and forced the Catholic scouting organisations to participate in the Catholic Action Pope Pius XI had initiated in the early 1930s. Moreover, the clergy remained hostile to anything resembling naturalness, natural development or any other sign of a diminishing awareness of the sinfulness of the human flesh:

> The naturalist... is unable to speak coherently about the reigning of
> the passions.... No wonder that... the complaints about profligacy,

lust and unrestrainedness of the modern youth are growing louder every day in all countries. What do the statistics learn about the increasing criminality of the youth on ALL terrains?... All in all, we long for a Spartan education, an education for simplicity, severity and habituation to afflictions [*smartgewenning*].[47]

The same hostility to naturalness and the unrestrained development of the innate capacities of the youth was voiced by the Protestant leaders of youth organisations. Although they also criticised the bias towards the intellectuality of the previously dominant liberal conception of education, and considered natural development compatible with God's predestination, they continued to reject the celebration of the youthful force of the youth movement.[48]

The situation was rather different in the socialist youth movement. To begin with, socialists had no interest in the existing social order. They were as worried as others about the unruliness and criminality of the youth, but they interpreted this as the consequences of the materialism and alienation of capitalist society. Young people did not need to be disciplined; rather they had to be liberated. Moreover, socialists lacked their own social work organisations. They had set up friendly and mutual societies on a limited scale. Yet, for social care that could not be expressed in financial support, they depended on local or national government organisations. The social democrats also met with strong resistance from vested denominational interests when they tried to create their own organisations. For instance, this was the case in 1911, when they tried to achieve official recognition and funding for the society *Zedelijke opvoeding* (Moral education), directed at the moral education of non-religious children.[49]

The socialist youth movement whole heartedly embraced the critical stance of new youthfulness against society as it was: 'Ever greater become our ranks, of those who consciously turn away from the bourgeoisie fake civilization, who are no longer attracted by the fair, the pub, the cinema and the dance hall.'[50] Instead, the new youth celebrated nature and naturalness, to be expressed in walks, dances, and clothes. Moreover, there was a close connection with the teetotalers, vegetarians and followers of the ideals of *Rein-Leven*, Tolstoi and other wandering birds. As one of the main departments of the socialist *Arbeiders Jeugd Centrale* (AJC) stated in their *Rode Valkenwet*, 'We, Red Falcons, aim at sobriety and simplicity. We do not use any alcohol and no tobacco. We, Red Falcons, take care of our body by purity, exercise and endurance. We, Red Falcons, are friends and protectors of nature.'[51]

The leaders of this new movement also considered themselves to be the avant garde: 'Behold the Dutch youth: while the most forceful joy and wonderful hard-sought revelations make our heart-beat shiver through our whole body, they never had any emotion, their questions are smothered and overgrown by the soulless worries of everyday life... Behold the Dutch youth – it awaits *our* education.'[52] Yet this elite outlook caused irritation among the ranks of the socialist movement. The AJC had a troubled relationship with the rest of the socialist movement. By 1926, most of the youngsters who had entered the AJC through the socialist labour unions had left the organisation. And in 1924 the leadership of the social democratic party, which financed the AJC, complained that 'we get a youth movement *of* the youth, instead of *for* the youth'; 'the cracking up of the youth has to stop'.[53]

Youth movements had a considerable membership, by the 1930s probably making up one-third of the 1.4 million youngsters aged between 12 and 20.[54] However, it did not include the majority of the lower class youth; that is, the category causing most concern in connection with rising crime rates, alienation and unhealthy habits. The criticism of the leaders of the youth movement about the bad influence to which all youngsters except their happy few were exposed, even reinforced abhorrence of what was called the 'majority youngster'. He was 'tall yet weakish. His knees are turned to the inside and his back is bent, as if he walks on a rope. If he stands, he leans, and if he sits, he hangs. His arms flutter along his body like empty sleeves and his hands are purple, wet or neglected... He is unspeakably clumsy... things no one ever imagined they could break, he breaks. I am not even talking here about his wantonness and lack of restraint.'[55]

This description was written by W.E. van Wijk, one of the founders of the *Tucht-Unie* (Discipline Union, established 1908). It brought together not only private members, but also organisations such as scouting groups, unions of police-officers and schoolmasters and *Volksweerbaarheid*. The union aimed at a return to discipline and increasing the moral, spiritual and physical force of the nation, by promoting such diverse activities as scouting and sports, singing and traffic safety, and protesting against alcohol abuse, maltreatment of animals and brutality against tourists.[56] Other organisations were concerned with the alienated youth. Labour unions not only objected to the elitism of the socialist youth movement, but also contributed to the development of activities for young workers in their neighbourhood. Most importantly, lower class boys were organised in sporting clubs. While before 1900 most of these clubs were decisively upper-middle class, football clubs soon became very popular, growing from 7,500 participants in 1910 to 150,000 in 1940.[57] From the perspective of the socialist youth movement, this was just as bad as the other pleasures of capitalist society: 'We don't want to be sports maniacs and waste our precious time on a hot football field. We only promote physical exercise as a means, not as a goal.'[58] This harsh judgment applied not just to football, but also to all other sports. They are 'a training for national and international champions, which is useless and even dangerous for the general physical education', the AJC-leader Koos Vorrink stated in 1928.[59]

Increasingly, the most important institutional environment for unorganised youth became the network of state, semi-state and private organisations concerned with the health, discipline and punishment of children. Although much of the work of the multifarious and barely coordinated organisations was aimed at neglected, orphaned, or unruly children, care soon became available to other sections of the population as well. For example, after a visit to the United States, in 1928 the criminologist and social worker Mrs E.C. Lekkerkerker set up the first 'medical-pedagogical bureau', which was meant to take care of the not yet criminal, but mentally criminality-prone young child. Within ten years all major cities had their own bureau.[60]

A whole series of 'randdiensten', surrounding services, were developed around the school. The Society for School Physicians, established in 1908, eventually succeeded in the 1930s in developing a more systematic surveillance of the health of children at school. They reported on eating habits, contributed to the fight against tuberculosis, for which a legal framework was created in 1934, and participated in regular check-ups for other contagious diseases and physical inconveniences, such as head-louse. Attempts to create systematic dental care at school by the Dutch Society for Social Dental Care, established in 1933, were less successful. The Dutch *Zuivelcentrale* obtained better results when they tried to create a national milk distribution system for children. In 1937 the minister of agriculture agreed to subsidise milk distribution through a *Centraal Schoolmelkcomité*, which was established in the same year.[61]

Infant welfare is a further example of gradual centralisation. After the first bureaus were established in 1901, the state agreed in 1932 to finance and support provincial and denominational organisations involved in infant care.[62] Finally, the development of this network both benefited from and contributed to the professionalisation of child care. This had important consequences, not only for the clients, but also for the mostly female workers who staffed these organisations. The organisations for child care offered new opportunities for women, who could now claim a larger public and professional role. In 1927, for instance, Cornelia de Lange became the first female university professor in paediatrics. Other women, like Mrs Lekkerkerker, found equally prominent positions, albeit that their influence remained limited to the occupations that could be connected to supposedly female characteristics, care, compassion and self-sacrifice.[63]

In this period, the road to citizenship for children was routed mainly through the body. The demise of liberal citizenship at the end of the nineteenth century created a conception of youth as a separate category, which soon came to be understood as an alternative to the alienated life of the adults. Children represented a resilience older people had lost. Their common activities, which were part of a third environment alongside school and family, became the locus of this alternative conception. The core of this conception was a natural development, inherited from the critique on the intellectualism of the liberal conception of citizenship. True, citizens did not need discipline, but a liberal growth of their natural potentialities in a natural environment. This notion applied to both boys and girls, and co-education was one of the fundamental and, according to its opponents, repulsive characteristics of the new youth movement. However, many children, and especially adolescent boys who were feared the most for their criminal vitality, did not participate in this environment and remained exposed to the pathological influence of modern urban life. Yet they were also objects of intervention, which mainly targeted their bodies, rather than their souls. The network of institutions for child care that began to develop after 1900, was based on the same critique of intellectualism and the pedagogical conception in which disciplining the body was equally, or even more valuable, than educating the mind.

The most vulnerable citizens, post-1950

The youth movement did not survive the Second World War. It was largely discredited after the downfall of the Nazis. Not only had the atrocities of war and persecution undermined faith in the goodness of the human race, but also many of the ideals and symbols were contaminated through their use by national socialist youth organisations. Before the War, some members of the socialist youth movement had had even made a switch to national socialism, including W. van Tiel, former president of the NBAS, the Dutch union for teetotal students, who died in 1943 as an SS-soldier at the Eastern Front. Although the AJC was re-established after 1945, its membership soon dropped until the organisation was disbanded in the late 1950s.[64]

Anxiety about lack of discipline amongst the youth, however, had not abated. On the contrary, it reached an all-time high directly after the German surrender. A moral panic developed, a result of the combination of various issues: social and sexual intercourse between Canadian soldiers and young Dutch women; vandalism, excessive dancing, drinking and smoking amongst young men; black market trading; work-avoidance; and violence against former collaborators, especially women who had been involved with German soldiers.[65] Although not all of these issues directly involved children, the solutions were mainly concerned with recreating the moral bonds that were needed to educate or re-educate the youth. As one of the many theologians and moralists who participated in this debate, H. van Oyen, stated: 'All bonds of family and school are now unbearable for the youngsters after years of man-hunts and dissolution of all social ties like schools and clubs.' Against the 'vital-instinctive reactions', which the untying of these bonds had unleashed, the main solution was the reconstruction of the family.[66] A national campaign under the banner of *Gezinsherstel brengt volksherstel* (Family reconstruction creates popular reconstruction) combined the need for reconstruction of the devastated country with a renewed appeal for discipline, and was aimed primarily at the 'majority youngsters', the lower-class boys in the urban areas, since the 1930s commonly called the 'mass youth'.[67]

The moral panic of the immediate post-war years caused a shift in the dominant conception of citizenship in relation to child health, from an emphasis on physical aspects back to the mental well-being of the child. Again, the mind became the direct object of intervention, with on the physical condition of children being affected only indirectly.

This is not to say that the physical health of children was forgotten after 1945. After a major increase in infant mortality in 1945 (which correlated not only with the lack of food and medical care, but also with the baby boom after the end of the war) the statistics soon showed a continuation of the steady decline in infant mortality that had already started in the 1920s.[68] The pre-war network of institutions for infant care was soon reconstructed and quickly expanded to become a standard item in the fabric of the welfare state. As a result, classic childhood diseases appeared less frequently. The arsenal of childhood vaccination gradually expanded. Child health care became more specialised and focused increasingly on complex diseases, such as cancer and heart disease.[69] In recent years, these developments have gained in visibility, as the heroic fights of sick children in apparently lost causes have become a central ingredient of reality television. This has served to confirm the dominant ideology of medical modernisation that has swept the world since 1945.

There are only a few counter-tendencies against this medical success story. One is resistance to vaccination, which has remained controversial in the Netherlands as it interferes with religious freedom.[70] Only in recent years, after resistance to vaccination has been taken up by parents with a Steinerian orientation, has opposition to vaccination lost some of its image of a rearguard battle against the invincible forces of modernity.[71] Nevertheless, the highest standards of child health care now appear to be considered an inalienable right, to which children can also appeal.

However, the most important objectives of the post-war period concerned the mental rather than the physical well-being of children. They soon became objects of a series of investigations undertaken by private and state organisations. Initially, these investigations were still influenced by fear of the mass youth. As the title of the report of a state commission chaired by the prominent pedagogue M.J. Langeveld indicated, the first concern was with the *maatschappelijke verwildering van de jeugd*, the social degeneration of the youth. Yet in the second half of the 1950s, the tone and perspective began to change, leading to a more positive evaluation of what now came to be viewed as 'the new adults', as a report written by the sociologist J. Goudsblom in 1959 was entitled.[72]

According to first approach, the core of the problem was identified as deficiencies in the family. Anti-social behaviour resulted from deviation from what was considered a desirable family life, based on the three R's of 'reinheid' (cleanliness), 'rust' (rest) and 'regelmaat' (regularity). Irresponsible parents did not clean the house, did not play with their children, did not give good examples of civilised behavior, did not observe school attendance, and consequently: 'the indispensable cornerstone of a healthy family bond, the authority of the parents, is completely lacking'.[73] These social deficiencies were often interpreted in medical terms: 'Every child in custody is by definition a mentally neglected child', claimed the psychiatrist Trimbos in 1953.[74] The deficient family was sick, or even itself a source of sickness. As stated in the official report of a state commission, established in 1948 to investigate 'onmaatschappelijke gezinnen' (anti-social families): they are 'an intolerable source of contagion for their environment, which causes the downfall also of other families and in particular, of the children from other families'.[75] Therefore, solutions had to be radical. Until 1960, anti-social families were locked up in 'gezinsoorden', family compounds, where they were subjected to intense surveillance. These compounds were eventually closed, as much for financial as for ethical reasons. Even more radical, eugenicist solutions were considered. Eugenic ideas were not immediately discredited despite the national-socialist policies in this area, but proposals for the systematic sterilisation of women in anti-social families were never implemented, although sterilisation was suggested as a solution.[76]

According to the alternative approach, the behaviour of the youth was not considered pathological or deviant, just different. In an influential report of 1959, the sociologists Krantz and Vercruijsse observed 'a contradiction between the lack of a real problem of the youth and the need to make the youth into a problem'. According to their analysis, 'the adult generation has an ideal of a youth which actively and convincingly participates in youth movements... To *their* standards these youngsters fall short. But these criteria themselves are of limited value, time-bound and therefore unjust.'[77] Instead, the new adolescents were assumed to have chosen their own path, and should only be urged to follow it as successfully as possible.

This re-orientation in the approach to the problems of childhood were part of a larger shift in the functioning of the state. After 1945, the state assumed a greater responsibility for the well-being of citizens. Its guarantee of social security did not imply 'a soft bed for everyone and an invitation to laziness and negligence'.[78] But it did involve the idea that material welfare had to be in reach of every citizen and that all citizens had to be enabled to develop personal responsibility. This applied especially to children, whose enjoyment of the growth of luxury and leisure was difficult to reject, once the rise of consumption was stated to be an official goal of public policy. There was also little reason for a negative judgment, once it was officially recognised that 'there is an increasing emphasis on the personality, its individual disposition, nature, intellectual and moral capacities, its self-reliance and inalienable responsibility for its own life and that of the communities of which it is part'.[79]

The recognition that children and adolescents created their own world with its own values did not result in less intervention. Since it was assumed that the development of the personality required a stimulating environment, acknowledgement of the self-developing child invited a new wave of institutionalisation and regulation of child care. In 1955 the government created a new Council for Youth Affairs, and in 1956 the Ministry of Education established a section for *Jeugdvorming en Volksontwikkeling*, youth formation and national development. Both contributed to the planning of the *jeugdwerk*, or juvenile work.[80]

These efforts soon ran into trouble. The reasons were partly financial, but there was also a more fundamental problem. Child care had always been a joint effort between the state and denominational private organisations, and this had not changed after 1945. However, the legitimation of the religious influence on child care, and of the fabric of the welfare state in general, began to erode, as a result of the expansion and concomitant professionalisation of the social welfare institutions. The more the workers in these institutions adopted professional standards, and that implied in this case notions of individual development and personal responsibility, the less they were able to justify their work in terms of religious adherence.[81] In the case of child education, this contradiction was aggravated by the paradox of paternalism: the impossibility of ordering people to be independent. As a result, many of the new policies were unsuccessful, because the youth for which it was intended had different ideas about what made sense and what was enjoyable. The result was that child care workers and policy makers gradually handed over the initiative to the youth itself, and tried to answer to what they thought were the demands of a new generation.[82]

The radical changes of the 1960s were in the Netherlands perhaps more radical than elsewhere in terms of secularisation, a decline in birth rates and marriages, the rise in divorces, and acceptance of post-materialist values.[83] But they did not emanate from a more vigorous new generation. They came about as the result of a particular set of conditions in the dominant culture, which led leading politicians, cultural spokespersons and public moralists to invite radical change, carried out by the youth.[84] Again, the future lay with the young, but this time it was not as part of a unified political movement representing a new form of citizenship, but as an aggregate of individuals, each looking for a way to self-realisation.[85]

Older traditions within the youth movement did revive, for instance in the cultural criticism of the Provo-movement against the bourgeois mentality of the majority of the population and the romantic rejection of urban life by the Kabouters.[86] The ideology of natural development was also revived, but this time it was connected much more with the free development of sexuality than the old youth movement had ever dreamed of. The latter example not only indicates a difference from the earlier youth movement (or better, since there was little collective movement: culture) in the attitude towards sexuality. The discussions about sex after sexual liberation also made it clear that the notion of human development had become more procedural. Everyone had to work on self-realisation; what one's self was, one had to find out for oneself.[87]

The lack of substance in the notion of self-realisation paradoxically reinforced the criticism of the influence of family and society on the well-being of children. One may have expected the criticism to become fuzzier, since the self that was wrongly influenced, and thus the potential damage to mental health, had become more vague. Yet criticism became sharper, since now all aspects of social life potentially had a pathological effect. Since the self-development of the child was such a precarious process, every interference could lead to disaster. In other words, the child was no longer a bundle of potentialities, but became increasingly an intersection of infringements: a victim.

Again, this is part of a larger shift. After 1945, citizenship became increasingly identified with a set of entitlements. This set itself also expanded: an increasing range of aspects of personal and social life became subject to regulations and entitlements. This also meant that the quintessence of citizenship was now exercised by protesting against the infringement of rights, by claiming the position of the victim of injustice. Citizenship thus became increasingly identified with vulnerability.[88]

As a consequence, children became once again model citizens. It was no longer the vitality and resilience of the youth, but the vulnerability which created this equation. As a result, attention shifted from boys to girls, and from older juveniles to younger children. While in most of the developments discussed so far, the implicitly assumed child was male, it now became female. The vulnerable child, whose health was threatened by the family and society at large, was the young girl. The typical childhood diseases are no longer measles or rubella, but child abuse, anorexia nervosa and sexual traumatisation.[89] At first sight, this seems to undermine the claim that it is the mind, more than the body, which is now the object of intervention. However, in all cases it is not the body that is unhealthy and in need of a cure, but the mind: 'Women who want to be sick, beautiful or different acquire a new identity by not eating... they want to be noticed in a culture that is dominated by the male vision and by the visual'.[90] Citizenship in this context is pre-eminently exemplified by the young girl. She is a victim, not primarily of physical distress or disease, but of cultural pathologies, and her fate depends, not on somatic treatment, but on psychotherapy.

Conclusion

A remarkable aspect of the development outlined in this paper is the change in the relationship between citizenship and the state. At the end of the nineteenth century, citizens were considered a potential asset, a productive entity, capable of contributing to the national wealth and military strength. This implied also a criterion for exclusion from citizenship: only productive members of the nation could be citizens. It was therefore in the nature of things that children, at least boys, could only be potential, yet never actual citizens. At the end of the twentieth century, this relationship has almost become reversed. Citizenship is now defined, not in terms of the contribution of citizens to the commonwealth, but the other way around, by the entitlements the state should guarantee and that citizens can make a claim to: 'Ask not what you can do for your country, but what the country can do for you', to reformulate a well-known dictum. Since citizenship has become equated with vulnerability, children, and especially girls, now function as model citizens.

Paradoxically, this shift is coupled with a change in emphasis, from the body back to the mind. Together with the growing worries about the vulnerability of the child, its actual physical condition has greatly improved, and mortality rates have dropped dramatically. The increasing vulnerability of the child thus refers mainly to its mental stability, and, even within this field, attention has shifted from the most severe and visible pathologies, like suicide, to the less obvious cases of mental illness, such as depression, which were earlier considered 'normal adolescent turmoil'.[91]

The crucial episode in this development was the first half of the twentieth century, when childhood came to be viewed as a separate sphere of life. At the time, this was accompanied by the expectation that the youth also represented an alternative to the dominant conception of citizenship. Furthering a healthy youth could therefore be considered way of improving the health of the nation. After 1945, this expectation was lost: children remained a central concern, but this was no longer a result of a positive conception of the nation's future, but in a sense followed from a negative conception. Children became model citizens by virtue of their 'negative' quality; by the fact that they were the most vulnerable to harm. Consequently, this is what the health of the nation now implies: the absence of illness and a strongly increased sensitivity to the ways in which people can be ill.

Acknowledgements

I want to thank Marijke Gijswijt-Hofstra, Frank Huisman and Gary Price for their comments on earlier drafts of this article.

Notes

1. M. Foucault, 'Governmentality', *Ideology and Consciousness*, 6 (1979), 5–21; *idem*, 'Omnes et Singulatim. Toward a Critique of "Political Reason"', in S. McMurrin (ed.), *The Tanner Lectures on Human Values II* (Cambridge: Cambridge University Press, 1981), 222–55; G. Oestreich, *Neostoicism and the Early Modern State* (B. Oestreich and H.G. Koenigsberger, eds; translated by D. McLintock) (Cambridge: Cambridge University Press, 1982); C. Tilly, *Coercion, Capital, and European States, AD 990–1990* (Cambridge, Mass./Oxford: Basil Blackwell, 1990).

2. See, on Dutch liberalism, S. Stuurman, *Wacht op onze daden. Het liberalisme en de vernieuwing van de Nederlandse staat* (Amsterdam: Bert Bakker, 1992); H. te Velde, *Gemeenschapszin en plichtsbesef. Liberalisme en nationalisme in Nederland, 1870–1918* (Den Haag: Sdu Uitgeverij, 1992); S. Dudink, *Deugdzaam liberalisme. Sociaal-liberalisme in Nederland 1870–1901* (Amsterdam: IISG, 1997); R. Aerts, *De letterheren. Liberale cultuur in de negentiende eeuw: het tijdschrift* De Gids (Amsterdam: Meulenhoff, 1997).

3. G.W. Brands-Bottema, *Overheid en opvoeding. Onderzoek naar de motivering door politieke partijen van formele wetgeving of poging daartoe, betreffende de overheidsbemoeiingen met de verzorging en opvoeding van kinderen door hun ouders, in de periode 1870–1987* (Arnhem/Deventer/Gouda: Quint/Kluweris, 1988), 20–7.

4. Rineke van Daalen, 'Openbare hygiëne en privé-problemen: het ontstaan van de Amsterdamse gezondheidszorg', *Amsterdams Sociologisch Tijdschrift*, 9 (1983) 568–605: 571.

5. E.S. Houwaart, *De hygiënisten. Artsen, staat en gezondheidszorg in Nederland 1840–1890* (Groningen: Historische Uitgeverij, 1991), 97–117, 193–6.

6. B. Kruithof, *Zonde en deugd in domineesland. Nederlandse*

protestanten en problemen van opvoeding. Zeventiende tot twintigste eeuw (With a summary in English) (Dissertation University of Amsterdam, 1990), 233.

7. J.J.H. Dekker, *Straffen, redden en opvoeden. Het ontstaan en de ontwikkeling van de residentiële heropvoeding in West-Europa, 1814–1914, met bijzondere aandacht voor de "Nederlandsche Mettray"* (Assen/Maastricht: Van Gorcum, 1985), 122.

8. Th. Wijsenbeek, *Zieke lieverdjes. 125 jaar kinderzorg in het Emma Kinderziekenhuis* (Amsterdam: Ploegsma, 1990), 24–31, 53–62.

9. Rineke van Daalen, 'Het begin van de Amsterdamse "zuigelingenzorg": medicalisering en verstatelijking', *Amsterdams Sociologisch Tijdschrift*, 8 (1981), 461–98.

10. Dekker, *op. cit.* (note 7), 97–101; B. Kruithof and P. de Rooy, 'Liefde en plichtsbesef. De kinderbescherming in Nederland rond 1900', *Sociologisch Tijdschrift*, 13 (1987), 637–68.

11. J.C. Vleggeert, *Kinderarbeid in Nederland 1500–1874. Van berusting tot beperking* (Assen: Van Gorcum, 1964), 71 ff.; Houwaart, *op. cit.* (note 5), 274–8.

12. Rapport der Commissie belast met het onderzoek naar den toestand der kinderen in fabrieken arbeidende (1869), quoted in Vleggeert, *op. cit.* (note 11), 89.

13. Stuurman, *op. cit.* (note 2), 189; Vleggeert, *op. cit.* (note 11), 109 ff.

14. Th. Veld, *Volksonderwijs en leerplicht. Een historisch sociologisch onderzoek naar het ontstaan van de Nederlandse leerplicht 1860–1900* (Dissertation University of Leiden, 1987), 83–98.

15. A. Postma. *De mislukte pogingen tussen 1874 en 1889 tot de verbetering en uitbreiding van de kinderwet-Van Houten* (Deventer: Kluwer, 1977); Brands-Bottema, *op. cit.* (note 3), 68–9.

16. I. Weijers, 'Het pedagogisch tekort van de strafrechtelijke kinderwet', *Comenius*, 18 (1998), 12–27; Brands-Bottema, *op. cit.* (note 3), *passim*; Dekker, *op. cit.* (note 7), 150 ff.; Kruithof and De Rooy, *op. cit.* (note 10).

17. The standard account on pillarization in English is A. Lijphart, *The Politics of Accommodation: Pluralism and Democracy in the Netherlands* (Berkeley: University of California Press, 1968).

18. The debate on pillarization in the Netherlands is almost boundless. For an overview see J.C.H. Blom, 'Onderzoek naar verzuiling in Nederland. Status quaestionis en wenselijke ontwikkeling', in J.C.H. Blom and C.J. Misset (eds), *'Broeders sluit U aan'. Aspecten van verzuiling in zeven Hollandse gemeenten* (Den Haag: De Bataafsche Leeuw/Stichting Hollandse Historische Reeks, 1985), 10–29. For data on the growth of denominational organisations in the area of

health care, see P. Pennings, *Verzuiling en ontzuiling: de lokale verschillen. Opbouw, instandhouding en neergang van plaatselijke zuilen in verschillende delen van Nederland na 1880* (Kampen: Kok, 1991), 92.

19. See, for instance, S. Collini, *Public Moralists: Political Thought and Intellectual Life in Britain 1850–1930* (Oxford: Clarendon Press, 1991).

20. Weijers, *op. cit.* (note 16), 19–20.

21. Ido de Haan, 'Een gevelde Goliath? Liberale onderwijspolitiek 1848–1920', in T.J. van der Ploeg *et al.* (eds), *De vrijheid van onderwijs, de ontwikkeling van een bijzonder grondrecht* (Utrecht: Lemma, 2000), 35–57.

22. N. Bakker, 'Een gezamenlijk karwei. Nederlandse pedagogen over de inbreng van moeders en vaders in de gezinsopvoeding, 1845–1920', *Comenius,* 18 (1998), 115–30.

23. W.H. de Beaufort, *Onderwijs en maatschappij (een voorlezing)* (Utrecht: Gebr. van der Post 1880), 37; Te Velde, *op. cit.* (note 2) , 104–17.

24. See, for instance, D. Bos, *Onze volksopleiding* (Groningen: J.B. Wolters, 1898).

25. N. Bakker, 'Dokter Allebé: de negentiende eeuwse Dokter Spock', *Jeugd en samenleving,* 25 (1995), 243–53.

26. G.A.N. Allebé, 'Beweging en rust', in *Twee hygiënische studies* (Amsterdam: P.N. van Kampen 1878 [1859]), 35-90: 75.

27. Quoted in R. Stokvis, 'De school en de ontwikkeling van de sport- en spelbeweging in Nederland', in M. D'hoker and J. Tolleneer (eds), *Het vergeten lichaam. Geschiedenis van de lichamelijke opvoeding in België en Nederland* (Leuven/Apeldoorn: Garant, 1995), 69.

28. D. Bos, 'Onderwijshervorming', *Vragen des Tijds,* 37 (1911), 1-32: 1.

29. G.A.N. Allebé, *Onderzoek naar de waarde van kunstmatige oefeningen voor de vrouwelijke jeugd* (Amsterdam: P.N. van Kampen, 1857), *passim.*

30. J.T.T.C. van Dam van Isselt, *Volksopvoeding en volksweerbaarheid. Voordracht gehouden in de Vereeniging tot beoefening van de Krijgswetenschap. Nieuwe uitgave* ('s-Gravenhage: Gebr. Belinfante, 1895), 8, 12, 33.

31. Te Velde, *op. cit.* (note 2), 78–82.

32. Quoted in K. Neuvel, 'Schoolbanken, gymnastiek en klassikaal onderwijs in de tweede helft van de negentiende eeuw', *Amsterdams Sociologisch Tijdschrift,* 10 (1983), 479–94: 484.

33. Allebé, *op. cit.* (note 26), 74.

34. Quoted in [N.M. Graafland], *Na vijf-en-zeventig jaar. Gedenkboek*

uitgegeven bij het 75-jarig bestaan der Vereeniging van Leeraren en
Onderwijzers in de Lichamelijke Opvoeding in Nederland 1862–1937
(n.p.: Jan Luiting Fonds, 1937), 67.

35. [F.W.C.H. van Tuyll van Serooskerken], *Rapport aan den minister*
van onderwijs, kunsten en wetenschappen betreffende de hoofdlijnen,
waarlangs de overheidsbemoeiing met de lichamelijke opvoeding zich zal
hebben te bewegen (Amsterdam: Ridderinkhof, Ruijs & Co.,1921), 3.

36. J.J. de Ruijter, *Lichaamsoefeningen en volksweerbaarheid* (Rotterdam:
Meindert Boogaerdt, 1906), 18.

37. See N. Bakker, *Kind en karakter. Nederlandse pedagogen over*
opvoeding in het gezin 1845–1925 (Amsterdam: Het Spinhuis, 1995),
87.

38. *Verslag van de Staatscommissie tot onderzoek naar de ontwikkeling der*
jeugdige personen van 13–18 jaar ('s-Gravenhage, 1919), quoted in
M. Lunenberg, *Geluk door geestelijke groei. De institutionalisering van*
de jeugdzorg tussen 1919 en het midden van de jaren dertig, uitgewerkt
voor Amsterdam (Zwolle: Waanders, 1988), 49.

39. N. Bakker, 'Een lastige levensfase. Nederlandse gezinspedagogen over
puberteit en adolescentie in het gezin, 1916–1950', *Comenius,* 45
(1992), 3–15.

40. J. Peet, *Het uur van de arbeidersjeugd. De Katholieke Arbeiders Jeugd,*
de Vrouwelijke Katholieke Arbeidersjeugd en de emancipatie van de
werkende jongeren in Nederland 1944–1969 (Baarn: Arbor, 1987),
76.

41. J.R. Gillis, *Youth and History. Tradition and Change in European Age*
Relations, 1770–Present (New York: Academic Press, 1974).

42. *Kweekelingen Almanak* (1911), quoted in G. Harmsen, *Blauwe en*
rode jeugd. Ontstaan, ontwikkeling en teruggang van de Nederlandse
jeugdbeweging tussen 1853 en 1940 (Assen: Van Gorcum, Prakke &
Prakke, 1961), 86.

43. Kruithof and De Rooy, *op. cit.* (note 10), 658.

44. Kruithof and De Rooy, *op. cit.* (note 10).

45. P. Selten, *Het apostolaat der jeugd. Katholieke jeugdbewegingen in*
Nederland 1900–1941 (Dissertation Catholic University Nijmegen,
1991), 130.

46. P. Selten, 'Tussen Patronaat en Instuif. Dux en de katholieke
jeugdorganisatie, 1927–1958', in *Tussen jeugdzorg en*
jeugdemancipatie. Een halve eeuw jeugd en samenleving in de spiegel
van het katholieke maandblad Dux 1927–1970 (Baarn: Ambo, 1979),
179-91: 181, 185.

47. G. Lamers SJ, 'Moderne opvoeding' (1914), quoted in Selten, *op.*
cit. (note 45), 119.

48. B. Kruithof and E. Mulder, 'Natuurlijk, dus christelijk. Nederlandse gereformeerden en de reformpedagogiek', *Comenius*, 42 (1991), 142–54; see, on the Protestant youth movement, J.C. Sturm, *Een goede gereformeerde opvoeding: over neo-calvinistische moraalpedagogiek (1880–1950), met speciale aandacht voor de nieuw-gereformeerde jeugdorganisaties* (Kampen: Kok, 1988).

49. Kruithof and De Rooy, *op. cit.* (note 10), 659.

50. AJC-leader K. Vorrink, 1924, quoted in Harmsen, *op. cit.* (note 42), 188.

51. Quoted in L. Hartveld, F. de Jong Edz. and D. Kuperus, *De Arbeiders Jeugd Centrale AJC. 1918–1940 / 1945–1959* (Amsterdam: Van Gennep, 1982), 111.

52. *KGOB-Almanak* (1915), quoted in Harmsen, *op. cit.* (note 42), 101.

53. SDAP-leader B. Schaper in 1924, quoted in Hartveld *et al.*, *op. cit.* (note 51), 77.

54. P. de Rooy, *Kinderbescherming en jeugdbeweging* (Amsterdam: Pedagogisch-Didactisch Instituut, [1981]), 29.

55. W.E. van Wijk in *Volksontwikkeling* (1924–1925), quoted in Lunenberg, *op. cit.* (note 38), 79.

56. Te Velde, *op. cit.* (note 2), 218 ff.

57. H. Dona, *Sport en socialisme. De geschiedenis van de Nederlandse Arbeiderssportbond 1926–1941* (Amsterdam: Van Gennep, 1981), 126.

58. NBAS-brochure, n.d., quoted in Harmsen, *op. cit.* (note 42), 248.

59. Quoted in Dona, *op. cit.* (note 57), 131.

60. E.C. Lekkerkerker, 'Geschiedenis', in *Het moeilijke kind. Tien jaren medisch-opvoedkundige bureaux* (Eibergen: Heinen, 1938), 7–22.

61. A.H. Bergink, 'De ontwikkeling der randdiensten', in J.W. van Hulst, I. van der Velde and G.Th.M. Verhaak (eds), *Vernieuwingsstreven binnen het Nederlandse onderwijs in de periode 1900–1940* (Groningen: Wolters-Noordhoff, 1970), 317–42.

62. N. Knapper, *Een kwart eeuw zuigelingenzorg in Nederland* (Amsterdam: Scheltema & Holkema, 1935), 23.

63. Wijsenbeek, *op. cit.* (note 8), 99; N. Wiegman, '"De verpleegster zij in de eerste plaats vrouw van karakter": ziekenverpleging als vrouwenzaak (1898–1998)', in R. van Daalen and M. Gijswijt-Hofstra (eds), *Gezond en wel. Vrouwen en de zorg voor gezondheid in de twintigste eeuw* (Amsterdam: Amsterdam University Press, 1998), 125–40; H. Marland, '"A Woman's Touch": Women Doctors and the Development of Health Services for Women and Children in the Netherlands 1879-c.1925', in H. Binneveld and R. Dekker (eds), *Curing and Insuring: Essays on Illness in Past Times* (Hilversum:

Verloren, 1993), 113-33.

64. See H. van Setten, *Opvoeding in volkse geest. Fascisme in het onderwijs 1940–1945* (Bergen: Octavo, 1985); H. Malschaert, 'Sport, opvoeding en nationaal-socialisme. Lichaamsoefening en opvoeding bij de Nationale Jeugdstorm', *Comenius*, 25 (1987), 27–48; Geertje Beerenhout-Naarden, '"De wereld omspannen met vriendschap". De Arbeiders Jeugd Centrale na de bevrijding', in H. Galesloot and M. Schrevel (eds), *In fatsoen hersteld. Zedelijkheid en wederopbouw na de oorlog* (Amsterdam: SUA, n.d.), 47–62; Harmsen, *op. cit.* (note 42), 292–3.

65. H. de Liagre Böhl, 'Zedeloosheidsbestrijding in 1945. Een motor van de wederopbouw', in Galesloot and Schrevel (eds), *op. cit.* (note 64), 15–28; G. Dimmendaal, 'Over "deraillerende meisjes". De opvang van ontspoorde jonge vrouwen in een Groningse inrichting rond 1945', in Galesloot and Schrevel (eds), *op. cit.* (note 64), 115–34; H. de Liagre Böhl and G. Meershoek, *De Bevrijding van Amsterdam. Een strijd om macht en moraal* (Zwolle: Waanders, 1989).

66. H. van Oyen in *De reactie van ons volk op de bevrijding* (1946), quoted in De Liagre Böhl, *op. cit.* (note 65), 18.

67. F. van der Wel, 'Het onmaatschappelijke kind en de massajeugd', *Comenius*, 25 (1987), 63–82.

68. D. Hoogendoorn, *De zuigelingensterfte in Nederland* (Assen: Van Gorcum, Prakke & Prakke, 1959); H.W.A. Voorhoeve, 'De situatie van het kind in de eeuw van het kind', in *idem* (ed.), *75 jaar Kinderhygiëne in Nederland. Van zuigelingenzorg tot jeugdgezondheidszorg* (Assen/Amsterdam: Van Gorcum, 1977), 24-32: 27.

69. See, for instance, Wijsenbeek, *op. cit.* (note 8), 126 ff.

70. P.F. Maas, *Parlement & polio* (Den Haag: SDU, 1988).

71. See, for instance, 'Kinderziekten', *Orthomoleculair: tweemaandelijks bulletin van de Survival Stichting*, 12 (1994), 156–63.

72. See P. de Rooy, 'Vetkuifje waarheen? Jongeren in de jaren vijftig en zestig', in H.W. von der Dunk (ed.), *Wederopbouw, welvaart en onrust. Nederland in de jaren vijftig en zestig* (Houten: De Haan, 1986), 119–46; R. Abma, 'Nuchterheid en nozems', in G. Tillekens (ed.), *Nuchterheid en nozems. De opkomst van de jeugdcultuur in de jaren vijftig* (Muiderberg: Coutinho, 1990), 31–45; J. Kennedy, *Nieuw Babylon in aanbouw. Nederland in de jaren zestig* (Meppel/Amsterdam: Boom, 1995), 42–9.

73. A.A.M. Dercksen and L.H.J. Verplanke, *Geschiedenis van de onmaatschappelijkheidsbestrijding in Nederland 1914–1970* (Meppel: Boom, 1987), 93.

74. Quoted in S. van 't Hof, J. Broerse and L. de Goei, *Tulpenburg en Amstelland 1951–1994. Bladzijden uit de geschiedenis van de Nederlandse kinder- en jeugdpsychiatrie* (Utrecht: Trimbos-instituut, 1997), 23.

75. Commissie-Eyssen, *Rapport Onmaatschappelijke Gezinnen* (1951), quoted in Dercksen and Verplanke, *op. cit.* (note 73), 103.

76. J. Noordman, *Om de kwaliteit van het nageslacht. Eugenetica in Nederland 1900–1950* (Nijmegen: SUN, 1989), 140; Dercksen and Verplanke, *op. cit.* (note 73), 144.

77. D.E. Krantz and E.W. Vercruijsse, *De jeugd in het geding* (Amsterdam: De Bezige Bij, 1959), 143.

78. A.A. van Rhijn, *Sociale zekerheid* (Amsterdam: Uitgeverij Vrij Nederland, 1947), 13.

79. Handelingen der Staten-Generaal 1959–1960, quoted in S. Gerritsen and I. van der Zande, 'Met beleid omgeven. De afdeling Jeugdvorming en Volksontwikkeling', in Tillekens (ed.), *op. cit.* (note 72), 104-22: 121.

80. Gerritsen and Van der Zande, *op. cit.* (note 79).

81. See, for instance, E. Simons and L. Winkeler, *Het verraad der clercken: intellectuelen en hun rol in de ontwikkelingen van het Nederlandse katholicisme na 1945* (Baarn: Arbor, 1987); I. Weijers, *Terug naar het behouden huis. Romanschrijvers en wetenschappers in de jaren vijftig* (Amsterdam: SUA, 1991); H. Oosterhuis, *De smalle marges van de Roomse moraal. Homoseksualiteit in katholiek Nederland 1900–1970* (Dissertation University of Amsterdam, 1992).

82. Gerritsen and Van der Zande, *op. cit.* (note 79); De Rooy, *op. cit.* (note 72).

83. H. Righart, *De eindeloze jaren zestig. Geschiedenis van een generatieconflict* (Amsterdam: De Arbeiderspers, 1995), 59–70.

84. See I. de Haan, *Zelfbestuur en staatsbeheer. Het politieke debat over burgerschap en rechtsstaat in de twintigste eeuw* (Amsterdam: Amsterdam University Press, 1993), 100–10; *idem*, 'De eindeloze jaren zestig', *De nieuwste tijd*, 5 (1995), 37–45.

85. I. Weijers, 'De slag om Dennendal. Een terugblik op de jaren vijftig vanuit de jaren zeventig', in P. Luykx and P. Slot (eds), *Een stille revolutie? Cultuur en mentaliteit in de lange jaren vijftig* (Hilversum: Verloren, 1997), 46–50.

86. V. Mamadouh, *De stad in eigen hand. Provo's, kabouters en krakers als stedelijke sociale beweging* (Amsterdam: SUA, 1992), 106; Kennedy, *op. cit.* (note 72), 126.

87. J.W. Duyvendak, 'De constructies van de andragologie versus de waarheid van zelfkennis. Of: waarom de andragologie ten onderging

aan "autonomie"', *Krisis,* 63 (1996), 38–49: E. Tonkens, *Het zelfontplooiingsregime. De actualiteit van Dennendal en de jaren zestig* (Amsterdam: Bert Bakker, 1999).

88. See H. Boutellier, *Solidariteit en slachtofferschap. De morele betekenis van criminaliteit in een postmoderne cultuur* (Nijmegen: Sun, 1993); I. de Haan, *Na de ondergang. De herinnering aan de Jodenvervolging in Nederland 1945–1995* (Den Haag: SDU, 1997), 146–50.

89. See Rineke van Daalen, 'Aantekeningen over kindermishandeling en incest. De medische definitie, de feministische definitie en hun onderlinge relatie', in G. Hekma *et al.* (eds), *Het verlies van de onschuld. Seksualiteit in Nederland* (Groningen: Wolters-Noordhoff, 1988), 151–68; N. Draijer, *Seksuele traumatisering in de jeugd. Gevolgen op langere termijn van seksueel misbruik van meisjes door verwanten* (Amsterdam: SUA, 1990).

90. A. van Lenning, *Het vege lijf. Anorexia nervosa: kwijnen, lijnen of hongeren* (Dissertation University of Utrecht, 1992), 165.

91. See M. Ruiter, *Preventie van depressie bij jongeren. Probleemanalyse, ontwikkeling en evaluatie van de cursus 'Stemmingmakerij'* (Dissertation Catholic University of Nijmegen, 1997), 9.

3

Child Health, National Fitness, and Physical Education in Britain, 1900–1940

John Welshman

The emphasis on the 'third way' that characterises contemporary health policy attempts to create a new paradigm and overcome the earlier dichotomy between Left and Right on behavioural and structural causes of ill-health. In addition, debates on such issues as unmarried mothers tend to be couched in terms of international league tables, with references to the relative position of Britain compared to other developed countries. And so it is not surprising that recent policy documents have linked physical education for young people with broader objectives in the field of public health. The recent White Paper, *Saving Lives: Our Healthier Nation* (1999), for example, argues that 'good physical education and school sports provision are essential to the foundation of lifelong positive attitudes towards health and fitness'.[1] And this emphasis is evident in other policy initiatives. The Girls in Sport Partnership Scheme, for instance, run by the Youth Sport Trust and Nike, was prompted by evidence that 40 per cent of girls drop out of sport by the age of 14, and aims to encourage them back into sport at school. Playing sport, it is claimed, increases the confidence of girls, making them less likely to have eating disorders, unplanned pregnancies, or to leave school early.[2] Thus it is clear that sport in schools, for both boys and girls, continues to be linked with important concepts of health, citizenship, and fitness.

This return to the concept of national fitness has interesting echoes with the period 1900–40, when it is recognised that the movement for national efficiency was a key influence on the development of child health and welfare. In what remains an important study, Geoffrey Searle has argued that the 'efficiency group' thought that men and women formed the raw material for national greatness, and argued these resources should not be squandered. This concern with organisation and with eliminating waste brought a new urgency to the work of social reform.[3] This has been an influential interpretation, so much so that the Report of the Inter-Departmental Committee on Physical Deterioration (1904) is still credited with playing a major part in the creation of the School Medical Service. At the same time, later writers have often missed the subtlety of Searle's original argument and have reproduced it in bowdlerised form. In fact, Searle noted that 'national efficiency' was not a homogeneous political label, but one under which a complex series of beliefs, assumptions, and demands could be grouped. Furthermore with the return of peace in 1918, the mood evaporated, indicating that movements for 'national efficiency' tended to emerge at periods of imagined national crisis – as in the early-1900s and in the 1930s – when a mood of introspection was prompted by economic crisis.[4]

This chapter seeks to look more closely at the usefulness of the concept of national efficiency as an influence on child health and welfare in Britain in the period 1900–40. Whether national efficiency can be equated with national fitness is an interesting question. Here we try to examine the connections that were made in the context of the development of physical education, in part through the writings of one contemporary observer, Sir George Newman (1870–1948). As is well-known, Newman was Chief Medical Officer (CMO) to the Board of Education, 1907–35, and the Ministry of Health, 1919–35. But unlike his contemporary Sir Arthur Newsholme, Newman's work has not as yet attracted the attention of a biographer. What is clear is that Newman was particularly interested in physical education – he was an active chairman of the Dartford Physical Training College – and in his annual reports *The Health of the School Child* he provides an interesting summary of the ways in which child health was conceptualised.[5] While well-known and often cited, these have usually been analysed more for the information they provide on the development of medical services, and less for the wider insights they offer into the ideological background to health policy. This chapter argues that while the concept of national fitness was an important influence on the development of physical education in schools, it was not the only one. Moreover the influence of these ideas was mediated by both political traditions and practical problems, creating a significant mismatch between policy rhetoric and the provision of facilities on the ground.

City and countryside in debates about physical education

In the late-nineteenth century, there had been attempts to provide physical education for children in schools, though these had been based predominantly on drill. After 1900 on the other hand, physical education came to play a larger role in official writings on the operation of health services for children, though its relationship with key services such as medical inspection and treatment was always somewhat tangential. Work by historians has already revealed aspects of this story. The early research examined the expansion of courses for teachers, the employment of specialist staff, and the increasing provision of playgrounds and playing fields, and also revealed how influential athleticism was as an ideology in the Victorian public school.[6] More recent studies have examined the growth of physical education in countries including the Republic of Ireland and Scandinavia, and have shown how it developed as a school subject in the years after the Second World War.[7] The role of women in the history of physical education has received some attention, though this remains a neglected area.[8] And medical sociologists have drawn on physical education in order to support a Foucauldian interpretation of the influence of power and surveillance on the body. David Armstrong, for instance, writes that 'instead of bodies being confined in homes and hidden by clothing, physical culture enabled them to be legitimately and publicly viewed'.[9]

It is clear that the concept of national fitness was only one important theme among many shaping the emergence of physical education before 1940. Older, but still deeply-held, ideas about the effects on child health of living in cities also influenced the debates on physical fitness. In the late nineteenth century, drill and physical education in the open-air was regarded by social reformers as a means of alleviating the allegedly debilitating effects of urban life. As is well-known, the theme of 'physical deterioration', while its impact may well have been exaggerated by earlier writers, was essentially a debate about the effect, on child and adult health, of living in the city. Concerns about such issues as juvenile smoking relied heavily on the image of the urban 'loafer'.[10] And while this emphasis was to an extent less apparent in the interwar period, it is also arguable that it continued up to and including the Second World War. The supposed value of fresh air was seen in such innovations as open-air schools, and more widely in other public health institutions, including tuberculosis sanatoria.[11] Indeed, this was expressed with particular force in September 1939 when the cultures of urban and rural Britain were compelled to meet head-on with the evacuation of schoolchildren from the cities to the countryside.[12]

Although rarely explicit, there was an implicit assumption in Newman's thought, as in that of many interwar social reformers, that rural life was superior to that of the towns. The rural idyll was a reference point for all that was assumed to be healthy and wholesome – a point that was to an extent timeless, but which perhaps reached its apogee in interwar advertising. A number of reasons can be advanced to account for this. One was simply the technological advances in printing which, along with increasing demand on the part of consumers, stimulated a rapid growth in the advertising industry.[13] A second was the rate of suburban growth that led numerous contemporary observers to write of the countryside being eroded by persistent ribbon development. Another was perhaps that, paradoxically, at a time of important scientific research into nutrition and such areas as vitamins, manufacturers perceived that references to the 'natural' might have a heightened appeal.[14] Certainly physical fitness was almost always seen in terms of the city child. As Newman wrote in 1920 of Wales, 'in the industrial areas and in the larger towns there is a special need for vigorous and active physical exercise of a recreative character... so that an interest in physical training for its own sake may be aroused and lasting effects on character and habit produced'.[15]

One example of this theme being translated into practical health policy is provided by the increase in school journeys, which for administrative purposes came to be subsumed under the umbrella of physical education. In some ways, these were a logical extension of developments in transport, and of the opening up of the countryside to the motor car that has previously been noted as having been a characteristic feature of the interwar period. But there was a particular move to provide school journeys for children attending schools in urban areas, where they tended to head out to the countryside or to seaside resorts. In 1918, for example, children attending schools in the London area visited small towns such as Guildford in Surrey and Loughton in Essex, and the resorts of Shanklin and Ryde on the Isle of Wight. It was believed that these would literally transform the outlook of the city child. As the School Medical Officer (SMO) for the London County Council (LCC) wrote in 1928, 'the escape from the smoke pall of the city, the breathing of pure air, and the country regime puts new life into the city-bred child'.[16]

The LCC was the most prominent Local Education Authority (LEA) in this area, in conjunction with voluntary organisations that were set up for this purpose, such as the Children's Country Holiday Fund.[17] But school journeys were also organised for children attending schools in the cities of economically depressed regions.

The extent of these was limited by the low level of rates which, it has been argued, acted as a drag on health expenditure in these areas. But the deficiencies of state funding created an opportunity for voluntary organisations, and on those occasions when these LEAs were able to organise school journeys, it is clear that they were regarded as having a beneficial effect on both health and citizenship. The SMO for West Hartlepool, for instance, noted in 1928 of visits to York and Warwick that 'if the chief aim of education be the "formation of character", then the school journey, especially for the town child, renders the greatest possible assistance'.[18]

The demonising of urban life, and corresponding idealisation of the rural, was also arguably at its most apparent in the attempts to develop school camps. It is well-known that Robert Baden-Powell had laid down careful guidelines for them in *Scouting for Boys*, and the appeal of the camp was one of the reasons for the rapid success of the Scouting movement. Not surprisingly, this attracted the attention of educational reformers. E.A. Impey for example, wrote in 1913 that the various activities associated with camping 'make the school child resourceful, fearless, and fit in himself, and a thousand times more helpful and unselfish at home'.[19] What is not perhaps so well known is that Newman was an admirer of the Scouting movement. This raises interesting questions about the relationship between voluntarism and the state. More specifically, Newman's comments support the view that in this period Scouting was less about militarism and much more about introducing boys to the outdoors.[20]

As with school journeys, there was a particular focus on London in the case of camps, in part because it represented the 'problems' of urban life in their most intense form, but also because the LCC was relatively 'progressive' in terms of health policy. The best-known of these school camps was the King's Canadian Camp School at Bushey Park where children thought to be suffering from anaemia or malnutrition were sent for four-week periods. There were various attempts to assess the beneficial effects of such camps through alleged increases in such indices as the haemoglobin content of the blood. Although these comparisons had little scientific value, Newman was in no doubt about the value of these activities. He wrote that 'to boys whose horizon is bounded by a slum environment, [the camp] must create an oasis in the desert of their daily lives' – a striking metaphor which, like much of the language used in this context, is worthy of further analysis.[21] LEAs either organised camps themselves or contributed to others run by the Scouts and the Boy's Brigade. But the emphasis on school camps also became wider than this since LEAs were given new powers to provide them through the 1918 Education Act.

The model adopted for the ideal school camp drew closely on the earlier examples provided by the Scouting movement. Here ideals of health and citizenship were closely linked. The recommended form of camp life was marked by a stress on work – 'pioneer' work such as the making of camp furniture – while there was also firm discipline and an emphasis on personal cleanliness. There are parallels here with the belief in 'work therapy' that characterised the tuberculosis sanatorium in this period – as Newman observed in 1917, 'there must be plenty of occupation and no loafing in camp'.[22] And as with the sanatorium there was no mistaking the aim of the camp, or of its perceived value in introducing the working-class child to both the pleasures of the countryside, and to increased contact with middle-class mores. As an editorial in the *Times Educational Supplement* argued in August 1929, the task of the teacher was 'to create a tradition in the light of which these lads – splendid material, but crude and ignorant – will come to see the advantages of higher standards'.[23] Overall, the appeal of physical education, and of such activities as school journeys and camps, can be seen as a means of providing a suitable hobby for the urban youth, and of solving the 'problem' of leisure in a mass, industrial society.

Physical education, discipline, and public health

If the urban/rural dichotomy was one theme in the development of physical education for schoolchildren, another was the belief that gymnastics and drill could both prevent and cure more serious health problems. In this sense, physical education came to be incorporated in the move, after 1900, from environmental health to an emphasis on personal health services. There were many reasons why physical education featured so prominently in official reports. On the one hand, while a system of medical inspection had been created in 1907, it was only more gradually that a network of clinics was established to actually treat the various 'minor ailments' that inspection had revealed.[24] Physical education proved increasingly attractive to the Board of Education as it came to be faced, in the interwar period, with critics who argued that much of the statistical evidence derived from medical inspections was worthless, particularly with respect to malnutrition. And since physical education was regarded as a particularly cheap way of improving children's health, it was to an extent protected from the financial retrenchment that hampered expenditure as a whole in the early-1920s and early-1930s. But physical education was also in the vanguard of more 'modern' aspects of education policy, as for example a means of incorporating blind and deaf children, as well as those regarded as mentally or physically 'defective'.

There were some areas where officials were cautious. The whole question of physical education for girls, for example, was regarded as presenting something of a special case. On the one hand, policy-makers recognised that girls should not be excluded from physical education lessons. In an era when eugenics was influential, the health of women was important – possibly even more so than that of men, since 'on them devolves the duty of producing and rearing a strong and healthy race'.[25] But it was also thought that girls had no experience of vigorous exercise, possessed little stamina, and were particularly vulnerable to physical exhaustion. At some schools, it was claimed, girls were 'not infrequently under-nourished, anaemic, flabby, unaccustomed to exercise and readily fatigued'.[26] The solution therefore, was to adapt physical education and games – by reducing the size of the pitch or making the equipment less heavy – so that girls could participate. Direct competition with boys in games demanding strength and stamina, for example, was particularly discouraged. In contrast it was more feminine sports that were favoured – or other forms of exercise such as dancing.

But this hesitancy was unusual, and the association between physical education and improved health was apparent in Newman's annual reports from the early years of the School Medical Service. It was most obviously true in the special case of remedial gymnastics, and in the focus on posture. In 1916, for example, Newman claimed that where children were suffering from minor cases of 'bodily deformities', the result of treatment based on nothing more than suitable exercise and correct posture was that 'the incipient deformity frequently disappears'.[27] To an extent this was translated into practical reality at the local level where 'progressive' LEAs such as Bradford appointed remedial gymnasts. The link between posture and improved performance in the classroom was amplified in contemporary photographs. And it was associated with the general expansion of orthopaedics as a medical specialism in the interwar period. But the direct association between physical education and improved health was also apparent in comments on physical education for schoolchildren as a whole. In a way this also paralleled the stress on the 'normal' child, who was regarded as being more important to the nation and the future than his 'deficient' counterpart.

In 1908 for example, Newman had written that physical education and games would 'do much to improve the physique of all children, and some of the brightness and happiness so essential to healthy childhood can be introduced in this way'.[28] Sport and exercise could not only improve nutrition, and increase the body's natural resistance to disease, but could also prevent a wide range of specific ailments – among them flat feet, curvature of the spine, adenoids, deafness, and mental 'backwardness'. Newman was careful to point out that in certain cases teachers should seek medical advice and consult the SMO – anaemic children, for example, should rest in the fresh air during the games lesson.[29] But other children (such as those with 'minor' heart disease) could participate, so long as exercises like running, jumping, and skipping (that would leave them out of breath) were omitted. Thus by 1912 Newman was able to argue that physical education had become 'a preventive measure of substantial value', and, indeed, that it was only through this that child health could be improved.[30]

The fact that physical education appeared to guarantee improved health with little financial outlay meant that it was particularly attractive to the Board of Education (and its political masters) in periods of financial retrenchment. Thus in March 1922, for example, shortly after the Geddes Axe on public expenditure, one civil servant noted that more attention should be paid to games and exercise since 'the work is of primary importance; it is the first line of defence in preventive medicine; and it is absurdly cheap'.[31] Annual reports and circulars issued at this time urged those LEAs considering cuts in health services for schoolchildren to give 'very careful attention' to the particular merits of this area of spending. Similarly, in 1931, following the publication of the May Committee on public expenditure, it was observed that no one who had witnessed the effects of physical education could doubt its efficiency in preventing illness and making the body more resistant to disease.[32] Indeed, this argument was taken further so that physical education became a cheap solution to the effects of unemployment on health – a convenient way of killing two birds with one stone. In the new syllabus published in 1933 for instance, the Board of Education claimed that physical education was particularly important in periods of high unemployment, poverty, and economic dislocation.[33]

Certainly the emphasis on physical education as a branch of public health was particularly noticeable during the 1920s – as Newman argued at the beginning of the decade, 'to prevent infection is good; to build healthy and resistant bodies is better'.[34] As has already been noted, exercise had the character of a kind of general panacea or universal remedy, and it was not surprising that physical education was put forward as the solution to the 'mental stress' to which teenage children attending secondary schools were thought to be particularly susceptible. Indeed, in Newman's own words, physical education had become 'the supreme method of medicine in behalf [sic] of the normal school child'.[35] Once the appointment of trained teachers and specialist staff ensured that it was generally available at the local level, there would be a corresponding reduction in the need for formal health care – a point that echoes the claim frequently made about the early National Health Service. Thus Newman wrote that as physical culture became more firmly established in schools 'the less shall we need formal and corrective work in physical training, *and the less shall we need medical treatment*' (Newman's italics).[36]

It is instructive to see why some forms of exercise were favoured at the expense of others. Swimming, for example, was regarded as being one of the best forms of physical education since it was enjoyable, provided exercise without over-developing any one group of muscles, made full use of the heart and lungs, and encouraged the general development of the body. An additional benefit was its practical contribution to 'habits of bodily cleanliness'.[37] Although swimming was cheap in terms of access and kit, building new pools demanded high capital expenditure. But there is also perhaps a danger of exaggerating the dichotomy between the supposedly 'reactionary' and 'radical' aspects of physical education. In reality the picture was more complex that a simple binary opposition would imply. It is worth noting that in the 1930s, for instance, physical education was recommended (though belatedly) for children who were blind and deaf, and for those deemed to be 'defective'. This focus had been absent in earlier years, perhaps because physical education was aimed at the 'normal' child who, as we have seen, was always juxtaposed with his 'deficient' counterpart. But certainly it came to be recognised that physical education could have an important role in the curriculum of special schools.[38] Thus by the 1930s, some of the arguments that had been advanced earlier in support of physical education had been turned on their head.

There were other ways in which the focus on physical education changed in the 1930s, possibly as a reaction to shifts in the debate on citizenship, but perhaps also as a response to wider changes in expectations about the potential scope of health services. The emphasis placed on physical education, and the claims advanced on its behalf, led to controversy in relation to the parallel issue of school meals and milk. In the interwar period, as is well known, nutrition came to have an increasingly prominent place in the battle between the Board of Education and its critics. On the one hand, the new knowledge that resulted from scientific research into areas such as vitamins threatened to expose the ineffectiveness of the school medical inspection as a means of assessing the nutritional status of schoolchildren. On the other, it was pointed out that LEAs in depressed regions seemed unable to provide free school meals and milk for those children who most needed them.

Given its central role in official propaganda, it was inevitable that physical education would be drawn into this debate. Thus in 1923 Newman had written that 'nutrition implies more than feeding.... besides proper food, we must make sure of suitable exercise, because without the stimulation of exercise we cannot expect satisfactory building up of the tissues'.[39] Similarly in 1929, he argued that, as a factor in nutrition, the value of exercise could not be overestimated, especially in the case of the 'weakly' child. This reflected in part the rival arguments about whether malnutrition was more an issue linked to structural factors such as income and unemployment, or a problem associated with ignorance that would best be solved by educational measures. Although Newman conceded that meals and milk were essential for schoolchildren to have perfect health, health education was also important, in inculcating a 'right habit of living'. Health was not so much a right, but an individual responsibility. Thus physical education made healthy children stronger, but also gave those who were less robust 'an opportunity of removing or reducing their disabilities'.[40]

Even so, although the Board of Education's critics had never had access to the resources available to official propagandists, these arguments had never gone entirely unchallenged. A few SMOs had always been critical of the emphasis on physical education and the failure, as they saw it, to expand other health services. In 1904, for example, Norman Bennett, later an influential figure in the British Dental Association, had written 'how impossible it is to remedy by physical exercise in adolescence and early manhood the physical defects which are the result of unhygienic environment and neglected minor diseases in childhood'.[41] Moreover by the late 1930s, there were signs that the claims earlier advanced in support of physical education were more difficult to sustain. Dr Henry Herd, SMO for Manchester, for example, argued in 1937 that 'while the object of physical education is to produce fitness, we must not forget that the community must be made fit for physical education'. At the same time, he went on to state that 'physical education must be recognised by medical officers as ranking with other measures such as housing, nutrition, sanitation, etc, in making a contribution to the health of the nation'.[42]

The British Medical Association's report on physical education, issued in 1936, stressed that 'unfit' children should not participate in unsuitable exercises or games, and that malnourished children should receive school meals.[43] This was particularly the case in relation to nutrition, a point that comes across strongly in the debates leading up to the 1937 Physical Training and Recreation Act, and in the work of the Advisory Committee on Nutrition. It is important not to exaggerate this point – there was of course a 'keep fit' campaign in the autumn of 1937. But there was also greater defensiveness, so that Neville Chamberlain, for example, was careful to make sure that nutrition experts such as Frederick Gowland Hopkins, Edward Mellanby and Sir John Boyd Orr were not associated with his campaign.[44] Newman had of course retired as CMO in 1935, and under his successor, Sir Arthur MacNalty, there were subtle changes in the stress placed on physical education. Physical education was clearly associated with national fitness and linked to more general objectives in the field of public health. At the same time, this remained a controversial policy aim, which met with resistance.

Physical education and the making of citizens

In reality, the various arguments that were advanced in support of physical education, and the links that were made with the concept of national fitness, are not easy to separate. Much of what was written about physical education was less about international competitiveness, and more about using sport as a means for social integration. And this is particularly evident when one comes to the theme of citizenship, which is a tenuous and slippery concept at the best of times. As with the rural/urban dichotomy, this was an aspect of the debate that went back to the late nineteenth century, if not further, and which incorporated many of its other elements. As is well-known, drill and games had frequently been advanced by earlier social reformers, such as Charles Russell, who were involved in the settlement movement and in the growth of boys' clubs in areas such as London's East End.[45] But the debate about physical education and citizenship also had elements that were more definitely located in the particular milieu of the interwar period.

Although George Newman did not often use the term

'citizenship', this was again a recurring theme in the *Health of the School Child* reports. In 1916, for instance, he wrote that physical education was important, not only for its impact on health status, but also because of its effect on 'the address, discipline, character and general outlook of those who come within its influence'.[46] Some of these alleged advantages were of direct value in the classroom – it was said that exercise introduced 'those elements of freedom, elasticity and enjoyment which make education a living power and a vital interest to the child'.[47] But physical education also embodied assumptions that working-class children were destined to be the factory workers of the future. Drawing on a military metaphor, it was claimed that with habits of exercise, knowledge of health, sufficient rest, adequate food, a love of fresh air, and an interest in games, the young citizen was 'equipped with weapons' that would be valuable in the 'struggle' with exhaustion, the 'insidious attacks' of disease, and other 'strains' likely to undermine health.[48] In many ways, this showed how economic concerns underlay educational policy, since there clearly was concern about the future employment prospects of these children. In the case of gymnastics in junior technical schools, for example, Newman claimed that this had direct benefits since 'it teaches precision of movement and economy of effort, and helps to cultivate the habit of assuming the appropriate posture for the work in hand....in short, it is an invaluable basis for manual efficiency and working capacity'.[49]

But while physical education was seen to be of value to the future factory worker, it also reflected more general anxieties. As was noted earlier, one belief was that the period of adolescence that coincided with leaving school and starting work was marked by 'physical stress', and that it was important to take preventive action. But possibly more influential was concern about the leisure time of the young worker, again a return to the moral panics about youth of the early 1900s. The hope was that through physical education, working-class children might come to see the value of making more constructive use of their leisure time, and would be directed away from unsuitable activities. As Newman wrote in 1919, games and exercise should 'offer welcome means of occupation for leisure hours and point the way to a host of interests undreamed of by the town-bred child'.[50] While some of these desirable qualities were of direct relevance to work, others were of more general significance – including such virtues as a spirit of 'healthy' rivalry, co-operation, courage, endurance, public-spiritedness, fair play, loyalty, and the ability to work together. A further list published in 1930 numbered 'promptitude of action, close attention, instant obedience, persistence and continuity, co-operative team work, sportsmanship in losing as well as in winning'.[51]

In some respects, physical education was regarded as a potential solution to old problems – there were echoes, for example, with the late nineteenth-century debates about the challenge of 'boy labour'. But physical education, and the qualities associated with it, were also seen as a means of tackling some of the newer threats to child health and welfare. By the 1930s, these included concerns about the impact, on young people, of the Americanisation of British culture. In his report for 1933, for example, Newman quoted approvingly from an address to the National Union of Teachers by Dr Cyril Norwood, former headmaster of Harrow and then President of St John's College, Oxford. Norwood had advocated physical education at a time when 'we are surrounded by ugliness on so many sides, and trans-Atlantic vulgarities are corrupting the cinema and the music and the dance halls and the newspapers to which the public as a whole has access'. The need was to regain the value of 'real craftsmanship' and to return to the courage and resourcefulness of primitive man – a belief with which Newman agreed.[52]

In many ways, Newman's thinking echoed the approach of organisations such as the National Council of Social Service (NCSS). Groups like its New Estates Community Committee (1928), with its chairman Sir Ernest Barker, sought to civilise the inhabitants of large council estates by building community centres, and, in rural areas, to recapture the neighbourliness of an earlier age through the construction of village halls.[53] Another aspect of the work of the NCSS was with the unemployed in the economically depressed regions. Indeed in the 1930s the Board of Education co-operated with the NCSS to train men to become physical training instructors in the Special Areas – it was claimed that these were making 'a direct contribution to the national well-being of the unemployed'.[54] It has been argued that in the case of the community centres, the NCSS failed to understand the nature of working-class housing estates such as Becontree, and offered solutions to the imagined 'problem' that were unlikely to meet with much success. Something of this is also true of Newman's approach to physical education, where the recurring reference to the ideology of the Victorian public school was unlikely to have much appeal for the working-class child.

A further link between Newman and the NCSS lay in the reference to solutions drawn from the classics, and from Greek and Roman culture. As Jose Harris has noted, classical Greek philosophy was one of the most potent sources of idealist social thought in this period, since it was seen as providing a series of clues, principles, and practical solutions with which to approach mass, urban, class-based industrial civilisation. She has argued that Plato was the most influential thinker for four reasons – on account of his emphasis on society as an organic spiritual community, his vision of an ethical citizenship, a focus on justice as the basis for the state, and his mysticism and anti-materialism.[55] There was a cyclical element in this – references to the fall of Rome had been made in the 1900s. But it was also noticeable that the *Health of the School Child* report for 1934 referred at length to classical Greek culture. Indeed, it was claimed that 'the old Greek spirit has been recaptured and the harmony between training of the mind and training of the body has been re-established'.[56]

The political context for physical education

If physical education was regarded as a means of bringing classes together, it is also the case that the values it embodied often reflected wider concerns and anxieties about Britain's declining international status. This was particularly true in the early 1900s when the development of child health and welfare in other countries acted as both a stimulus and a model for subsequent British efforts. A typical commentator then was George Shee, Secretary of the National Service League from 1902.[57] And of course the whole notion of 'physical deterioration' was predicated on the fear that Britain was being overtaken by other nations. During the First World War, for instance, there certainly was much reference to the usefulness of exercise and games as a means of preparing soldiers for military training. In his report for 1914, Newman wrote that, apart from its benefits as far as health was concerned, physical education was useful since it 'makes the man quick, alert, keen, and steady, and inculcates a true sense of discipline'.[58] It was not coincidental that the 1918 Education Act gave LEAs new powers to develop school journeys and to introduce children to the countryside through camping. The experience of wartime had served to demonstrate the value of child health, and it was well-known that physical education and games had been useful for training soldiers.

In the early-1920s, these anxieties were more implicit than explicit, and there was little direct debate about equivalent movements for child health in other European countries. However, this changed in the late 1920s and early 1930s when there was increasing reference to the physical training schemes that had been set up in Germany, Italy, Czechoslovakia, and Russia. The evidence that the continental dictatorships had set up more systematic ways of providing physical fitness for their children and youth did force a reappraisal of this approach. While Newman noted that England had tended to provide physical education through its schools, and in voluntary movements such as the Scouts and Guides, he admitted in 1933 that 'the time may have come for some subsidising or constructive action by the State itself'.[59] The approach taken by Russia to physical education was well-known in Britain, not least through some of the Gollancz publications that were selected for the Left Book Club. Moreover, Board of Education officials saw facilities at first hand in Russia in November 1935. One of its civil servants noted in a confidential minute that 'starting from very much behind us Russia has outstripped us in the realisation of the value of collective action with regard to physical training'.[60]

But it was the 1936 Olympics, held in Berlin, that provided the most dramatic illustration of the progress of other nations in this area, since Germany came first and Britain tenth in terms of the overall medal table. The implications of this for Britain's international ranking were immediately picked up in newspapers and periodicals. Moreover another group of civil servants from the Board of Education saw German facilities for themselves on a visit in November 1936. In cities such as Berlin, they observed physical training in schools, the Hitler Youth, the Labour Service Corps, the *Kraft durch Freude* (Strength through Joy) movement, and in the Siemens industrial firm. Their report noted that schools were better provided with gymnasia than their British counterparts, and more time was spent on physical training. Of the Hitler Youth for example, it was written that 'much of its training is valuable from the physical, mental and character-training points of view'. Similarly, the group concluded that physical education in Germany as a whole was 'novel, far reaching, highly interesting and often very instructive'.[61] Many observers, including Newman, remained in awe of this aspect of German health policy up to the outbreak of war.

However, there were other ways in which the emphasis on national fitness in policy rhetoric were mediated by other political traditions, including the relationship between central and local government. The *Health of the School Child* reports only served as a means of encouraging LEAs to make provision in certain areas, and the statutory obligations represented very much a minimum level of provision. In fact, Newman frequently expressed his frustration at what he perceived to be the slow rate of progress at the local level. It was partly for this reason that he put much emphasis on voluntarism and on such bodies as the Boy Scouts and Girl Guides. This was particularly the case in the years before and after the First World War. In 1914, for example, Newman had argued that the Scouting movement had been 'successful in obtaining an exceptional degree of individual development in the direction of resourcefulness, self-reliance, inter-dependence and mutual aid'.[62] Indeed he wrote that the activities associated with this and similar movements were 'the expression of the underlying principles which should guide us in the education of the boy and girl'. In this, he reflected ideas that were shared by local SMOs. The SMO for Hertfordshire, for example, claimed in 1919 that a comparison of the health of children in two towns revealed the beneficial effects of being in the Scouts.[63]

But despite concern about the physical training schemes set up by the continental dictatorships in the 1930s, there was also a strong sense of the British tradition as being one of games playing, embodied in the voluntarist and amateurish character of the 1937 Physical Training and Recreation Act. Thus in 1923 Newman had emphasised that the aim in the development of physical education should be to start from scratch, and to build a system 'suitable to our conditions, climate, habits, physique, and in harmony with our general attitude towards exercise'. This approach was to be characterised by what he termed 'an enlightened and progressive conservatism'.[64] And in this at least, Newman was clearly articulating a more widely shared sense. The *Sunday Times* newspaper, for instance, reacted strongly in August 1926 to the idea of physical education talks on the radio, arguing 'What next! Shall we have State breakfast hints, or tooth-cleaning drill, or possibly Government golf. We may be a C3 nation, but at least we preserve our individuality'.[65]

This emphasis on the distinctive British tradition of voluntarism persisted alongside the concern with the physical training schemes that characterised the early 1930s. In January 1936, for instance, a circular issued by the Board of Education argued that a centralised system of the continental type would not be appropriate, and that 'organised local development' would be more suitable.[66] And this was essentially the approach taken in the debates on the 1937 Physical Training and Recreation Bill. In the course of the second reading, for example, in April 1937, Aneurin Bevan, MP for Ebbw Vale, argued that Britain should 'try to prevent any lopsided development of our national health, and certainly not imitate the absurdities we see across the water'.[67] This was borne out in the membership of the National Advisory Council, whose members included Dorothy Round, winner of the women's singles at Wimbledon in 1934, Stanley Rous, Secretary of the Football Association, and Prunella Stack, leader of the Women's League of Health and Beauty.[68]   In fact the 1937 Act made little impact on facilities for physical education at the local level before the outbreak of war.   What was perhaps more interesting was what the debates about physical education revealed about attitudes to the state.   Proposals were put forward by civil servants to take physical education in a new direction, to use military instructors to direct physical education, and to set up a national badge scheme.   But these were nearly always resisted as being inappropriate and likely to meet opposition – a point which is again important in terms of the way that the concern about national fitness was mediated by older and more deeply-held political traditions.   It was only later, for example, that the idea for badges (which owed much to Kurt Hahn) was reborn as the Duke of Edinburgh's Award Scheme.

In fact, developments on the ground suggested that physical education made slow progress in the period before the Second World War.   The content of lessons only moved gradually away from an emphasis on drill, in part because the development of team games and swimming was dependent on playing fields and pools that required heavy capital expenditure.   LEAs were slow to appoint the organisers that were regarded as the best means of developing physical education at the local level.   By 1938, for example, only 249 of the 315 LEAs employed specialist organisers for their physical education schemes, in most cases a single man and woman for what could be major cities or large county areas.[69]   And statistics indicated that physical education comprised a relatively small proportion of LEA expenditure on the School Medical Service.   If we take 1932–33 as a typical year, for example, expenditure by LEAs on physical training represented only £58,773 of a total of £4,626,395 (1.27 per cent).[70]   In this sense there was an important gap between what was advocated as the ideal and what was really happening on the ground.

The inadequacy of facilities for physical education is apparent from the Political and Economic Planning (PEP) report on health services (1937), one of the few objective reports on medical services in this period.   PEP found that there were great local variations in the adequacy of the service, and the shortages of trained teachers were matched by the lack of facilities, equipment, gymnasia and playing fields.   The report concluded that 'evidently the state of physical education in Great Britain is far from satisfactory'.[71]   There was no way that these problems could be solved through the grants available through the 1937 Physical Training and Recreation Act.   Moreover, it is clear that in the short-term at least, progress was further retarded by the Second World War. Teacher training courses closed, halls were requisitioned for military use, playing fields were used for the growing of crops, male instructors were called up, and deficiencies in equipment were exacerbated. Even the Ministry of Education conceded that 'physical education, especially on the boys' side, suffered a severe regression'.[72]

It is also arguable that the stress on national efficiency that characterised the 1900s and 1930s evaporated after the Second World War. As eugenics declined as a potent current in social thought, the analogy between individual and national fitness appeared less appropriate, and lost much of its intellectual appeal. In a practical sense, the content of physical education widened to include a much broader range of team sports and individual pursuits. Physical education came to be permeated by a more individualistic character, and there was greater emphasis on activities such as abseiling, and on the outdoors in general. Furthermore, it is possible that at the level of popular culture, there was a deeper sense of scepticism about, and resistance to, the public-school games playing tradition than previously. One thinks, for instance of Alan Sillitoe's short story, *The Loneliness of the Long Distance Runner* (1959). And similar themes are expressed in the football match in the film *Kes*, where Brian Glover memorably played the part of the games teacher, in the adaptation of Barry Hines' *A Kestrel for a Knave* (1969). Perhaps the changes in schools that followed the 1944 Education Act, along with the creation of the welfare state, simply meant that the concerns previously expressed through the preoccupation with national fitness were articulated in different ways. Much more research is needed, on these and other points, at the local and voluntary organisation level. But the fact that the concept of national fitness could not be sustained in the changed climate of the postwar years suggests that the ideology had always been sporadic and contested.

Conclusion

In many respects, this study only serves to problematise some themes and to raise a number of further questions. One is the extent to which the ideas expressed in the *Health of the School Child* reports can be ascribed to Sir George Newman himself. Since it seems likely that these would have been drafted for him by civil servants, it is perhaps safer to say that these were views that he certainly shared. A notable feature of the reports is the way in which they conflate children with boys, and in fact say very little indeed about physical education for girls. Possibly this indicates that national fitness was seen in terms that were themselves very gender specific, but also points to the need for further research in this area. Regional variations are also a missing dimension – it remains unclear how these ideas were received on the ground, how influential they really were, and how they might have been interpreted by SMOs at the local level. And the extent to which the Second World War may have marked a turning point, and more specifically the influence of the Youth Service on the development of physical education, both require further analysis.

These questions aside, it is clear that part of the appeal of physical education lay in the ways that it appeared to support a wider concern with national fitness. This built on the ideals of athleticism that had been such an important aspect of ideology in the nineteenth-century public school, and drew strength from the emergence of eugenics as a theme in health policy. Activities like school journeys and camps that were bracketed with physical education appeared to offer a means of countering the allegedly debilitating effects of urban life. In addition, sport and exercise seemed to provide a cheap method of improving the health of children, in such areas as their ability to resist disease, raising their nutritional status, and in inculcating a self-help philosophy that linked with the parallel emphasis (for both young and old) on health education. Physical education was regarded as a powerful force for inculcating ideals of citizenship among working-class children, and here, as in organisations like the NCSS, there was frequent reference to models drawn from classical Greece. Debates embodied a kind of social and economic accounting, where physical education was seen to improve the employment prospects and efficiency of working-class children as future industrial workers. And there was a clear reference, in both the 1900s and the 1930s, to the wider international context. The force of these arguments was all the more powerful since the delay in developing facilities for physical education at the local level meant that the claims advanced in its favour remained essentially untested.

However, although it is clear that concepts of national efficiency and national fitness were important influences on child health and welfare in the first half of the twentieth century, it is arguable that these provide a narrowly functional view of health policy. National fitness was only one influence on the development of physical education, and citizenship was also an important aspect. Physical education was not just about international rivalry, but also concerned with social integration between classes. There were aspects of the

British political tradition – including the relationship between central and local government, and the role of voluntarism – that served to mediate the effectiveness of this vision. It was partly because of this that there was an important gap between what was advocated in policy rhetoric and what actually happened on the ground in terms of the provision of facilities. There were hints of resistance on the part of local SMOs and other organisations to the emphasis that was placed on physical education and national fitness, and evidence that the concern with national fitness evaporated after 1945. Overall, these emphases in debates about child health and welfare have served to oversimplify what is a complex story, and have obscured the ways in which variations in class, region and gender shaped the reception of these ideals. At the same time, at the start of a new century, there is evidence that New Labour continues to see issues such as physical education for children in terms of national fitness.

Acknowledgements

I would like to express my thanks to Mick Carpenter who provided the commentary on an earlier version of the chapter when it was given as a paper at the Warwick conference, to Hilary Marland, and to the other conference participants who put forward suggestions for ways in which it might be improved. Allen Warren also kindly read an earlier draft.

Notes

1. Department of Health, *Saving Lives: Our Healthier Nation* (Cm 4386) (London: Stationery Office, 1999), para. 4.19. See also Anthony Giddens, *The Third Way and its Critics* (Cambridge: Polity Press, 2000).
2. 'Gym-Shy Girls Tempted with Fun and Games', *The Times*, 18 March 1999, 9.
3. G.R. Searle, *The Quest for National Efficiency: A Study in British Politics and Political Thought, 1899–1914* (Oxford: Basil Blackwell, 1971), 60–7.
4. *Ibid.*, 54, 259–63.
5. On Newman, see, for example, *Who Was Who 1941–1950*, 843; *Dictionary of National Biography 1941–1950*, 624–5.
6. See, for example, P.C. McIntosh, *Physical Education in England Since 1800* (London: Bell, 1952); P.C. McIntosh, J.G. Dixon, A. D. Munrow, and R. F. Willetts, *Landmarks in the History of Physical Education* (London: Routledge and Kegan Paul, 1957, 2nd edn,

1968); W.D. Smith, *Stretching their Bodies: The History of Physical Education* (London: David and Charles, 1974); J.A. Mangan, *Athleticism in the Victorian and Edwardian Public School: The Emergence and Consolidation of an Educational Ideology* (Cambridge: Cambridge University Press, 1981).

7. Thomas A. O'Donoghue, 'Sport, Recreation and Physical Education: The Evolution of a National Policy of Regeneration in Eire, 1926–48', *British Journal of Sports History*, 3 (1986), 216–33; Henrik Meinnader, 'Towards a Bourgeois Manhood: Nordic Views and Visions of Physical Education for Boys, 1860–1930', *International Journal of the History of Sport*, 9 (1992), 337–55; David Kirk, *Defining Physical Education: The Social Construction of a School Subject in Postwar Britain* (London: Falmer Press, 1992).

8. Sheila Fletcher, 'The Making and Breaking of a Female Physical Tradition: Women's Physical Education in England 1880–1980', *British Journal of Sports History*, 2 (1985), 29–39.

9. David Armstrong, *Political Anatomy of the Body: Medical Knowledge in Britain in the Twentieth Century* (Cambridge: Cambridge University Press, 1983), 34–5; David Kirk, 'Foucault and the Limits of Corporeal Regulation: The Emergence, Consolidation and Decline of School Medical Inspection and Physical Training in Australia, 1909–30', *International Journal of the History of Sport*, 13 (1996), 114–31.

10. See, for example, John Welshman, 'Images of Youth: The Issue of Juvenile Smoking, 1880–1914', *Addiction*, 91 (1996), 1379–86.

11. See, for example, Linda Bryder, '"Wonderlands of Buttercup, Clover and Daisies": Tuberculosis and the Open-Air School Movement in Britain, 1907–39', in Roger Cooter (ed.), *In the Name of the Child: Health and Welfare 1880–1940* (London: Routledge, 1992), 72–95.

12. See, for example, John Welshman, 'Evacuation and Social Policy During the Second World War: Myth and Reality', *Twentieth Century British History*, 9 (1998), 28–53.

13. See, for example, Stephen Constantine, *Buy & Build: The Advertising Posters of the Empire Marketing Board* (London: Public Record Office, 1986).

14. Sally M. Horrocks, 'The Business of Vitamins: Nutrition Science and the Food Industry in Inter-War Britain', in Harmke Kamminga and Andrew Cunningham (eds), *The Science and Culture of Nutrition, 1840–1940* (Amsterdam: Rodopi, 1995), 235–58.

15. Board of Education, *Health of the School Child, 1920* (London, 1921), 165.

16. Board of Education, *Health of the School Child, 1928* (London,

1929), 38.

17. H. Llewellyn-Smith (ed.), *The New Survey of London Life and Labour* (London: P.S. King and Son, 1935), vol. 9, 85–6.

18. Board of Education, *op. cit.* (note 16), 39.

19. E.A. Impey, *Military Training Considered as Part of General Education* (London, 1913), 5.

20. On this debate, see, for example, J. O. Springhall, *Youth, Empire and Society: British Youth Movements 1883–1940* (London: Croom Helm, 1977); Allen Warren, 'Sir Robert Baden-Powell, The Scout Movement and Citizen Training in Great Britain, 1900–1920', *English Historical Review*, 399 (1986), 376–98.

21. Board of Education, *Annual Report of the CMO, 1919* (London, 1920), 142.

22. Board of Education, *Annual Report of the CMO, 1917* (London, 1918), 122. See also Linda Bryder, *Below the Magic Mountain: A Social History of Tuberculosis in Twentieth Century Britain* (Oxford: Oxford University Press, 1988).

23. Board of Education, *op. cit.* (note 16), 41. On the reality of school camps, see Jerry White, *Rothschild Buildings: Life in an East End Tenement Block 1887–1920* (London: Routledge and Kegan Paul, 1980), 186; Ralph Glasser, *Growing Up in the Gorbals* (London: Chatto and Windus, 1986), 54–5.

24. See, for example, Kirk, *op. cit.* (note 7), 126-31; Bernard Harris, *The Health of the Schoolchild: A History of the School Medical Service in England and Wales* (Buckingham: Open University Press, 1995).

25. Board of Education, *Annual Report of the CMO, 1909* (London, 1910), 183.

26. Board of Education, *op. cit.* (note 15), 158. For a cautious interpretation of the involvement of women in the development of sport, see Neil Tranter, *Sport, Economy and Society in Britain 1750–1914* (Cambridge: Cambridge University Press, 1998).

27. Board of Education, *Annual Report of the CMO, 1916* (London, 1917), 136.

28. Board of Education, *Annual Report of the CMO, 1908* (London, 1909), 76.

29. Board of Education, *op. cit.* (note 25), 62.

30. Board of Education, *Annual Report of the CMO, 1912* (London, 1913), 345.

31. Public Record Office, Kew (hereafter PRO), ED 50/104: A. H. Wood to G. Newman, 27 March 1922.

32. Board of Education, *Health of the School Child, 1921* (London, 1922), 22; Board of Education, *Health of the School Child, 1931*

(London, 1932), 111.

33. Board of Education, *Syllabus of Physical Training for Schools 1933* (London, 1933), 6–7.
34. Board of Education, *op. cit.* (note 32), 73.
35. Board of Education, *Health of the School Child, 1925* (London, 1926), 144.
36. Board of Education, *op. cit.* (note 16), 44.
37. Board of Education, *Health of the School Child, 1930* (London, 1931), 79.
38. Board of Education, *Health of the School Child, 1935* (London, 1936), 50–2.
39. Board of Education, *Health of the School Child, 1923* (London, 1924), 108.
40. Board of Education, *op. cit.* (note 27), 125.
41. Norman G. Bennett, 'Dental Hygiene and the National Physique', *British Dental Journal,* 25 (1904), 687-8: 688.
42. Henry Herd, 'Physical Education', *Public Health,* 50 (1937), 251–7: 251, 256.
43. British Medical Association, *Report of the Physical Education Committee* (London: British Medical Association, 1936), 37.
44. George Newman papers, Wellcome Institute London, Neville Chamberlain to George Newman, 12 October 1936.
45. See, for example, Charles E.B. Russell, *Manchester Boys: Sketches of Manchester Lads at Work and Play* (Manchester: Manchester University Press, 1905); Alexander Paterson, *Across the Bridges: Or Life by the South London Riverside* (London: Edward Arnold, 1911).
46. Board of Education, *op. cit.* (note 27), 125.
47. Board of Education, *Annual Report of the CMO, 1919* (London, 1920), 183.
48. Board of Education, *op. cit.* (note 35), 105.
49. Board of Education, *Health of the School Child, 1933* (London, 1934), 40.
50. Board of Education, *op. cit.* (note 47), 172.
51. Board of Education, *op. cit.* (note 37), 70.
52. Board of Education, *op. cit.* (note 49), 33–4.
53. See, for example, Andrzej Olechnowicz, *Working-Class Housing in England Between the Wars: The Becontree Estate* (Oxford: Clarendon Press, 1997); John Welshman, 'Evacuation, Hygiene, and Social Policy: The *Our Towns* Report of 1943', *Historical Journal,* 42 (1999), 781–807.
54. Board of Education, *Health of the School Child, 1934* (London, 1935), 44–7.

55. Jose Harris, 'Political Thought and the Welfare State 1870–1940: An Intellectual Framework for British Social Policy', *Past and Present*, 135 (1992), 127–31.
56. Board of Education, *op. cit.* (note 54), 8.
57. See, for example, George F. Shee, 'The Deterioration in the National Physique', *Nineteenth Century and After*, 53 (1903), 797–805.
58. Board of Education, *Annual Report of the CMO, 1914* (London, 1915), 198.
59. Ministry of Health, *On the State of the Public Health, 1933* (London, 1934), 254.
60. See, for example, N.A. Semashko, *Health Protection in the USSR* (London: Victor Gollancz, 1934), 60–2; PRO ED 50/243: A.F. Birch-Jones to Captain Parker, November 1935.
61. PRO ED 121/92: 'Physical Education in Germany', 2, 34, 71; Board of Education, *Physical Education in Germany* (London: HMSO, 1937), 75. See also Hajo Bernett, 'National Socialist Physical Education as Reflected in British Appeasement Policy', *International Journal of the History of Sport*, 5 (1988), 161–84.
62. Board of Education, *op. cit.* (note 58), 197.
63. Board of Education, *op. cit.* (note 47), 35.
64. Board of Education, *op. cit.* (note 39), 110.
65. PRO ED 50/244: cutting from the *Sunday Times*, 1 August 1926.
66. Board of Education, Circular 1444, *Administrative Programme of Educational Development*, 6 January 1936, 10.
67. *House of Commons Debates*, vol. 322, no. 85, 7 April 1937, c. 257.
68. PRO ED 136/76: 'Physical Recreation Committees'.
69. Ministry of Education, *Health of the School Child, 1939–45* (London, 1947), 113.
70. Board of Education, *Health of the School Child, 1932* (London, 1933), 165, table XV.
71. Political and Economic Planning, *Report on the British Health Services: A Survey of the Existing Health Services in Great Britain with Proposals for Future Development* (London: PEP, 1937), 8, 340, 349–50.
72. Ministry of Education, *op. cit.* (note 69), 113–19.

4

Educational Reform, Citizenship and the
Origins of the School Medical Service

Bernard Harris

In recent years, there has been a growing interest in the origins and growth of the school medical service, and in the relationship between the state and the welfare of children generally.[1] This literature has often tended to focus on the extent to which it was in the state's *own* interests to pay greater attention to the needs of the coming generation. The aim of this contribution is to examine the extent to which the introduction of measures such as the Education (Provision of Meals) Act (1906) and the Education (Administrative Provisions) Act (1907) may have also reflected a conscious desire to serve the child's own interests as well.

In approaching this topic, I have chosen to concentrate on the growth of the school medical service as a branch of the public education service, rather than as a medical service which happened to be located in schools. This is partly because of the way in which T.H. Marshall identified the growth of public education in the latter part of the nineteenth century as an early manifestation of what he called 'the social rights of citizenship'.[2] In what follows, I intend to begin by examining the relationship between the idea of citizenship and the introduction of the Forster Education Bill in 1870. I shall then examine the debates which preceded the passage of the Education Acts of 1876, 1880 and 1891, which between them extended the principle of compulsory education to the whole of England and Wales, and established a national system of free education for the vast majority of children attending public elementary schools.[3] Finally, I shall consider the part played by ideas about the rights and duties of citizenship, and the needs of both the individual and the community, in relation to the introduction of school meals in 1906, and school medical inspection in 1907.

Whilst this chapter is concerned primarily with the history of social policy, it is also bound up inescapably with the history of childhood itself. In 1977, Jacques Donzelot argued that the main

85

reason for the development of child welfare policies lay in their capacity to reinforce the role played by the working class family in acting as a bulwark against social change, whilst Harry Hendrick has argued that they were really designed to counter the 'uncontrollability' of children themselves.[4]   However, as Hugh Cunningham has shown, child welfare policies were also influenced by a growing belief in the separation of childhood from adulthood, and by the perceived need for the state to step in as the guarantor of children's rights in an adult world.   As Cunningham himself has concluded, it was the convergence between these different sets of imperatives, allied to the growing interest in national efficiency, which lay behind the development of a new set of child welfare policies in the late-nineteenth and early-twentieth centuries.[5]

The origins of public education:
The Forster Education Act of 1870

As W.B. Stephens has recently pointed out, Britain was not entirely bereft of educational institutions at the beginning of the nineteenth century. It is likely that a significant number of children attended what have traditionally been known, somewhat pejoratively, as 'dame schools'.   From the first decade of the nineteenth century, these schools were joined by a growing number of so-called 'voluntary schools', generally associated with either the Non-Conformist British and Foreign Schools Society, founded in 1808, or the National Society for Educating the Children of the Poor in the Principles of the Established Church, founded in 1811. In 1833, Parliament took the first steps towards the creation of a state-funded education service when it awarded a grant of £20,000 to the two societies to support the construction of new schools in the north of England. However, it was not until 1870 that the Liberal government decided to establish the machinery for the creation of schools which were provided and maintained by local rates.[6]

The subject of public education provides a particularly good illustration of the ambiguities underpinning the concept of citizenship itself because, as Marshall himself noted, the concept of citizenship has always included an element of rights and an element of duties.[7] In 1848, when John Stuart Mill wrote the *Principles of Political Economy*, he argued that it was an 'allowable exercise of the powers of government' to provide a publicly-funded education service in the interests of the children themselves, and of the community to which they belonged.[8] Just over a hundred years later, when Marshall delivered his famous lecture at the London School of

Economics, he argued that children had a right to be educated 'because the aim of education during childhood is to shape the future adult', and that the state had a right to expect children to be educated, because 'the social health of a society depends upon the civilisation of its members'.[9]

In his recent study, W.B. Stephens has suggested that, whilst an earlier generation of educational historians had been accustomed to regard the growth of public education as 'a development benevolently contrived and part and parcel of the democratisation of society, bringing benefits to all', more recent historians have preferred to emphasise the role of education as an instrument of 'social control'.[10] In a series of articles, Richard Johnson argued powerfully that 'the early-Victorian obsession with the education of the poor is best understood as a concern about authority, about power, [and] about the assertion (or re-assertion?) of control',[11] whilst both Philip Gardner and Kevin Stannard have claimed that the growth of state intervention in the field of education was deliberately intended to undermine the autonomous working-class tradition of private venture schools.[12] However, other writers have questioned at least some of the assumptions on which these arguments are based. W.B. Stephens has pointed out that 'working-class attendance at private schools was in decline long before 1870', whilst Jonathan Rose has argued that, even if some children (and some parents) resented the imposition of compulsory education, the vast majority were happy to attend school, and felt that they had derived considerable benefit from the tuition they received.[13]

If one looks at the arguments used by the Liberal MP, W.E. Forster, when he introduced the Education Bill in 1870, it is difficult to avoid the conclusion that arguments about social control, allied to considerations of national and economic efficiency, were indeed at the heart of the Government's desire to expand educational provision. Forster began by arguing that the aim of public education was to remove 'that ignorance which we are all aware is pregnant with crime and misery, with misfortune to the individual and danger to the community',[14] before going on to suggest that 'an education rate would save the prison rate and the pauper rate'.[15] He also said that education was necessary in order to ensure industrial prosperity, and to guarantee 'the safe working of our constitutional system'.[16] Finally, he concluded, educational reform was also necessary in the interests of 'national power. Civilised communities throughout the world are massing themselves together, each mass being measured by its force; and if we are to hold our position among men of our own race or among the nations of the world, we must make up the smallness of our number by increasing the intellectual force of the individual'.[17]

However, although Forster was content to stake his case on the grounds of national interest, other speakers did focus on the individual interests of the children themselves, or, to put the matter more simply, on the basis of the children's rights as individuals, rather than on the nation's interest in their capacity to labour as adults. George Melly, the Liberal MP for Stoke-on-Trent, argued that the Bill was 'one of the noblest messages of peace and goodwill to all classes' which any government had ever offered 'to the people it was called on to govern'.[18] Henry Fawcett, one of the leading lights of mid-Victorian liberalism,[19] argued that 'to provide ... was not enough. Parliament should guarantee to every child an education',[20] and the Conservative MP for Droitwich, Sir John Pakington, claimed that 'I do not believe that without compulsion we can have anything like a satisfactory national education system that will bring, as it ought to do, education to the door of every citizen of this country, however humble'.[21]

Towards compulsion:
The Education Acts of 1876 and 1880

The previous section has shown that questions about children's rights did play an important part in the debates which accompanied the passing of the Forster Education Bill in 1870. However, it was certainly noticeable that these arguments were advanced most forcefully by those calling for education to be made compulsory across the whole country. Consequently, it is not surprising to find that these arguments emerged much more strongly in the debates which preceded the passing of the Elementary Education Act of 1876, and the further Elementary Education Act of 1880.

Although the Education Act of 1870 is rightly regarded as the major landmark in nineteenth-century educational legislation, it is important to realise that it failed to establish an elementary education system which was either compulsory or free. The main aim of the Act, as introduced by Forster, was to 'fill up gaps' by facilitating the creation of school boards in those parts of the country where the existing level of provision was deemed to be inadequate.[22] It was only in those areas where such a school board was set up that it would have the power to make school attendance compulsory. Consequently, there was no power to make education compulsory in areas where the existing level of voluntary educational provision was not deemed to be inadequate.[23]

The first attempt to address this issue in areas where school boards were not set up was made in 1876. The Elementary Education Bill which was introduced in May of that year sought to make education compulsory first of all by prohibiting employers from offering work to children who were under the age of ten, or to children over the age of ten who failed to produce a certificate to show that they had either attended a public elementary school, or attained recognised standards of proficiency in reading, writing and elementary arithmetic; and, secondly, by empowering either the local Borough Council or the Board of Guardians to 'make bye-laws respecting the attendance of children at school under section 74 of the Elementary Education Act, 1870, as if such councils and guardians respectively were a school board'.[24] However, it was not until the passage of the Elementary Education Act of 1880 that education was made compulsory for all children of elementary school age. This Act imposed a duty on all local authorities to pass bye-laws making education compulsory in their districts, and gave the Department of Education the power to frame its own bye-laws if the local authorities failed to do so.[25]

The 1876 Education Act was, in many ways, an attempt to build on the foundations laid in 1870, and therefore it is not surprising to find that many of the same types of argument were advanced in its favour. However, if one looks at the arguments put forward by the Conservative spokesperson, Viscount Sandon, when he introduced the Bill, it is possible to detect a certain change of emphasis. Whereas Forster, in introducing the first Bill, had chosen to place the greatest weight on the benefits to the community of providing education to the children, Sandon chose to pay much more attention to the interests of the children themselves. He argued that the whole question 'was of far too much importance to the interests of the working class and the employers of labour ... and to the interests of the country to be treated as a party question', but he went on to say that 'the Lord President [i.e. the President of the Privy Council] and himself had given the question their most anxious, careful and constant attention', and 'had looked at it primarily in the interest of the children; and, secondly, in the interest of the country as a whole'.[26]

One of the most interesting features of Sandon's speech was the way in which he sought to link a child's educational opportunities, and the state's obligation to provide those opportunities, with traditional concerns about the diminution of pauperism and crime. In 1870, when Forster had introduced the first Education Bill, he had claimed that 'an education rate should save the prison rate and the pauper rate', but he did not spell out the ways in which this might be accomplished. By contrast, Sandon argued that if a child was allowed to grow up without being equipped with the skills needed to earn a living, society could hardly complain if that child resorted to crime or the Poor Law in order to survive. The community therefore had an obligation to ensure 'that no child in the country should hereafter enter on the struggle of life without those simple tools needed by our civilisation to enable him to make his way hereafter'.[27] He also argued that 'it was the settled sentiment of this country that sound elementary instruction should be provided for ordinary children, and that all talent and merit should have an opportunity of rising',[28] and, although he was at pains to emphasise how the Bill was designed to reinforce rather than undermine parental responsibility, he was forced to concede that it also constituted existing local authorities 'as protectors and guardians of children' if their parents failed, or were unable, to ensure they were educated.[29]

Whilst Sandon's was the most important speech to be made in favour of the Bill, it was not the only one, and it is certainly true that a number of the other speakers chose to express their support for its provisions in more traditional terms. W.E. Forster, speaking from the Opposition benches, urged that 'it was most important that children should be trained to a love of virtue and of God, and ... that the school boards deserved credit for what they had done in that way'.[30] Edward Hermon, the Conservative MP for Preston, 'thought it was important that political economy should be taught in the schools, as the masses were liable to fall into error on that subject'.[31] However, the Conservative MP for Manchester, Hugh Birley, 'was of opinion that what was proposed in the Bill as to poor districts would really be a just measure of relief; and he trusted that they would all, on whatever side they sat, cooperate with a view to make the measure practical, useful and satisfactory, not merely to the working classes, but to the nation at large'.[32]

Towards free education:
Proposals for education reform 1886-91

Although the 1870 Education Act was designed to improve access to education, it did not abolish school fees, nor did it establish a free system of elementary education. However, Forster did include a proposal to establish a limited number of free schools in the most impoverished areas, and he gave school boards the power to remit a child's fees if the parents were found to be unable to pay.[33] In 1876 Viscount Sandon extended the opportunities for free education to other areas (that is, to areas not covered by school boards) by stating that if a parent was unable to pay the school fees, then it should be the duty of the Board of Guardians (and not the School Board) to pay them on the parent's behalf.[34] However, although the measure was probably designed to overcome the limitations of the 1870 Act rather than anything else, its impact was limited, because many parents resented the association with the Poor Law, and thus refused to apply for the remission of fees which they were unable to pay.[35]

During the first half of the 1880s, a series of attempts were made in Parliament to amend the legislation regarding school fees and to extend the principle of free education, but none succeeded. In 1886 E.H. Llewellyn, the Conservative MP for Somerset North, introduced a Bill under which Boards of Guardians would delegate their power to pay school fees on behalf of parents to a separate school fees committee, in order to lessen any possible association between the payment of school fees and the stain of pauperism.[36] In 1887 a second group of MPs submitted a Bill which said that any pupil who attended 75 per cent or more of the sessions in one school year should be granted exemption from fees for the whole of the next year.[37] E.H. Llewellyn also made further attempts to move his original Bill (or a very slightly amended version thereof) in 1887 and 1888.[38] However, it was not until 1891 that a successful attempt was made to introduce legislation leading to the abolition of school fees for the vast majority of elementary school children.

Although the 1891 Act was in many ways a measure of considerable importance in the history of state welfare provision, it has received relatively little attention from historians of either education or welfare, possibly because it has tended to be overshadowed, in educational history, by the Acts of 1870 and 1902, and in welfare history by the Liberal reforms of 1906-11. However, it is clear that it was the focus of considerable controversy at the time of its introduction.[39] George Bartley, the Conservative MP for Islington North, predicted that the Bill would undermine parental responsibility and authority, and that 'the social mischief of this measure would be very far-reaching'.[40] The Conservative MP for Christchurch, C.E. Baring-Young, claimed that the measure was nothing less than 'a step towards state socialism'.[41] However, other speakers regarded it as an act of considerable political opportunism. They noted that the Conservative party had campaigned against the abolition of school fees in the 1886 general election, and they attributed its leaders' conversion to the cause of free education to the imminence of the 1892 election.[42] W.P. Sinclair, the Liberal MP for Falkirk, suggested that the real reason for introducing the Bill was that 'political power in this country has shifted; the governing power is now handed over to the people. There is a change from parental to national responsibility, and that is a great reason why the Government are to be congratulated upon the action they have taken'.[43]

However, while some speakers suspected the Government of political opportunism, or of having been forced into action by the tide of history, the debate also provided some of the clearest examples of educational arguments based on ideas about the rights of the child, as opposed to the duties of the future adult and the needs of the wider community. Some of the most powerful of these arguments also concerned the relationship between the child, the adult and the state. George Dixon, the Liberal MP for Edgbaston, argued that 'it is the duty of the state and of educationists to protect children against the poverty or selfishness of parents, and if under this Bill we make all our schools free irrespective of age, we can effectually do this'.[44] The 'progressive and independent Conservative' MP for Islington South, Sir A.K. Rollit, also urged the House 'not [to] forget the claims of the children themselves. If parents cannot pay, and the education of the child is neglected, the consequences to the latter may be disastrous and lifelong. The primary duty of the House in this matter is to provide for the welfare of the children'.[45]

In addition to the educational needs of the children themselves, the 1891 Bill was also seen by a number of speakers as part of a larger programme of social reform. A number of speakers, including C.W. Gray, the Conservative MP for Maldon, and H.R. Farquharson, the Conservative MP for Dorset, believed that the abolition of school fees would make an enormous difference to the welfare of agricultural families, because of the disproportionate burden which the obligation to pay school fees placed on households with very low incomes.[46] Others argued that the abolition of school fees represented a major advance in the social rights of poor families. Sir George Trevelyan, the Liberal MP for the Bridgeton division in Glasgow, believed that the abolition of fees would enable the poor parent to feel that 'if his child needs education he gets it as the child of a citizen, and not as the child of a pauper'.[47] Others, such as Thomas Ellis, Liberal MP for Merionethshire, argued that measure could be justified 'on the ground of social justice.... Relatively to their income, the working classes contribute more to Imperial

Revenue than any other class, and it [is] only fair in the matter of education that they should as soon as possible receive a grant from the Imperial Exchequer. The parents will also be relieved of a heavy burden which presses upon them at the time when it is most difficult to be borne'.[48]

The introduction of school meals and school medical inspection

The previous section has shown that arguments about the rights and entitlements of the working class, as well as those of the individual child, did indeed play an important part in the development of educational legislation after 1870. Although the main supporters of the 1870 Act justified the measure primarily in terms of the state's interest, there was a noticeable shift in the arguments used by their successors when they extended the terms of the original legislation in the Acts of 1876, 1880 and 1891. However, it is difficult to avoid the conclusion that there was a further shift in emphasis, and a renewed concentration on the interests of the state, in the debates which accompanied the introduction of free school meals and school medical inspection in 1906 and 1907 respectively.

As John Burnett has recently argued, the movement for the provision of free school meals really took off in the 1870s, when the introduction of compulsory education brought many of the poorest children into contact with formal education for the first time. During the 1880s a number of religious and voluntary organisations began to make arrangements for the provision of free school dinners to schoolchildren in London and elsewhere, and organisations such as the Social Democratic Federation and the Independent Labour Party campaigned for the introduction of free schools meals as a statutory responsibility. Nevertheless, it was not until 1906 that legislation permitting local education authorities to provide such meals entered the Statute Book.[49]

The Education (Provision of Meals) Bill was introduced in the House of Commons by a Labour backbencher, W.T. Wilson, in 1906. Although the provision of free meals had long been supported by socialist and labour organisations, Wilson preferred to argue his case, not so much on the grounds of the rights of the child (although he did not entirely neglect these) as on the needs of the state. He argued that 'the children of a nation were its best assets' and that it was important to ensure that 'those assets [were] made as valuable as possible'. He urged the House 'to look at the matter from a purely business standpoint', and claimed that the money spent on school meals 'would be well invested, because not only would the children be better equipped for fighting the battle of life, but ... the expenditure on prisons, workhouses and asylums [would be] considerably reduced'.[50] However, when he came to the end of his speech, he made a direct attempt to couple his appeal to the nation's self-interest with an appeal on behalf of the child's own interest. He argued that the Bill would 'be to the best interests and the welfare of the nation', and he urged the House to adopt it 'in the name of humanity and Christianity'.[51]

In the debate which followed, several speakers chose to echo the cautious way in which Wilson had sought to balance the claims of humanity with those of national efficiency. The Liberal MP for Chester-le-Street, J.W. Taylor, argued that 'the proposals in the Bill were in the first instance humane, and in the second place they were on economic grounds such as would promote the best interests of the nation'.[52] However, the Liberal MP for Market Harborough, Rudolf Lehmann, said that 'if it was important that we should equip for the race of life the rising generation, it was necessary that we should feed them if they could not feed themselves, and it was for that reason that he so heartily supported the Bill'.[53] The Liberal MP for North Camberwell, Thomas Macnamara, who was himself a former teacher, argued that the Bill reflected 'the best and truest interest of the highest Imperialism - the Imperialism which began at home'. He concluded, in what one must imagine were suitably ringing tones, that 'they must not only sing "Rule, Britannia", but they must weave the chorus into every clause of our social statutes for the betterment of the people ... it was not out of the mouths of knitted gun nor the smoothed rifle, but out of the mouths of babes and sucklings, that the strength is ordained that would still the Enemy and the Avenger'.[54]

One of the most interesting speeches in support of the Bill was made by the Labour MP for West Bradford, Benjamin Jowett. Jowett did not question the extent to which the provision of school meals would serve the nation, but he nevertheless managed to combine an appeal to the 'national interest' with a scorching critique of existing social arrangements. He argued that the only way to improve the condition of the population was 'to say to the parents, "You are not responsible for the system of society under which you live; the economic conditions have not been created by you; your children must be looked after, and they must be fed, if we are to lift our heads among the nations of the earth, and if we desire to keep our place in the civilised world"'.[55] He also tackled head on the extreme individualist arguments advanced by MPs such as Sir Harold Cox, the Member for Preston, and by the Charity Organisation Society, which believed that the introduction of free school meals would undermine parental responsibility and demoralise the working class:[56]

> It seemed to him that, underlying some remarks made during the discussion by previous speakers, there was an idea that if they were to do something to relieve the material necessity under which people had to struggle, the desire to struggle would cease, and that, therefore, a greater mistake could not be made. But what was civilisation if it was not directed to freeing the people from material necessities; and if they could do that, surely the result would be that the struggle would be transferred to a higher plane, and the people would have the opportunity to fight for better things.[57]

The Provision of Meals Bill was not the only Education Bill to be presented to Parliament in 1906. On 2 April, the Labour MP, Will Thorne, introduced the state Education Bill, which included provisions calling for local education authorities to publish annual returns showing the height, weight and chest measurement of school entrants, and to appoint Medical Officers 'whose duty it shall be to medically examine and … test such children as the teachers may consider in need of medical advice'.[58] Thorne then agreed to withdraw his Bill, following representations from the Government, when the President of the Board of Education, Sir Augustine Birrell, introduced his own Bill one week later. This Bill was primarily concerned with religious questions, but it included a clause which was designed to give local education authorities the power to make arrangements for attending to the health and welfare of elementary schoolchildren. In July 1906 Birrell agreed to amend his own clause, in order to ensure that all local education authorities would be compelled to make arrangements for medical inspection, although not for medical treatment. The Bill as a whole was eventually withdrawn at the end of the year, but the amended version of the clause dealing with medical inspection won widespread support, and the Government agreed to reintroduce it when it presented the Education (Administrative Provisions) Bill to Parliament at the beginning of 1907. This Bill passed through Parliament with relatively little difficulty, and the clauses which led to the establishment of the school medical service passed into law at the end of August.[59]

If one compares the debates which took place around the question of medical inspection with those which preceded the introduction of free school meals, a familiar pattern emerges, although it is certainly arguable that the proponents of medical inspection were inclined to be at least a little more forward in basing their claims on the rights of the child as well as the needs of the state. The backbench Liberal MP, H.J. Tennant, argued that thousands of children were suffering from physical ailments which made it difficult for them to profit from the education they were receiving, and that since the state compelled local education authorities to provide education, it should also compel them to make arrangements for the medical inspection of the children who were obliged to be educated.[60]   Although he followed W.T. Wilson in urging that children whose bodies were stunted and whose education was underdeveloped were more likely to drift into the 'asylums, workhouses, and … ranks of the unemployed', he managed to present this in a way which suggested that it would be at least as great a source of misfortune to the child as it was a source of expense to the state. He concluded that the provision of school medical inspection was an elementary right of childhood, as well as a form of elementary justice to the nation, a formulation which was immediately echoed by the Liberal MP for West Ham, North, Charles Masterman.[61]

However, while some MPs presented the case for medical inspection in terms of children's rights, others continued to emphasise the overriding importance of national needs. The Conservative MP for Glasgow and Aberdeen Universities, Sir Henry Craik, who had been a vocal opponent of the plans to introduce school feeding, argued that 'if the children were to be properly equipped for the work of education, medical inspection must be carried out as part of the educational work of the schools'.[62] The Conservative spokesperson on education, Sir William Anson, who had been responsible for the establishment of the Interdepartmental Committee on Medical Inspection and Feeding in the previous year, said that 'the question of the medical inspection of the children lay at the root of all the questions relating to the physical condition of the people, and it was a matter of national importance'.[63] The MP for North Camberwell, Thomas Macnamara, repeated a claim he had made earlier in the year:

> As one who had spent many years of his life in daily touch with some
> of the poorest children in one of our great cities … he used literally
> to shudder in contemplation of the fact that it was upon these
> ricketty shoulders that the burden of the Empire in time to come
> would have to rest.[64]

Many of the arguments which were used to support the introduction of compulsory medical inspection in the House of Commons resurfaced when the amended clause was debated by members of the House of Lords later in the same year. The Bishop of Ripon thought that the country had a moral obligation 'to take care that the weak children, who would not have been in the school but for the compulsory provision, should be protected against undue strain by some careful medical examination'.[65] The Earl of Crewe, speaking on behalf of the government, urged his colleagues to consider 'merely from an economic point of view, what a waste it is to teach a great many of these children … in the condition in which they are'.[66] However, it was left to the Conservative Earl of Meath, whose concerns over the physical condition of Scottish schoolchildren and army recruits had played a large part in the appointment of the Interdepartmental Committee on Physical Deterioration, to make the most dramatic appeal:

> It was of the most vital importance to this country that our children should be strong and full of vitality, and money could not be spent better than on raising a healthy and Imperial race, which should carry on the traditions of this great Empire.[67]

Conclusions

By looking at the origins of the school medical service as an aspect of educational legislation, rather than as a piece of medical legislation, and by examining the history of educational reform over a longer period, this contribution has tried to shed new light on the relationship between the origins of the school medical service and the concept of citizenship. One of the main aims of the contribution has been to emphasise that the concept of citizenship has always involved notions of both rights and duties, and these were reflected, in a variety of ways, in all the legislation we have studied. It is certainly true that the language of children's rights was most apparent in the debates which accompanied the passage of the Elementary Education Acts of 1876, 1880 and 1891, but it was also apparent in connection with the other reforms as well. However, it would be difficult to argue that the more 'humanitarian' arguments for the introduction of school meals and school medical inspection would still have prevailed, if they had not been reinforced by arguments about national efficiency.

Although this contribution has concentrated primarily on the history of education policy in the late-nineteenth and early-twentieth centuries, it is not without relevance to more recent debates. In recent years, the concept of citizenship has played an increasingly important part in political discussions, and politicians of all shades have sought to emphasise the responsibilities which the citizen is supposed to owe to the community, as well as the responsibilities which the community owes to the citizen. In this respect, the different emphases placed on the rights of the child and the needs of the community in the history of educational reform between 1870 and 1907 show that there is nothing new in present-day dilemmas.

Notes

1. See e.g. J.D. Hirst, 'The Origins and Development of the School Medical Service 1870-1919', unpublished PhD thesis, University of Wales (Bangor), 1983; *idem*, 'The Growth of Treatment through the School Medical Service, 1908-18', *Medical History*, 33 (1989), 318–42; *idem*, 'Public Health and the Public Elementary Schools, 1870-1907', *History of Education*, 20 (1991), 107–18; A.J. Welshman, 'The School Medical Service in England and Wales, 1907-39', unpublished D.Phil. thesis, University of Oxford, 1988; *idem*, 'School Meals and Milk in England and Wales, 1906-45', *Medical History*, 41 (1997), 6–29; R.J. Cooter (ed.), *In the Name of the Child* (London: Routledge, 1992); H. Hendrick, 'Child Labour, Medical Capital and the School Medical Service, c. 1890-1918', in *ibid.*, 45–71; *idem*, *Child Welfare: England 1872-1989* (London: Routledge, 1994); B. Harris, *The Health of the Schoolchild: A History of the School Medical Service in England and Wales* (Buckingham: Open University Press, 1995).
2. T.H. Marshall, *Citizenship and Social Class and Other Essays* (Cambridge: Cambridge University Press, 1950), 25.
3. This contribution will concentrate exclusively on legislation affecting England and Wales. Separate Acts were passed governing the provision of public education in Scotland and Ireland.
4. J. Donzelot, *The Policing of Families: Welfare versus the State* (London: Hutchinson, 1979); Hendrick, *Child Welfare* (note 1), xi-xii.
5. H. Cunningham, *Children and Childhood in Western Society since 1500* (London: Longman, 1995), 159–62.
6. W.B. Stephens, *Education in Britain 1750-1914* (Basingstoke: Macmillan, 1999).
7. A.M. Rees, 'The other T.H. Marshall', *Journal of Social Policy*, 24 (1995), 341–62.
8. J.S. Mill, *Principles of Political Economy and Chapters on Socialism*,

edited with an introduction by Jonathan Riley (Oxford: Oxford University Press, 1994 [first published 1848]), 339–42.

9. Marshall, *op. cit.* (note 2), 25–6.

10. Stephens, *op. cit.* (note 6), 81.

11. R. Johnson, 'Educational Policy and Social Control in Early-Victorian England', *Past and Present*, 49 (1970), 96–119: 119.

12. P. Gardner, *The Lost Elementary Schools of Victorian England* (London: Croom Helm, 1984); K. P. Stannard, 'Ideology, Education and Social Structure: Elementary Schooling in Mid-Victorian England', *History of Education*, 19 (1990), 105–22.

13. Stephens, *op. cit.* (note 6), 82; J. Rose, 'Willingly to School: the. Working Class Response to Elementary Education in Britain, 1875-1918', *Journal of British Studies*, 32 (1993), 114–38.

14. *Parliamentary Debates*, 3rd series, vol. 199, col. 438.

15. *Ibid.*, col. 455.

16. *Ibid.*, col. 465.

17. *Ibid.*, cols. 465–6.

18. *Ibid.*, cols. 478–9.

19. See S. Collini, *Public Moralists: Political Thought and Intellectual Life in Britain 1850-1930* (Oxford: Clarendon Press, 1991), 170–98.

20. *Parliamentary Debates*, 3rd series, vol. 199, col. 482.

21. *Ibid.*, col. 487.

22. *Ibid.*, col. 444.

23. 33 & 34 Vict. C. 75, *An Act to provide for public elementary education in England and Wales*, section 36. In his speech to the House of Commons on 17 February 1870, Forster explained that if school boards were not given the power to make education compulsory, they would have less incentive to make educational facilities available (*Parliamentary Debates*, 3rd series, vol. 199, col. 462).

24. PP 1876 (155) ii, 231, A Bill to make further provision for elementary education, sections 4-6.

25. 43 & 44 Vict. C. 23, *An Act to make further provision as to byelaws respecting the attendance of children at school under the Elementary Education Acts*, section 2.

26. *Parliamentary Debates*, 3rd series, vol. 229, cols. 929–30.

27. *Ibid.*, col. 931.

28. *Ibid.*, col. 933.

29. *Ibid.*, col. 948.

30. *Ibid.*, col. 955.

31. He explained that their error 'was in the nature of a struggle between labour and capital'. See *Parliamentary Debates*, 3rd series, vol. 229,

col. 959.

32. *Ibid.*, col. 960.

33. *Parliamentary Debates*, 3rd series, vol. 199, cols. 454–5; *An Act to provide for public elementary education in England and* Wales, sections 17, 25.

34. 39 & 40 Vict. C. 79, *An Act to make further provision for elementary education*, section 10.

35. See also B. Simon, *Education and the Labour Movement 1870-1920* (London: Lawrence and Wishart, 1965), 127.

36. PP 1886 (114-I) v, 473, A Bill to amend the provision of the Education Act, 1876, so as to enable parents of children being non-paupers to obtain payment of school fees without having to apply to the Guardians or their officers; *Parliamentary Debates*, 3rd series, vol. 303, cols. 1721–6.

37. PP 1887 (295) ii, 265, A Bill to enable children to earn exemption from school fees by regularity of attendance, and to amend the Elementary Education Acts in other respects.

38. PP 1887 (106) vi, 53, A Bill to amend the law relating to the payment of school fees of non-pauper children; PP 1888 (13), vi, 571, A Bill to amend the law relating to the payment of school fees of non-pauper children (not printed).

39. Simon, *op. cit.* (note 35), 131, fn. 2.

40. *Parliamentary Debates*, 3rd series, vol. 354, col. 1110. Bartley was a noted authority on educational provision at the time (his study of *The Schools for the People* was published in 1871), and he founded the National Penny Bank, as a means of encouraging working-class thrift, in 1875. See M. Stenton and S. Lees (eds), *Who's Who of British Members of Parliament. Vol. II: 1886-1914* (Sussex: Harvester Press, 1978), 24.

41. *Parliamentary Debates*, 3rd series, vol. 354, col. 1117.

42. See *ibid.*, cols. 1110–1.

43. *Ibid.*, cols. 1153–4.

44. *Ibid.*, col. 1253.

45. *Ibid.*, col. 1348. For the description of Rollit as a 'progressive and independent Conservative', see Stenton and Lees, *op. cit.* (note 40), 309. Rollit contested the Epson division of Surrey in January 1910 as a Liberal, and became Consul-General for Romania in 1911.

46. *Ibid.*, cols. 1237–8, 1256; see also col. 1269.

47. *Ibid.*, col. 1133.

48. *Ibid.*, col. 1239.

49. J. Burnett, 'The Rise and Decline of School Meals in Britain 1860-1990', in J. Burnett and D. Oddy (eds), *The Origins and*

Development of Food Policies in Europe (Leicester: Leicester University
Press, 1994), 55–63; see also Simon, *op. cit.* (note 35), 133–7,
278–85; J.S. Hurt, *Elementary Schooling and the Working Classes,
1860-1918* (London: Routledge and Kegan Paul, 1979), 101–27.
The school boards which had been set up under the 1870 Education
Act were replaced by local education authorities in 1902. See
Harris, *op. cit.* (note 1), 40, for further details.

50. *Parliamentary Debates*, 4th series, vol. 152, cols. 1391–2. Wilson's
reference to the savings on expenditure on asylum, prisons and
workhouses echoed the arguments used by Forster 36 years earlier to
justify the creation of a public education system in the first place
(see *Parliamentary Debates*, 3rd series, vol. 199, cols. 438, 455).

51. *Parliamentary* Debates, 4th series, vol. 152, col. 1394.

52. *Ibid.*, col. 1428.

53. *Ibid.*, col. 1436.

54. *Ibid.*, cols. 1425–6.

55. *Ibid.*, col. 1411.

56. Hurt, *op. cit.* (note 49), 109–12; Burnett, *op. cit.* (note 49), 59;
Parliamentary Debates, 4th series, vol. 152, cols. 1412–20. Although
Cox was elected as a Liberal, he was strongly opposed to the
Government's social policies. His constituency party refused to re-
adopt him and he stood, unsuccessfully, as a Free Trade candidate in
the General Election of January 1910. See Stenton and Lees, *op. cit..*
(note 40), 79–80.

57. *Parliamentary Debates*, 4th series, vol. 152, cols. 1409-10; see also
ibid., col. 1441.

58. PP 1906 (143) ii, 199, A Bill to provide secular education,
periodical medical examination and food for children attending
state-supported schools, sections 7–8.

59. Harris, *op. cit.* (note 1), 44–7.

60. *Parliamentary Debates*, 4th series, vol. 160, cols. 1376–7.

61. *Ibid.*, col. 1379.

62. *Parliamentary Debates*, 4th series, vol. 152, cols. 1399–1404; vol.
160, cols. 1388-9.

63. *Parliamentary Debates*, vol. 160, cols. 1383–4.

64. *Ibid.*, col. 1382; see also *Parliamentary Debates*, 4th series, vol. 152,
col. 1425.

65. *Parliamentary Debates*, 4th series, vol. 165,col. 745.

66. *Ibid.*, col. 748.

67. *Ibid.*; see also Harris, *op. cit.* (note 1), 10.

5

Child Health, Commerce and Family Values: The Domestic Production of the Middle Class in Late-Nineteenth and Early-Twentieth Century Britain

Lyubov G. Gurjeva

The Mellin's Food advertisement in Figure 5.1 (overleaf) epitomises the commerce of health and offers a vivid visual image of healthy childhood in turn-of-the-century Britain. Our ability to relate to this image suggests that we share in the culture of child care represented by this advertisement. This paper will focus on that culture, analysing it in terms of the production of artifacts, children, and notions of health and childhood.

The Mellin's Food advertisement promoted the sale of one of the dozens of brands of infant food which were manufactured around the turn of the century in Britain as well as in other European countries and in the United States. The use of Mellin's Food envisaged a regime of child care involving rigorous preparation of the Food, regular feeding times and frequent weighing of the baby. References to these procedures are contained in the image: prepared food is in the bottle held by the baby, who is being weighed. Such child-care practices were justified in terms of scientific knowledge in chemistry, nutrition and physiology and were discussed at length in popular child-care manuals, targeted at mothers. Such manuals would lead us to believe that what is shown in the advertisement is a fine product of the combined effort of Mellin's Works, natural forces, and the baby's competent and committed mother. By celebrating the product of their mutual endeavour, this advertisement invited the viewers to emulate their fine performance.[1]

In Britain, child health was placed into the spotlight by the debate on physical deterioration triggered by the Boer War (1899–1902). The work of the 1904 Interdepartmental Commission on Physical Deterioration, which had been appalled by the infamous reports on the fitness standards of volunteers, has been well studied and analysed in relation to the provision of welfare services.[2] The Commission ruled that there was no national deterioration and

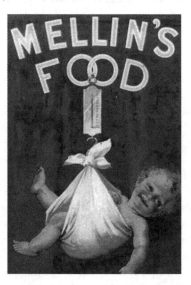

Figure 5.1
Mellin's Food advertisement, colour poster, 23 cm x 14 cm, no
date. This advertisement epitomises the commerce of health and
offers a vivid visual image of healthy childhood in turn-of-the-
century Britain. Source: Bodleian Library, University of
Oxford: John Johnson Collection; Food 8.

related ill health to living conditions, particularly in early childhood. It would be wrong, however, to directly relate the promotional and educational literature aimed at the middle classes to concerns about the fitness of volunteers, for the children of the readers of this literature were not seen as potential rank-and-file soldiers. What is, then, the connection between the middle-class project of scientific child care and the national fitness drive around 1900? The main protagonists in the discussions about efficiency and deterioration were professional experts, including doctors, scientists, military officers, and educated lay persons such as civil servants and journalists. I suggest that middle-class scientific child care, which dates back to the middle of the nineteenth century and which consolidated during the last decades of the nineteenth century, was a resource for the critique and the transformation of working-class child care through charity and welfare interventions during the twentieth century. Therefore, in order to understand the roots of many twentieth-century child health projects we need to understand middle-class scientific child care at the turn of the century.

Child health in middle-class daily life

Let us return to the Mellin's advertisement which trades on the traditional image of the stork delivering a baby in the nappy (Figure 5.1). This baby has been delivered from the hazards of early childhood by Mellin's Food. The balance confirms the progress of the child. But, on second thoughts, would you weigh a child with the feeding bottle? Would you hold the bottle at the tube? Would you use a 22lb scale if the child is heavier than 22lb? The answer to each of these questions is, obviously, 'no'. Therefore, this advertisement is saying that this balance and bottle are attributes of the past for this vigorous baby and her parents. The use of a joke in the advertisement indicates the familiarity of the advertiser and the target audience with the visual vocabulary of scientific child care, the central elements of which were weighing and feeding. It can be concluded from this that scientific child care was part of the everyday life of the middle classes. A description of common-sense assumptions and everyday practices encompassed by scientific child care will enable us to explore the subjective meanings of this activity and to appreciate it as a source of understanding oneself and others; it will also help us to discover its limitations.

Home as the site of analysis

Jane Panton confidently assumed in 1896 that readers of her child-care manual *The Way They Should Go* were upper-middle class and imputed to them a number of common characteristics, such as having servants and an eventful social life.[3] As with many other self-definitions of the middle class, this one was centred on the home. But the home was intimately connected with the work sphere and was itself a unit of production.[4] Therefore, it would be wrong to take the vision of an idealised home as a description of the actual state of affairs. The ideal, however, should be analysed as a powerful vision which affected child care practices.

The house was the physical setting and also an abstract map of family life.[5] Named spaces in the house - kitchen, day and night nurseries, bedrooms and so forth - represented various members of the household and practices associated with them. In the twentieth century family and house were integrated in the concept of 'home'. Houses embodied the self-sufficiency of the family and symbolised the interiority of their occupiers.[6] However, these homes also had a

Lyubov G. Gurjeva

display function. Fashionable houses afforded their inhabitants only as much privacy as lace curtains and privet hedges could provide.[7] One of the 'strongest strands' bringing together people of various incomes, locations, politics and religions into a middle-class population, was 'a commitment to an imperative moral code and the reworking of their domestic world into a proper setting for its practice'.[8] The social status of the family, as recorded in surveys, was primarily defined by the man's occupation, but it was displayed through female work.[9] Possessions and their management could point to politeness, wealth, modernity and the sophistication or otherwise of their owners.

Unlike the upper class, the middle-classes could not fall back on the legacy of the nobility, in opposition to whom professionals and industrialists had asserted themselves earlier in the century. Numerous books of hints and advice on how to manage the home were produced in the Victorian and Edwardian eras to assist families, who found themselves in a new financial situation, to acquire the attributes of the proper way of life.[10] Most of these books were addressed to women. 'Three main secular themes dominate books with "hints" or "home" in their title - how to start: how to manage: and how to improve - and by the very nature these three themes were calculated to appeal to a primarily middle-class public.'[11] Things, servants and children were the objects of appropriation, management and improvement. The absence of an established tradition offered a fertile ground for the appropriation and creation of new symbolic resources, one of which was scientific child care.

One of the consequences of high social mobility among the middle classes was that families changed houses as their incomes changed. A family would also normally move into a bigger house before a child was born. Thus, the birth of a child was integrated with the identity-creating and market-bound activity of buying or renting a house. Furnishing a new house was often accomplished with the help of one or more household manuals and magazines. Reading manuals and magazines and writing to them were, in turn, connected to such activities as going to exhibitions and shopping.[12] This connection was as much due to the hints and advice on shopping, as to the copious amounts of advertising published in mass-circulation periodicals. There was an essential connection between advertising and circulation: the mass late-nineteenth century press was largely financed by advertising income.[13]

106

Mass production as a vehicle of scientific child care

Consumption on behalf of babies and children distinguished upper- and middle-class families from their lower-class counterparts, and informed the notions of childhood articulated in child-care literature and fiction. In a sense, the child was constituted through specialised consumption. The range of consumer goods available included baby's layette, toiletries, infant foods and equipment for preparing and administering them, toys and educational material, clothes and shoes for older children, perambulators and medicines. Child-related products included goods for nursing women, baby diaries and advice books. Enumeration of groups of generic products hardly conveys the variety of brand names and the range of patented contraptions and gadgets that appeared on the market of child-care goods around the turn of the century.[14] Infant food brands numbered dozens and baby's layette could include a cap designed in a way that minimised the risk of baby's ears being folded between the cap and the head. If this misfortune occurred, a Claxton Patent Ear Cap for curing prominent ears could be purchased from W. H. Bayley and Son of Oxford Street, London, for 2 shillings 11 pence in 1913.[15] The explosion of brand names gave an impetus to the production of artifact-driven advice books, as well as magazines, which combined features of advertisements and instruction manuals. Many advertisers and manual writers appealed to scientific expertise. As science became fashionable, advertising departments of big companies hired researchers in order to have their products analysed and described in scientific terms.[16]

Many general British and American child-care magazines emerged during the last 15 years of the nineteenth century and in similar circumstances: the principle source of their income was advertising, and their editors included women established in literary and publishing careers as well as medical professionals.[17] Introducing the new magazine *Baby's World* in 1910, J. Johnston Macgregor did not deem it necessary to offer his readers and potential subscribers an apology for proclaiming the new world of the baby around them. He ushered them into his new publication filled with photographs of children, scientific explanations of child behaviour, and exposures of fallacious traditional ways of dealing with children. The new baby's world of special clothes, foods and child-care goods was already present in 1910, for the middle-class baby was a conspicuous consumer, although a consumer largely confined to the nursery. *Baby's World* (1910–1913) was subtitled *The Practical Magazine for*

Mothers. How could this glossy publication claim to be more practical than the more modest *Baby* (1887–1923), carrying parents' letters and clothes patterns? Possibly, the key was in *Baby's World's* approach to advertising. Like other child-care magazines, *Baby's World* published many advertisements in every issue, but unlike its competitors, it assured readers that every item was tested by its own employees against the claims contained in advertisements. Items which did not live up to what was promised were not accepted for advertising.

Concepts of advice and advertising were welded together in a special group of advice manuals, produced by manufacturers of child-care goods and distributed gratis. Some of the brochures accompanied child-care goods, others could be obtained separately. One of the earliest examples of such a publicity medium was the brochure *Baron Liebig and the Children* (1873). It launched a new line of Liebig's products, Malted Food Extract, which was advertised as an 'admirable substitute' for mother's milk. By the end of the century, there was a great variety of such brochures and even books. *Glaxo Baby Book*, covering a wide range of child-care issues, was also regarded as a successful advertisement device.[18]

The sciences and their attributes featured prominently in all promotional brochures. Thus, Liebig's Malted Food was described as 'artificially digested by chemistry'.[19] The most profuse references to science marked the *Infant Diet and Sterilised Milk* (1896) authored by 'a Physician' and fully dedicated to the promotion of Aymard's milk steriliser. While many doctors favoured formula feeding over patent foods, there seems to have been no shortage of doctors whose testimonies were used in infant food companies' publicity. An ironic protest of Mary V. Terhune, who co-edited the journal *Babyhood* (1888–1892) with a doctor, only underscored the ever increasing authority of science in child care: 'The author states, for the comfort of those whose quiet of mind is assured only upon authority, that so many of these chapters as are here reprinted, have passed the scrutiny of competent medical authority, and have been endorsed *Approved*.'[20]

Scientific child care

Some authors have suggested that the roots of scientific child care were in institutions and that the role of mothers was undermined by the joint efforts of the state, doctors and writers of manuals who had launched a crusade on maternal instinct.[21] However, the characterisation of scientific child care as an extension of hospital practices to homes and the imposition of professional views on to mothers has two flaws. First, many middle-class mothers were proponents of scientific child care and active counterparts of manual writers, scientists and manufacturers of child-care goods. Many manuals and advertisements were authored by women.[22] Second, the state, doctors and manual writers hardly formed a united front at the beginning of the twentieth century. Some doctors did act on behalf of the state in connection with vaccination or control of the quality of food stuffs, or, later, with maternal and infant welfare, but their position *vis-à-vis* the rest of the profession was problematic. Eric C. Pritchard, founder of the first infant welfare clinic in England, failed to reach the professional medical audience due to his association with a charity institution and a welfare clinic. Henry A. Allbutt was struck off the Medical Register in 1887 for the alleged underpricing of *Every Mother's Handbook* and for popularising contraception. Doctors used the British Medical Association to voice their concern about the future of private practice in the face of the employment of doctors by local government, claiming that this would deprive patients of choice and lead to a decline in the standard of medical care.[23] Doctors in private practice accommodated their clients' life styles. Thomas D. Lister, who edited the best selling *Chavasse's Advice to a Mother on the Management of Her Children* in 1906, recommended a wet nurse, which he considered a second-best feeding option for a baby after maternal breast-feeding, only if domestic conditions allowed for her residence.[24] Regimens of scientific child care had a class underpinning. The role of such institutions as hospitals in the communication of knowledge and practices to middle-class homes should not be exaggerated, for there was no direct transfer of hospital procedures to homes.[25]

Medical advice for the middle-classes drew on their traditions and conventions of domestic life, which was increasingly shaped by new goods. In the original edition of *Advice to a Mother* (1839), Chavasse recommended for the feeding of infants Robinson's Barley and 'Farinaceous Food for Infants', prepared by Hards of Dartford. The second posthumous edition of 1888 also included a positive reference to Cadbury's Cocoa. Ten years later, a new edition, revised by George Carpenter, had a 34-page advertising appendix, in which Robinson's advertisement proudly announced that 'Chavasse constantly recommends Robinson's Patent Barley, Oatmeal and Groats', and referred readers to pages 47, 150 and 286 of the *Advice*.[26] Advertisements became an important feature of all subsequent editions of *Advice to a Mother*. The core of advertisers remained the same: Robinson's, Mellin's, Allenbury's, Neave's and Frame infant

Figure 5.2
Information required on first page of <u>Baby's Diary</u>. Each child is identified by name, date of birth and date of vaccination. Hallmarks of the child's life comprise indicators of development and teething. The structure of column headings corresponds to the structure of the book. Source: Ada S. Ballin, <u>From Cradle to School: A Book for Mothers</u> (Westminster: A. Constable and Co., 1902), Appendix C.

BABY'S DIARY	TEETHING
Child's Name	
Date of Birth	**First Dentation:**
Date of Vaccination	Date first tooth cut
	Date completion of
DEVELOPMENT	first teeth
Date at which child	
first stood alone	**Second Dentation:**
Date at which child	Commenced
first walked alone	Finished
Date of first intelligible	
word	Remarks
Date of first sentence	

foods and Pears Soap. Not only were advertisements integrated with the text, through page references, but they were also revised to include new products and new themes. In 1906 Allenbury's advertisement stressed that their baby food was 'free from the dangerous organisms or the irritating products of decomposition, so frequently present in Cow's Milk as delivered in towns', referring to recent investigations of urban milk supplies duly reported in the artificial feeding section of *Advice to a Mother.*[27]

In 1906 Thomas David Lister substantially reorganised Chavasse's text, introducing new sections and revising and expanding most of the existing ones. The advertising appendix was also enlarged and indexed, which suggests that the publisher anticipated that readers might search it for information on particular brands. In the feeding section, Lister described two types of apparata for boiling baby milk produced by four different manufacturers. Some brand names became so entrenched in the child-care parlance that they almost became generic terms. Thus, a glass bottle with an opening at either end and with a teat on one end and stopper on the other was known by the name of a popular brand 'Allenbury'.

The work of manufacturers, advertisers and writers - only some of whom were doctors - was crucial for the introduction of science into child care. They reached wider audiences than scientists, and affected consumers and readers through changing their environments and life styles. A salient feature of scientific child care, conceived broadly as a way of life and propagated by these actors, is its continuity with other domestic practices and an almost inadvertent character of scientisation. Middle-class families were in many cases off-limits for the intervention of the state or medical profession. They were affected by the legislation on the registration of births, sale of foods and drugs, midwives and vaccination, but their relations with the doctors and scientists, who represented the state or acted on their own behalf, were symmetrical in terms of power and were based on exchange rather than coercion.

Production of healthy middle-class children: feeding and measuring

Popular child-care literature placed a strong emphasis on the physical development of children. Handbooks often included tables for recording various parameters of development. Ballin's *From Cradle to School* (1902), had several tables in appendices to be filled in by parents, so that the development of their own children could be compared with the norms in the book. One of the tables gave the following hallmarks of baby's life: name, date of birth, and date of vaccination (Figure 5.2). These were followed by the four indicators summing up development: dates at which the child first stood alone, walked alone, uttered the first intelligible word and first sentence. A separate section was devoted to teething. According to Ballin and many other authors, first dentition was one of the most troublesome periods. The special significance of this section of the table is underscored by the 'Remarks' column. Parents could note there which of their children gave them most trouble during teething and what remedies, if any, they used. As the structure of the column headings corresponded to the contents of the book, the table rekindled the memories of both reading the book and dealing with one's children, welding the two together.

Prefabricated baby diaries anticipated a far wider range of entries than Ballin's appendices, and were probably the most popular variety of the records of human development. Despite the ephemeral character of these publications, dozens of baby's books, baby's

111

Figure 5.3
Two record books: frontispiece and title page (a) and title page (b).
Sources: Record of Our Baby (London: Ernest Nister, 1905) and
H. N. M., Baby's Biography
(London: Simpkin Marshall and Co., 1899).

a)

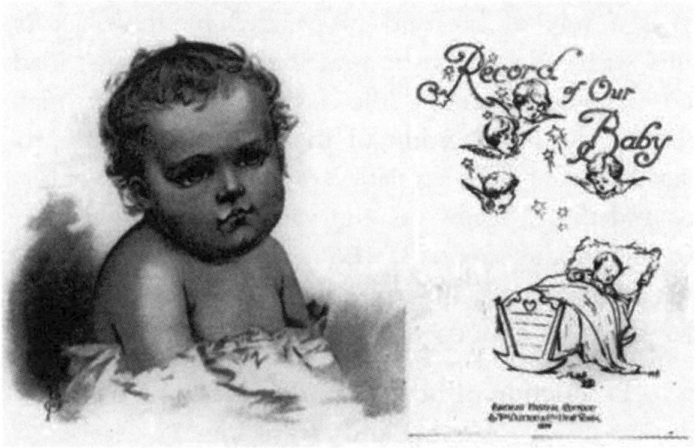

b)

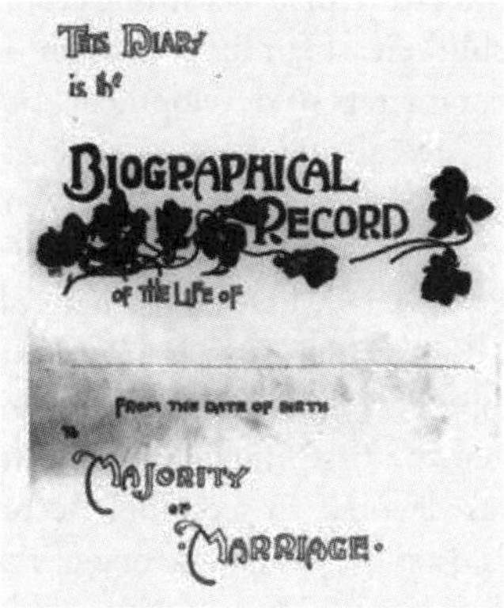

biographies, records of baby's life and such like are to be found in major libraries.[28] Being outlines of biographies, they included such entries as 'Lock of Baby's Hair', 'Baby's Photograph at Three Months', as well as 'Baby's Weight' and 'Baby's First Word', while catering to a variety of tastes and incomes. Their decoration ranged from baroque cherubs to *art nouveau* floral ornaments, which suggests that production and choice of diaries were influenced by taste and fashion (Figure 5.3). Most diaries were 'unisex' in that there were no differences between diaries for boys and girls. These differences became relevant as children grew up: according to one diary, boys stopped being children when they reached majority and girls when they got married.[29] The cheapest diaries were printed by the thousand, while more expensive ones came out in limited editions. All diaries were bound in hard covers and made to last, unlike, for example, some complimentary brochures on child management. Thus, while the quality of the diary that a family possessed can be read as a claim to taste and wealth, and, consequently, to a certain status within the middle or upper class, the very fact of possessing this expensive object was a demonstration of belonging to the better-off classes. Alongside all the ornaments and photographs, such entries as weight and height at different ages, first words and the age of the first walk, were included in most baby diaries. The usual records of child development became part of bourgeois family identity, which was increasingly connected with children.[30] In childhood records, the emphasis on physical development complemented and sometimes replaced parent's long-standing preoccupation with baptism and other events of religious life.

Artificial feeding

For young babies, the main factor of good health, according to child-care manuals, was feeding. Hence, a guide to adequate feeding was a compulsory section of advice books. Scientific feeding of infants was justified in terms of the results of milk analysis and the physiology of digestion. Such information was often provided by manufacturers of artificial feeding mixtures. With the introduction of feeding mixtures and the proliferation of prescriptions guiding their preparation and administration, the same questions were asked about breast feeding. The medical profession shared responsibility for publicising these questions with patent food manufacturers. It turned out that while the frequency of feeding was relatively easy to regulate in both bottle and breast feeding, the control of the intake was much more complex in breast feeding. It involved very precise weighing of the baby, which was more difficult to carry out than the measurement of the volume of artificial food. Control of the quality of breast milk, meanwhile, was almost impossible. Moreover, it was widely believed that the composition of breast milk was subject to constant variation, with the variation of woman's diet, environment and nervous state. 'Lactation', wrote Pritchard, 'is far more likely to "go wrong" in a woman than in the teetotal, vegetarian, nerveless cow. If the quality of the milk is to be constant, all the circumstances in the environment of the nursing woman must be constant also.'[31] Unchecked alterations in the woman's environment or regimen could lead to a deterioration of her milk and damage to the baby. In order to avoid detrimental consequences it was necessary either to strictly control the nursing woman's life, or to change the baby's diet to a more predictable product. And it was patented feeding mixtures that had the most predictable composition. The composition of infant foods was the most common subject of their advertisements, which alongside child-care manuals introduced the public to new scientific terms like 'peptonised' and new classifications of foods, like farinaceous and non-farinaceous, sweetened and unsweetened. New scientific knowledge on milk and lactation popularised through child-care literature must have swayed many middle-class women, who had already appreciated some of the benefits of bottle feeding, in favour of artificial feeding.[32]

Artificial feeding not only suited many women and met the anxieties of some sections of the medical profession, but also dominated images of childhood in public domains, of which the Mellin's Food poster is a prime example. Helen Campbell, like most doctors writing about child care, was compelled to discuss the latest commercial innovations in infant feeding, because her prospective readers were increasingly confronted with them in their homes, in shops and in the streets. A champion of breast-feeding, she considered milk formula a second best; nevertheless, she devoted several pages of *Practical Motherhood* (1910) to the description and classification of branded infant foods. Commercial goods shaped the regime of child care, in which measuring and weighing was central. Thus, Mellin's produced not only baby foods, but also weighing machines.

Compliance with the regime of scientific child care depended on leisured life style, literacy, numeracy and record-keeping skills, interest in this practice and access to at least some of its material trappings. The artificial feeding of infants at home, justified by appeals to science, was not imposed on to middle-class mothers, but neither was this process sheltered from the fluctuation of the market of infant foods, fashion, and so on. While health was a stable value, it was open to interpretation by advertisers, doctors and families.

Anthropometric measurement

Domestic record-keeping was central to the practice of scientific child care in general and scientific feeding in particular. Food manufacturers, like Mellin and Glaxo, printed their own tables of child development. In the context of this paper, the tables and diaries are interesting because they show that the scientific practices of record-keeping had a strong sentimental value. Family records of child development, however, were also of interest to turn-of-the-century students of evolution and human development. For late-nineteenth-century evolutionists, the child provided a missing link between the natural and human worlds. Continuity between nature and humans warranted the reception of humanity into the fold of evolution. Reasoning from the development of individual children to the path of the evolution of the human species was common: if human properties were gradually acquired by children, then it was likely that human properties were acquired by the human species gradually in the course of evolution. This pattern of reasoning was based on the biogenetic law or the law of recapitulation: individuals of every species repeat the evolutionary history of their species in a succession of brief stages.

Psychologists, ethnographers and other researchers wrote for parents' and child study magazines with a view to influencing the practices of child care and education, but not infrequently they also addressed readers with requests for information on their children and pupils. Relying on parents' observations, scientists incorporated into their studies elements of conventional child-care practices, such as the assumption that the mother's involvement with the child is an emotional and intellectual matter, that the relationship between parents and children is mediated by records of child development and by a multitude of child-care objects. Once these conventions were incorporated into the corpus of science, they lost their conventional character and acquired the status of regularities, if not natural phenomena. Thus research into human development naturalised culturally specific ways of child rearing of the middle classes.

Family values and scientific facts were closely intertwined in manuals. Writers reified the family unit through appeals to science, and exalted the female role through appeals to morality. Isabella Beeton, the author of the most famous domestic manual first published in 1861 and reissued for almost a century thereafter, and Dr Lister agreed that it was the duty and privilege of every healthy mother to breast-feed her child, and that expert scientific advice could help her fulfil this duty. Such uses of science were challenged by feminist and socialist critics of the bourgeois family. Even the alleged evolutionary foundations of the family and the division of labour were re-interpreted in the light of alternative values by such

Figure 5.4
Record card used at the Dublin Anthropometric Laboratory for noting personal information and the results of one series of measurements of one person. Similar cards have been used by Francis Galton in London anthropometric laboratories. Source: Daniel J. Cunningham and Alfred C. Haddon, 'The Anthropometric Laboratory of Ireland', Journal of the Anthropological Institute, 21 (1892), 39, 40.

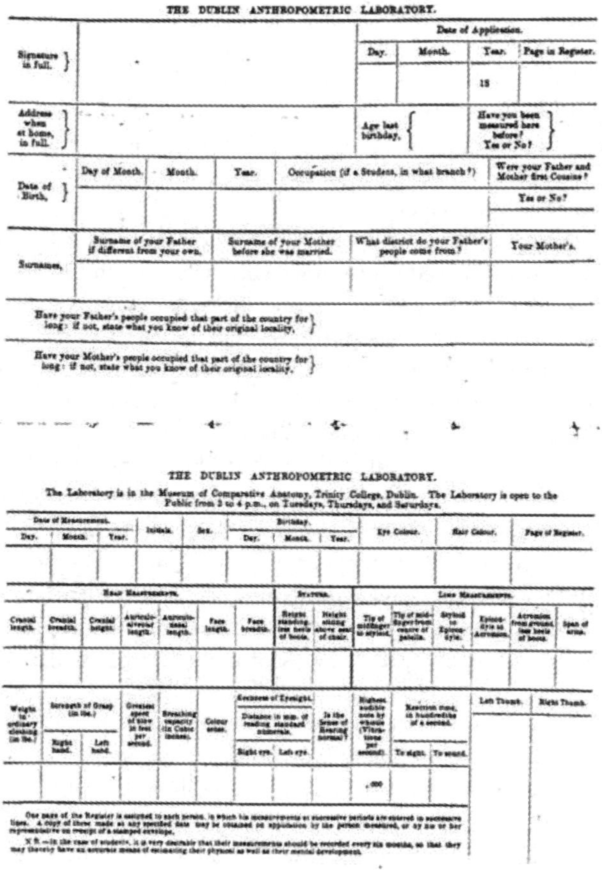

THE DUBLIN ANTHROPOMETRIC LABORATORY.

Signature in full.
Date of Application. Day. Month. Year. Page in Register.
18
Address when at home, in full.
Age last birthday,
Have you been measured here before? Yes or No?
Date of Birth, Day of Month. Month. Year.
Occupation (if a Student, in what branch?)
Were your Father and Mother first Cousins? Yes or No?
Surnames, Surname of your Father if different from your own. Surname of your Mother before she was married. What district do your Father's people come from? Your Mother's.
Have your Father's people occupied that part of the country for long: if not, state what you know of their original locality.
Have your Mother's people occupied that part of the country for long: if not, state what you know of their original locality.

THE DUBLIN ANTHROPOMETRIC LABORATORY.

The Laboratory is in the Museum of Comparative Anatomy, Trinity College, Dublin. The Laboratory is open to the Public from 3 to 4 p.m., on Tuesdays, Thursdays, and Saturdays.

Date of Measurement. Day. Month. Year. Initials. Sex. Birthday. Day. Month. Year. Eye Colour. Hair Colour. Page of Register.
Head Measurements. Cranial length. Cranial breadth. Cranial height. Auriculo-alveolar length. Auriculo-nasal length. Face length. Face breadth.
Stature. Height standing, less heels of boots. Height sitting above seat of chair.
Limb Measurements. Tip of midfinger to styloid. Tip of mid-finger from centre of patella. Styloid to Epicondyle. Epicondyle to Acromion. Acromion from ground, less heels of boots. Span of arms.
Weight in ordinary clothing (in lbs.) Strength of Grasp (in lbs.) Right hand. Left hand. Greatest speed of blow in feet per second. Breathing capacity (in Cubic inches). Colour sense. Keenness of Eyesight. Distance in mm. of reading standard numerals. Right eye. Left eye. Is the Sense of Hearing normal? Highest audible note by whistle (Vibrations per second). Reaction time, in hundredths of a second. To sight. To sound. Left Thumb. Right Thumb.
,000

One page of the Register is assigned to each person, in which his measurements at successive periods are entered in successive lines. A copy of these made at any specified date may be obtained on application by the person measured, or by his or her representative on receipt of a stamped envelope.

N.B.—In the case of students, it is very desirable that their measurements should be recorded every six months, so that they may thereby have an accurate means of estimating their physical as well as their mental development.

authors as Alfred Wallace and Edward Carpenter.[33] Such criticisms notwithstanding, the theme of maternal duties was regularly exploited in advertisements: in this genre, fulfilment of maternal duties was equated to choosing the best brand of infant food and purchasing the newest gadget.

Figure 5.5
Table of 'Heights in feet and inches of the family of Arthur A.
and Ellen C. West' prepared for Karl Pearson at University
College, London, c.1882. Source: Pearson Papers,
University College London Archives, file 139.

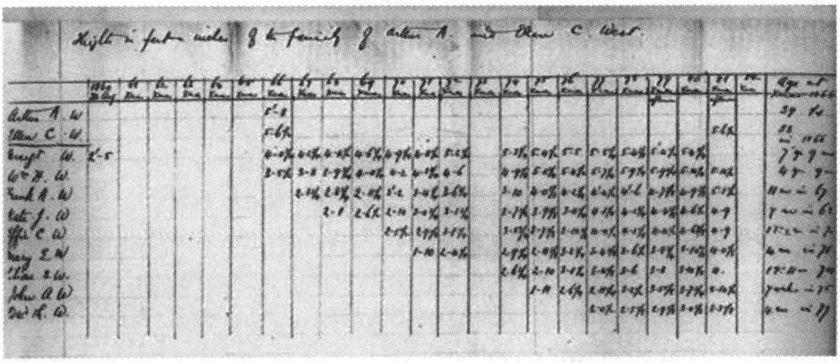

The other context of expert interest in middle-class childhood was created by the eugenics movement. One of its leaders, Francis Galton, collected anthropometric measurements at the International Health Exhibition in 1884 and at the University College, London in the late 1890s, where subjects paid for being measured. During 1884 the laboratory measured more than 9,000 people. Another anthropometric laboratory organised by Galton in South Kensington measured 3,678 different persons between 1889 and 1891. Galton's 'principal object in establishing the laboratory was to familiarise the public with the methods of anthropometry'.[34] The realisation of this objective furthered two related goals: to amass measurements and to generate eugenic awareness among the middle-class population. Record cards, which Galton reckoned were in many respects like his own, were presented to the British Anthropological Institute by the Dublin University Professor of Anatomy Daniel John Cunningham in 1891 (Figure 5.4). These cards were to be used at the Dublin Anthropometric Laboratory set up at the Trinity College Museum of Comparative Anatomy by Cunningham and Alfred Cort Haddon. The subjects also received a copy of the record of their measurements.

Anthropometrists also commanded techniques for producing one table of cumulative measurements without the aid of individual record cards. Artifacts from the archives of Karl Pearson, Galton's colleague at University College, shed light on these techniques. The hand-written table of the heights of the West children (Figure 5.5) and long narrow strips of paper with pencil marks illustrate two of the stages that height records of this family went through. Over 22 years the parents with their eldest son marked the children's heights on a steel rod at home. These marks were then transferred onto the paper strips. The height of each child at a particular date was marked with a pencil line and name. All subsequent operations occurred in the laboratory: paper strips were measured and results were recorded in the table specially drawn for this purpose.

Many of Ballin's tables belong to the same type as the table of the West children made for Pearson. They cover children of the same family and have time as one of the parameters. The difference between the two lies in the ways they were produced. Pearson's table was hand made for this particular set of measurements. Ballin's tables, on the contrary, were part of an industrially produced book. The history of Pearson's table illustrates the operations and elucidates the practices that would not have been very different from those involved in filling in Ballin's tables (Figure 5.2). Ballin's and other mass-produced tables show that by the beginning of the twentieth century these practices were increasingly standardised and technologised. On the one hand, the method of producing the tables was standardised, and they could be printed in inexpensive publications. On the other hand, the use of tables became part of the stock of the everyday skills of the middle classes: Ballin's tables had no instructions for users, besides the guidance that the table itself gave to a person familiar with its techniques.

While we can be reasonably certain that tables were kept at home, it is extremely difficult to find out how they were used. There was always a possibility that a table would never be used for recording measurements or, as in the case of a Virol weight chart, used just once and not in the exact way intended by the manufacturer (Figure 5.6). This table was designed for recording the weight of one child. The right hand side of the card, as it was printed, was identical to the left hand side. An adult appears to have used it to register his or her own weight and height on 16 May 1880. This person crossed out the column headings on the right hand side and inserted the word 'Height' where the date of another weight measurement was supposed to be written. He or she used two of the three columns originally assigned to the record of weight in stones, pounds and ounces, for noting height in feet and inches, having added appropriate column headings. Whoever filled this table in, did it in such a way that the record is transparent to us today. This means that we share the skills of using the table with that person adapting it in

Figure 5.6

Two sides of the Virol advertisement with weight chart, 6 cm x 9 cm when folded, cardboard, no date, c.1880. This card was devised for recording 16 weight measurements but was used only once for recording weight and height on 16 May 1880. Source: Bodleian Library, University of Oxford: John Johnson Collection; Patent Medicines 4.

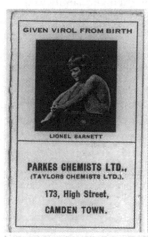

1880. While similar skills were needed for using tables in laboratories and homes, it is important to note that the aims of record-keeping in these locations were quite different. In laboratories, anthropometric records lost their sentimental meaning and acquired a new significance in relation to other similar records and as they were correlated with information on occupation, social class and place of origin. Mass studies of British populations, however, thrived on the middle-class interest in and the culture of record-keeping, and the first norms of human development were calculated on the basis of the records obtained from middle-class volunteers.

Conclusion:
Production of healthy children and family values

Child health was evidence of good parenthood, which was an important source of middle-class, particularly female, identity.[35] Child health, and parental care and emotions were embedded in child-care paraphernalia. Middle-class parents identified their care with possessing and handling these objects. Female authors drew explicit contrasts between themselves and aristocrats, who did not personally take care of their children, on the one hand, and between themselves and the poor, who used very few special child-care objects, if any at all, on the other hand. Middle-class charity workers were shocked to discover that working-class children had no clothes and cutlery of their own. 'With one saucepan in which to boil everything, a few odd cups and plates... how can a mother... with the best will in the world, prepare a really clean boracic lotion...?', bemoaned the author of a report on the North Kensington Baby Clinic.[36] Working-class parents who did not express their feelings and care for their children through consumption of child-care goods and did not share the obsession with baby weight, were constructed by many middle-class observers as bad parents. To an anonymous middle-class phrenologist, the precise knowledge of baby's weight showed 'that babies are carefully watched and looked after'.[37] At the same time, he or she noted that those who did not have children would not understand the obsession with the issue. In the eyes of middle-class experts, the poor who did not appreciate the importance of weighing babies and recording their growth, were, in some respects, like those middle-class people who did not have babies of their own and, who, therefore, could not comprehend habits and emotions of parenthood. Thus, the failure to exhibit certain attributes of child care effectively denied to the working classes subjective experiences of parenthood in the eyes of middle-class commentators. In Liverpool, government milk depots for the sale of sterilised milk to the urban poor were set up by E.W. Hope, the Medical Officer of Health, and his assistant and successor to the post, A.A. Mussen. They openly used their economic power over the poor in enforcing the regime of the depots modelled on middle-class child-care practices. Deploring the ignorance of the beneficiaries, they blackmailed them into co-operation, threatening to withdraw the supply of cheap clean milk if babies were not brought in regularly for check-ups and measurements.[38]

Working-class patterns of child care were particularly disturbing to middle-class observers because they undermined their notion of the child-centred nuclear family. In Northampton, two investigators of working-class neighbourhoods found that only 31 out of 693 households conformed to the standard definition of the family of man, wife and three children. The remaining 662 households fell into 330 'distinct groupings'.[39] These survey results demonstrate how alien these households seemed to the investigators, and how particular they were about defining the family as a paradigmatic social group. An appeal to seemingly universal values of health and family in practice excluded and dehumanised many people. Those who did not comply with the allegedly universal values were denied perceived attributes of humanity, such as parenthood and childhood.

Thus, before scientific child care became the basis for a universal notion of child health, it was a source of distinction and division along class lines. The adoption of various features of scientific child care by new welfare institutions, however, was a sign that these practices would develop into the norm encouraged and enforced nation-wide. As scientific child care expanded, the roles of its main protagonists changed. Parents became more passive, as their contributions to the discourse of scientific child care were marginalised by the strengthening alliance between private manufacturers and the state. Manufacturers of infant foods would not so much advertise directly to parents, as seek to secure orders from borough councils, and, later, from international development agencies and foreign governments. Through these more recent developments scientific child care acquired yet new meanings, but it did not loose the complexity it had at the turn of the century, and the analysis of its history can illuminate the intricate social relations it embraced later in the century.[40]

Domestic child care was never just consumption of whatever was produced outside the home, but a production in its own right. Infant foods, measuring instruments, child-rearing manuals and tabulated records, which are conventionally seen as consumer goods, were means of production. Processes of production inside and outside the home were mutually interlocked. Factory production would have been impossible without the domestic production which utilised its output. At the same time, knowledge produced in the University College laboratories depended on domestic measurements.

What are the advantages of viewing scientific child care as production rather than as consumption? As a description, it does justice to the work of many women as mothers and authors. As a heuristic tool, the notion of production directs our attention to the distribution of the means of production and products. The production of healthy children required various resources. The lack of adequate means deprived one of the possibility of producing healthy children in accordance with the middle-class blueprint. The products of this production process were not only children, but also class-specific notions of childhood and the child-centred family, which were to be universalised and internationalised through research and trade, and enforced through charities and welfare institutions.

Notes

1. On scientific motherhood in the US, see Rima D. Apple, *Mothers and Medicine: A Social History of Infant Feeding, 1890-1950* (Madison: University of Wisconsin Press, 1987).

2. See e.g. Deborah Dwork, *War is Good for Babies and Other Young Children: A History of the Infant and Child Welfare Movement in England 1898-1919* (London: Tavistock, 1987).

3 Jane Ellen Panton, *The Way They Should Go* (London: Downey and Co., 1896).

4. Amanda Vickery, 'Golden Age to Separate Spheres? A Review of the Categories and Chronology of English Women's History', *Historical Journal*, 36 (1993), 383-414. Even Leonore Davidoff and Catherine Hall, who largely embrace the separate spheres argument, stress this connection in *Family Fortunes: Men and Women of the British Middle Class, 1780-1850* (London: Hutchinson, 1987), 25–8.

5. Marilyn Strathern, *After Nature: English Kinship in the Late Twentieth Century* (Cambridge: Cambridge University Press, 1992), 90.

6. Raymond Williams, *Culture and Society 1780-1950* ((1958) Harmondsworth: Pelican Books, 1971).

7. F.M.L. Thompson, *The Rise of Respectable Society: A Social History of Victorian Britain, 1830-1900* (London: Fontana, 1988), 152.

8. Davidoff and Hall, *op. cit.* (note 4).

9. Cf. Deborah Gorham, *The Victorian Girl and the Feminine Ideal* (London: Croom Helm, 1982).

10. T.W. Heyck, *The Transformation of Intellectual Life in Victorian England* (London: Croom Helm, 1982), 28.

11. Asa Briggs, *Victorian Things* ((1988), Harmondsworth: Penguin, 1990), 217–8.

12. Ellen Gruber Garvey, *The Adman in the Parlor: Magazines and the Gendering of Consumer Culture 1880s to 1910s* (Oxford: Oxford University Press, 1996), 3–5. See also Thomas Richards, *The Commodity Culture of Victorian England: Advertising and Spectacle 1851-1914* (London: Verso, 1991); and J. McKenzie, *Propaganda and Empire* (Manchester: Manchester University Press, 1984), chapter 4, 'Imperial Exhibitions', 96–120.

13. James Curran and Jean Seaton, *Power Without Responsibility: The Press and Broadcasting in Britain* (London: Routledge, 1991).

14. See educational toys and layettes at the Museum of Childhood, Bethnal Green.

15. Selina F. Fox, *How to Take Care of Baby* (London: Women's Industrial Council, 1913), advertisement at the front of the book, no pagination.

16. See *The Advertiser's Guide to Publicity* (Birmingham: Moody's Printing Company, 1887); cf. Sally M. Horrocks, 'The Business of Vitamins: Nutrition Science and the Food Industry in Inter-War Britain', in Harmke Kamminga and Andrew Cunningham (eds), *The Science and Culture of Nutrition, 1840-1940* (Amsterdam: Rodopi, 1995), 235-58.

17. Kindergarten and child study journals were financed primarily through subscriptions and grants from founding organisations, such as the Froebel Society and Child Study Society.

18. Richard P.T. Davenport-Hines and Judy Slinn, *Glaxo: A History to 1962* (Cambridge: Cambridge University Press, 1992), 32–3; see also *Mellin's Fairy Booklet* (London: Mellin's Works, n.d.).

19. *Baron Liebig and the Children* (London: Lily and Co., 1873), 32.

20. Marion Harland (pseudonym of Mary Virginia Terhune), *Common Sense in the Nursery* (London, 1886), vi.

21. Christina Hardyment, *Dream Babies. Child Care from Locke to Spock* (London: Cape, 1983), 116. Rima Apple in *op. cit.* (note 1) also traces the roots of scientific child care to hospital routines.

22. Rima Apple shows that this was the case in the US up to about 1920. See *idem*, 'Constructing Mothers: Scientific Motherhood in the Nineteenth and Twentieth Centuries', in R. Apple and J. Golden (eds), *Mothers and Motherhood: Readings in American History* (Columbus: Ohio State University Press, 1997), 90-110:97.

23. See e.g. Report to the British Medical Association Medico-Political Committee on the Local Government Board circular concerning maternity and child welfare of July 30, 1914, British Medical

Association, *Maternity and Child Welfare Minutes*, I, 1914-1934, SA/BMA/J, 61-2, Contemporary Medical Archives Centre, Wellcome Institute for the History of Medicine, London.

24. Thomas D. Lister, *Chavasse's Advice to a Mother on the Management of Her Children and on the Treatment on the Moment of Some of Their More Pressing Illnesses and Accidents* (London: Churchill, 1906), 35. On American doctors, see Janet Golden, *A Social History of Wet Nursing in America* (Cambridge: Cambridge University Press, 1996), 56–7.

25. On the early twentieth-century debate on what sciences were relevant to clinical practice, and, particularly, on the role of paying patients in determining the style of clinical practice, see Christopher Lawrence, 'Incommeasurable Knowledge: Science, Technology and the Clinical Art in Britain, 1850-1914', *Journal of Contemporary History*, 20 (1985), 503–20.

26. Robinson's advertising in the end papers of G. Carpenter (ed.), *Chavasse's Advice to a Mother on the Management of Her Children* (15th edn, London: Churchill, 1898).

27. For a discussion of the issue of pure milk, see Dwork, *op. cit.* (note 2).

28. See, for instance, *Baby Life. With Spaces for Recording Notable Events* (London: E. Nister, 1895, new edn 1904); H.N.M., *Baby's Biography*, illustrated by Val K. Prince (London: Simpkin and Marshall, 1899); and *Baby O'Mine: An Anthologie and a Record for Mothers*, compiled by Cecil Charles (Hampstead, NW London: James Hewetson & Son, 1912). Such books remained popular throughout the twentieth century: see *Baby Mine [A Record Book]* (London: Fireside Press, 1946) and *Our Baby Album* (Bristol: Parragon, 1997).

29. H.N.M., *op. cit.* (note 28).

30. See also Ellen Key, *The Century of the Child* (New York: Putman, 1909), 44.

31. Eric Pritchard, *The Physiological Feeding of Infants* (London: Henry Kimpton, 1902), 93.

32. On women's preferences for bottle feeding, see Patricia Branca, *Silent Sisterhood: Middle Class Women in the Victorian Home* (London: Croom Helm, 1975), 95–113. For a contemporary view on the role of medical professionals, see David Forsyth, 'The History of Infant Feeding from Elizabethan Times', *Proceedings of the Royal Society of Medicine*, 4 (1910–11), 110–41.

33. See e.g. Edward Carpenter *et al.*, *Humane Science Lectures* (London: G. Bell and Sons, 1897) and *idem, Woman and Her Place in a Free*

Society (Manchester: The Labour Party Society, 1894).

34. Francis Galton, 'Retrospect of Work done at my Anthropometric Laboratory at South Kensington', *Journal of the Anthropological Institute*, 21 (1892), 31–9: 32.

35. See Branca, *op. cit.* (note 32).

36. *The Baby Clinic: First Annual Report, 1911-1912* (Keighley: The Rydall Press, 1912), 8.

37. *Chart No.1, What Baby Is Likely to Become According to the Rules Laid Down for Reading Head and Bodily Conditions* (Blackpool, no date, between 1891 and 1916), 17, Bodleian Library, Oxford.

38. E.W. Hope, *Report of the Medical Officer of Health for Liverpool* (1903), 171, and A.A. Mussen, *Report of the Medical Officer of Health for Liverpool* (1905), 144.

39. Arthur L. Bowley and Alexander R.Burnett-Hurst, *Livelihood and Poverty: A Study in the Economic Conditions of Working-Class Households in Northampton, Warrington, Stanley and Reading* (London, 1915), 62–3; quoted in Anna Davin, *Growing Up Poor: Home, School and Street in London 1870-1914* (London: Rivers Oram Press, 1996), 42–3.

40. On the costs of modern child care in the twentieth century, see Elizabeth Peretz, 'The Costs of Modern Motherhood to Low Income Families in Interwar Britain', in V. Fildes, L. Marks and H. Marland (eds), *Women and Children First: International Maternal and Infant Welfare 1870-1945* (London: Routledge, 1992), 257–80.

6

Health and the Medicalisation of Advice to Parents in the Netherlands, 1890-1950

Nelleke Bakker

In the Netherlands, as in other West European countries, an overall increase in concern about the quality of children's lives became manifest at the end of the nineteenth century. In the Dutch case it may have been inspired by the final take-off of industrialisation during the 1890s and the ensuing economic growth and social modernisation. Political and cultural integration into the nation of the rapidly growing urban middle classes and the new industrial working class proceeded along the lines of religion rather than class, in a process of so-called 'pillarization'. One of the effects of this was the relatively strong influence of the churches and their organisations in the social and cultural domain, especially on family life.[1]

As to the poor, the new interest in children's welfare expressed itself in laws restricting child labour, in pleas for compulsory education, and in a lively discussion about the best way of protecting neglected or abused children without the risk of punishing them instead of their drunken, absent or aggressive parents. In spite of the opposition of the recently organised denominational parties, who persisted in defending the father's authority against state intervention in the family, liberals succeeded in 1901 in having a series of laws passed which provided the conditions for a 'century of the child'. Compulsory schooling for children from six to twelve years of age was introduced and a legal basis was given to court custody of children whose physical and mental health was threatened at home. A rapidly growing number of privately organised re-education institutions took charge of society's responsibility for these victims of adults who could not stand up to the test of responsible citizenship.[2]

In the same year, the first infant welfare centre (*consultatiebureau*) was set up on a private initiative in a formula which immediately proved popular because medical advice was combined with free milk supplies for mothers who could not breast-feed their babies adequately on their own milk. By closely monitoring growth and feeding practices, these *bureaus* became the spearhead of the successful battle against infant deaths. Mothercraft courses and pamphlets on childcare supplemented the *bureaus'* work. From the late-1920s the *bureaus* also distributed cheap copies of small booklets on raising toddlers and schoolchildren, which promoted a slightly adapted version of the middle-class ideal of child rearing. For paediatricians these efforts to promote well informed or indeed 'scientific motherhood'[3] added to the carving out of a new specialist field among medical practitioners, as Hilary Marland has pointed out elsewhere.[4] Increasingly, other physicians shifted their attention away from normal family life and the prevention of unhealthy conditions of childcare to diagnosing, categorising, and treating physically or mentally handicapped children. This new specialisation developed in close relation to special education, another expression of society's increased sensitivity to the quality of children's treatment and environment.[5]

Although middle-class mothers also visited the *consultatiebureaus*, they did not figure particularly as targets of state or privately organised control and intervention as regards infants' health. However, they continued to be the audience of an older and less engaging means of influencing people's way of handling children: family guidance literature. Late nineteenth-century child-rearing books were addressed to middle-class readers as responsible citizens, capable of raising their children in the correct way without personal professional intervention. Whereas the patronage of working-class mothers focused particularly on promoting children's physical health, upper- and middle-class upbringing was not conceived of as high risk in this respect. Middle-class parents were expected to consult popular medical guides if necessary, or to be educated enough to know when to send for a doctor or visit a paediatrician. This, of course, does not deny that the very availability of a growing number of parents' manuals, itself an expression of the increased aspirations of professional groups, was interacting with middle-class ambitions to be the model citizens of society in yet another respect. Scientific motherhood or the expressions of the idea that parents, particularly mothers, needed experts' knowledge and advice in order to raise a child properly continued to include the physical aspects of childcare. At the turn of the century, however, Dutch physicians figured less prominently than their Anglo-Saxon counterparts.

The ascribed self-regulating capacity of the middle classes as regards children's physical health combined with the relatively strong position of clerics in the domain of family values to stimulate a shift of focus from infant's health to children's moral character. Gradually, medical aspects of child care were dealt with in popular paediatric handbooks, the most famous of which was Cornelia de Lange's *De geestelijke en lichamelijke opvoeding van het kind* (The Mental and Physical Care of the Child, 1908), which ran through seven editions.[6] Moral upbringing became the main subject of parents' manuals. Consequently, at the end of the nineteenth century teachers and clergymen took over physicians' role as leading authorities in matters of child rearing. At the same time, the new authorities stopped addressing mothers only. In their opinion, child rearing was a collective enterprise of mothers *and* fathers.

The turn-of-the-century climax of concern for working-class children's condition coincided with a rapid growth in the quantity of parental advice literature. This seems proof of a somewhat comparable anxiety about the quality of bourgeois and middle-class family life. Child-rearing literature stipulating the do's and don'ts of good parenting not only turned from an incident into a regular phenomenon; it became differentiated as well. As a consequence of pillarization, orthodox Calvinist dissenters and Roman Catholic revivalists added their own blueprints of strictly religious upbringing to the dominant liberal Protestant discourse. This is another reason why the child's moral character instead of its physical health became the main focus of the advice literature.[7]

However, the authority of teachers and clergymen to determine the ideal family upbringing appears to have lasted only until the 1920s. Since the 1930s mental health agents like psychiatrists and psychologists in turn seem to have been successful in pushing aside moral experts.[8] This shift from a predominantly moral to a principally medical approach to child rearing is most likely to have been part of a larger process of medicalisation, interpreted - according to Sol Cohen's definition - as 'the infiltration of psychiatric norms, concepts and categories of discourse' into virtually all aspects of education.[9] Up to the present, both in Britain and in the Netherlands, medicalisation of inter-war education has been observed primarily in relation to the rise of Child Guidance Clinics and their impact on other kinds of social work for children.[10] Moreover, in Britain inter-war advice to parents has been considered in terms of a transition from behaviourism to dynamic psychology and psychoanalysis as major sources of theoretical inspiration. This paradigmatic change, Cathy Urwin and Elaine Sharland have argued, was accompanied by a shift of focus from children's bodies and physical health to their minds and emotions.[11]

This chapter addresses the question as to whether these changes have been paralleled by similar developments in the Netherlands. More specifically, if morality instead of children's health was Dutch family advisors' first concern, how could a shift to mental hygiene as the dominant approach in children's welfare have possibly come about? In other words, which forces might explain a victory of the psychiatric perspective on child rearing in a society, in which the churches continued to be very influential, at least until the late 1950s, when the high tide of pillarization finally came to an end and secularisation began to break through.

The chapter commences by discussing the turn-of-the-century moral discourse on family upbringing. Next, it examines the medicalisation of the advice and its consequences for the relationship between parents and professionals. The transition is considered in terms of the experts' ideal of family upbringing, their theoretical assumptions, their concept of a normal or healthy child, and the roles and capacities they ascribed to parents. The advice of those experts whose conversion to the mental hygiene point of view was not particularly likely, that is orthodox Calvinists and Roman Catholics, is considered in more detail in the last section. Thus, the chapter clarifies the medicalisation of advice to parents in a modern democratic, industrialised and highly urbanised, but not yet secularised society.

A good character

Around the turn of the century liberal Calvinists defined child rearing almost exclusively in terms of moral education. Lack of trust in the school as an adequate milieu for character formation, inspired by Romantic reformist dislike of one-sided intellectualism, continued to be a source of inspiration for new ideals of child rearing in the family well into the new century. As a moral environment the home had to compensate for what went wrong at school. Parents were considered the foremost educators in forming a child's character. A well-bred child was a virtuous child and good parenting was defined to a large extent in terms of offering the right examples of self-control, responsibility, and good moral behaviour. Experts were confident that model parents would raise model children: obedient and morally autonomous, requirements that paved the way to adult citizenship in a democratic society.

These liberals agreed upon the Kantian notion that each child was born with a unique blend of good and bad qualities. A new-born child was nothing like a *tabula rasa*. It was the educator's task to turn

130

the bad seeds into good qualities and to let the good seeds flourish. Therefore, child rearing meant first of all knowing a child's individuality, cultivating the potentially good, and resisting the undesirable parts of its nature. That is why turn-of-the-century experts, like Friedrich Froebel in the Romantic era, often compared child rearing with gardening. Each plant had its own beauty, the experts explained. However, without regular parental weeding and lopping it would not last long. Like a botanical garden, a child's character needed constant supervision. Morality could only flourish in a child's heart if it had reached a certain level of self-denying control, a basic capacity to resist its inner drives and desires. Moreover, the child was considered to have no natural inclination towards the virtues that had to be instilled during the process: kindness, willpower and honesty, all based on moral autonomy. Fortunately, there was no opposite inclination either.[12]

The moral neutrality of the child was matched by the enormous positive power of education. This educational optimism was remarkable, and it reminds us of an important difference between the intellectual climates of continental Europe on the one hand and the Anglo-Saxon countries on the other hand.[13] The influence of Darwinian concepts was much more important in the latter. Although the origins of experimental child psychology are to be found in Germany, the new empirical and evolutionist child study was practised mainly in the Anglo-Saxon world.[14] In Germany and the Netherlands a traditional hermeneutic approach towards the child continued to dominate educational theory.[15] Whereas evolutionism did have a substantial impact on Dutch science, pedagogues preferred reformist optimism to any kind of determinism as regards parents' capacity to mould a child's character. So, belief in the power of education was closely linked with the liberal concept of the autonomous individual.

This is, for example, true of the most authoritative parents' manual of the time, *Zedelijke opvoeding* (Moral Education), which first appeared in 1894 and which had been reprinted eight times by 1919. The book is a fine example of Reform-inspired optimism. The author was the first female director of a teacher training college for girls, Ietje Kooistra. She emphasised the child's susceptibility to environmental influences, embodied first of all by the parents. Love, understanding, tact, trust, and patience, together with the child's conscience, were the most important tools in raising a child to moral goodness. The parents' good example was to invite the child to internalise crucial values like honesty and modesty. Indeed, she told

parents, 'the child becomes what you believe it to be'.[16] Her concept
of child rearing was first and foremost positive. Prevention of trouble
was better than redressing bad behaviour. If a child was lying, parents
were advised to scrutinise their own behaviour as the most likely
source of inspiration for this fault; mutual trust ought to be restored
as soon as possible. Stubborn children, she claimed, were the
products of weak parents, who spoiled their little darlings. Self-willed
children had not been used to obedience. Good parents used very
little and only mild punishments. Spanking or locking up a child in
a dark closet should be avoided, because it kept the little one from
feeling remorse. Guilt apparently played a central role in this model
of child rearing. Kooistra was more concerned about indulgence than
about neglect, and feared the dangers of weak parenting more than
those of strictness. She conceived of her middle-class audience as
tender, loving and caring parents, who lacked any natural tendency
to authoritarianism. Gradually, in her later work, she became less
optimistic and put more emphasis on the quality of parental
authority. She never ceased to insist that a child's will had to be
guided towards self-improvement and self-control with a gentle but
firm hand.[17]

At the time of World War I, in which the Dutch did not
participate except for aiding Belgian refugees, educational literature
in general paid more attention to parental authority. The first
academic pedagogue and editor of the first parents' journal, *Het Kind*
(The Child, 1900–55), the deeply religious but nonetheless liberal
Calvinist Jan Gunning, for example, did not stop repeating that
raising a child to moral autonomy did not mean raising it in freedom.
Parents had to rely on what he called tender strictness. The
punishment of children's misbehaviour was a useful means of child
rearing, he insisted, provided that it was not harsh or cruel, and
imposed out of love and in the child's interest. Beating was reserved
for rare cases and only for small children. Like God, parents had to
punish strictly and justly. As in the Calvinist religion, forgiveness out
of parental love was the reward for a child's sincere repentance.[18]

Among orthodox or Neo-Calvinist dissenters, who set up their
own churches from the end of the nineteenth century onwards, a
reversed tendency is discernible during the early decades of the
twentieth century. They indeed began to pay less attention to
parental authority, which used to be their central focus. Since the late
nineteenth century their clergymen had propagated an education 'in
the fear of The Lord' with a strong emphasis on authority and
discipline, especially punishment. The family was of divine origin

and parents were invested with absolute authority, they used to claim. Although these advisors had advocated the same educational goals as liberal authors, they had applied a different concept of childhood. For them the child was born with the curse of original sin. Education could eradicate sin and replace it with virtue. Therefore, parents were obliged to oppose their children's wickedness by all possible means. Post-1910 orthodox family manuals, however, insisted that this should not be done in the old biblical way, by breaking the child's will. The new generation of advisors insisted that it ought to be bent rather than broken.[19]

During the latter half of the 1920s orthodox advisors even showed a sudden ardour in warning parents against too much strictness in disciplining their children. Those were the old habits. Neo-Calvinist parents were now supposed to have a relationship of trust with their children. The new generation of orthodox manuals preferred the Gospel 'message of love and grace' to the Old Testament's regime of rules inspired by the Ten Commandments. Some innovators even took pains to explain that children's shortcomings were not a matter of sin. Parents could be severe, they claimed, but never harsh, so long as they followed the Christian principles of 'freedom, love and trust'. Since the late 1920s Neo-Calvinist parents' manuals advised their pious readers to create an enjoyable home, to pay attention to the individuality of their children, and to merit their confidence, just as liberal Calvinists did. When children feared their parents' severity, this would preclude a confidential relationship and consequently any real influence. Both were important, Calvinist parents now learned.[20]

The same was true of the two parents. Liberal protestants tended to value the male and female contributions as equal but different. Most often the difference was interpreted in terms of 'male' reason versus 'female' feeling. Orthodox Calvinists, however, had a clear concept of the father as head of the family; the mother was only his helpmeet. The patriarch was invested with earthly power over all members of the family. Therefore, he ought to admonish his wife to apply fixed rules. This warning was usually accompanied by a negative appreciation of the female contribution. So long as authority and punishment were most important for Neo-Calvinists, the mother was presented as constrained by deficiencies: a lack of calm resolution and an inclination towards indulgence. Gradually, however, as warnings against too much strictness began to dominate Neo-Calvinist manuals, fathers were disqualified as being incompetent to undertake more confidential parenting.[21]

Since the early twentieth century Roman Catholic moral authorities formulated their own versions of ideal family upbringing. Priests explained that it was Catholic parents' obligation to teach their offspring modesty and self-restraint as early as possible. Only strict discipline could teach the little sinners to fear His Majesty's 'ultimate punishment'. Although the 1920s witnessed pleas for more modest discipline and against the use of cruel punishments such as solitary confinement in a dark closet, Catholic family advisors continued to advocate a strict disciplinary regime. Catholics had to wait until the 1930s, when child psychologists and child psychiatrists replaced priests as leading authorities in family matters, before their child-rearing ideal was remodelled after the liberal one.[22]

A healthy mind

Since the early 1920s liberal Calvinist Dutch family advice came under the influence of subject-oriented, as opposed to the older function-oriented, psychological theories of development. German and Austrian theories, particularly the works of William Stern, Eduard Spranger, and Karl and Charlotte Bühler, were most influential. In turn, their ideas wore the imprint of biologically based theories of character, originating from current trends in psychopathology. Of the latter, only Ludwig Klages' vitalistic and anti-rationalistic characterology was widely acclaimed. In contrast with the Anglo-Saxon world, behaviourism had no substantial influence during the inter-war period. Dutch experts continued to prefer German hermeneutic theory to the Anglo-Saxon empirically based studies of child development. British theory, especially Anna Freud's psychoanalysis and John Bowlby's attachment theory, began to dominate Dutch child-rearing ideals only after 1950.[23]

A common element of the new subject-oriented theories of development was the acknowledgement of the uniqueness of the personality of the individual, not so much in terms of heredity but as the outcome of individual life history. Family advisors began to stress the influence of early emotional experiences on later patterns of behaviour and ways of coping with stress. That is why the 1920s saw the introduction of child-rearing manuals structured according to children's age, including separate chapters on babies, infants, toddlers, school-children, and adolescents. As children were changing constantly, the right way of handling them was just as variable. This acknowledgement of the natural development of the child as an important determinant of parenting was an expression of a more general tendency towards a dynamic approach to child rearing.

Moreover, it was a sign of progressive professionalisation, because henceforth parents needed to be informed about the psychological peculiarities of each of the stages their child would pass through. So, the ideal treatment of a child was not only dynamic and individualised, but also well informed by scientific knowledge. This made parents even more dependent on the advice literature.[24]

These changes are perfectly illustrated in the most authoritative child-rearing manual of the time, written by the liberal Calvinist and Leiden professor of Pedagogy Rommert Casimir. His *Langs de lijnen van het leven* (Along the Lines of Life) sold more than 10,000 copies within six weeks in 1927, and was reprinted eighteen times in just as many years. The manual also served as a textbook in all kinds of courses in the fields of childcare, development and education. In addition, it was the main source of wisdom for the popular pamphlets distributed through the *consultatiebureaus*. Casimir's manual was a plea for a loving, trusting, and respectful approach to the child in the different stages of development. Besides, the book echoed a wider shift in emphasis from the autonomous individual towards the community, which could freely be interpreted either as the nation or as one of the religious communities that constituted Dutch society. The child was not simply raised to individual moral goodness but to become a useful member of the community.[25]

The decisive step towards the introduction of the concept of a well-bred child as a mentally healthy child, however, must be attributed to dynamic psychology. Initially, leading educationalists showed a clear-cut disapproval of Freudianism, because of its 'pansexualism'.[26] They preferred the most conformist of psychoanalytic heterodoxies, Alfred Adler's individual psychology,[27] to Freud's iconoclasm of so many standards of nineteenth-century liberalism. Individual psychology, which in a sense upheld the notion of an autonomous individual, dominated Dutch child-rearing literature during the 1930s and 1940s, while orthodox psychoanalysis had only very limited influence. Compared with Freudianism, individual psychology was much more optimistic and consequently easier to apply in education.[28]

Adler, the disciple, had created his own theory after he had left the Vienna circle in 1911. He denied the sexual origins of mental illness and considered physical experiences during early childhood, especially diseases and infirmities, as the prime causes of neurosis. In his early work, physical distress was used to explain the development of feelings of inferiority and a compensatory pursuit of power. Later he attributed these feelings to every child, not only the disease-stricken. Throughout his work, the focus is directed at parent-child interaction, interpreted in terms of a power relationship. In a young child's mind a battle was fought between two opposite drives: one to defend the self and one to belong to the community. Frustration of either of the two could easily increase feelings of 'inferiority'. Parents could 'discourage' a child by making unrealistic demands or by failing to appreciate its true individuality. Extreme 'assertiveness' was one of the possible manifestations. In these cases, parents were to blame. Both spoiling and emotional neglect might be the cause. [29]

Dutch editions of Adler's work were published from 1930 onwards.[30] Within a few years several translations and a number of popular introductions to his work were produced.[31] Paradoxically, however, the best propaganda for individual psychology was an amendment of a disciple, Fritz Künkel, a psychiatrist from Berlin. By calling the infantile drives 'egotism' (*Ichhaftigkeit*) and 'realism' (*Sachlichkeit*), Künkel turned Adler's unconscious drives into normative categories of behaviour. This concept of the child was more consistent with the interpretation of growth as moral improvement and of growing up as submission to parental authority than was Adler's theory. Therefore, Künkel's version of individual psychology found an even warmer reception in the Netherlands, among both liberals and denominational groups. When he visited the Netherlands in 1931 and again in 1933 his lectures attracted large audiences.[32] His books were translated immediately after they were published in Germany. A popular synthesis of his theory, written together with his wife Ruth, was first translated in 1930 and sold over 17,000 copies by 1950.[33]

Not only the public but also leading pedagogues showed enthusiasm for individual psychology. Rommert Casimir reported extensively on the history of the theory and the ensuing movement in the German-speaking countries to establish clinics for child guidance. He valued the therapeutic qualities and educational optimism of Adler's approach but doubted its validity as a science.[34] Philip Kohnstamm, the Amsterdam professor of educational science, appreciated the way Künkel had 'deepened' his master's theory 'through combining it with the Christian interpretation of suffering'. He also liked the emphasis placed upon self-education, which happened to be a central theme in his own work.[35] Dick Daalder, the new editor of the influential parents' journal *Het Kind* (The Child) praised Künkel for his 'synthesis of the subject and the object'. According to him, his work succeeded in reconciling the contrast between science and religion and it could even help solve social problems like unemployment.[36] Many contributors to this journal used Künkel's theory to explain children's behaviour and the editor did the same in his answers to letter-writing mothers.

How did these theories and the corresponding interpretation of children's problems affect post-1930 child-rearing standards, as reflected in child-rearing literature? The first thing that strikes the historian, is that child rearing was no longer supposed to aim at self-control but at self-confidence, now a precondition for individual happiness, and, by implication, good citizenship. The parental role continued to be very important, but authority no longer mattered so much. Instead, the quality of the emotional parent-child interaction became the core issue. Parental love turned from a means of supporting their power into a source of mutual trust. Giving a perfect moral example stopped being considered as the parents' main task. Henceforth, good parents ought to scrutinise their children's 'real' emotions.

According to individual psychology, children's behaviour was to be interpreted in a symbolic way. Therefore professionals, especially psychiatrists, first had to interpret the symptoms and explain to parents the real nature of what was bothering their offspring. Behavioural problems were only symbolic representations of all kinds of feelings that made these children unhappy. Parents now had to understand that disobedience, bed-wetting or eating disorders were not the real problems. They were just expressions of all kinds of 'unconscious feelings' towards their parents, including 'discouragement' or frustrated 'assertiveness'. Consequently, in the advice literature moral condemnation of a child's bad habits was replaced by a medical account of mental illness.[37]

After 1930 the twin processes of professionalisation and medicalisation co-operated in pushing aside traditional moral experts such as teachers and clergymen as authors of parents' handbooks. Henceforth, child psychiatrists and psychologists claimed full authority to tell parents what a mentally healthy child looked like and, consequently, how to raise their children to emotional stability. They introduced the habit of sketching the ideal upbringing through the negative examples of clinical cases. One of the effects was to suggest that these disorders were indeed normal and could happen to every child and in every family. Even worse, parents who did not recognise any problems in their children's behaviour could easily be charged with a traditional or unreflective style of upbringing. These trends effectively blurred the line between parents' advice and parents' support, between prevention of trouble and actual intervention by professionals. Medicalisation and individual psychology co-operated in bringing about a process of normalisation in parents' manuals, drawing a clear line between normal or healthy and deviant child behaviour.

Thus, family manuals began to focus exclusively on emotional disorders. Experts explained what could go wrong in the parent-child relationship; this amounted to almost anything. They informed parents about ways of redressing their own faults in order to 'cure' the child, as the cause of the disorder was invariably found in the pattern of parent-child interaction, for which only the parents were held responsible. Whereas the 1920s saw the introduction of child-rearing manuals structured according to children's age, during the 1930s the type of problems parents were likely to meet became the alternative determinant of the table of contents of these books. For each manifestation of a troublesome or unhappy child - be it nervousness, fear, anger, bed-wetting, unruliness, refusal of food, or sleeping disorders - the possible causes of distress were analysed by the experts, who formulated corresponding advice. Parental responsibility was transformed from authority and control of children's behaviour into the management of the emotional parent-child relationship.

It was not only parents' handbooks that changed as a result of the narrowed interpretation of child rearing, which came to equal the prevention and correction of mental illness. From the 1930s parents' magazines also began to devote much more attention to parental anxieties about troublesome children. The number of published letters from readers grew at the expense of the volume and number of editorial articles. In these magazines a good deal of advice was now given through editorial answers to letter-writing parents, mostly mothers, presenting their worries to the experts.

Sins or symptoms

We still have to ask to what extent denominational groups were touched by the medical approach of the parent-child relationship and if they too embraced individual psychology. The most influential Roman Catholic educationalist of the time, Friar Sigebertus Rombouts, included separate chapters on psychoanalysis and on individual psychology in his well-known 1931 textbook *Nieuwste banen in psychologie en pedagogiek* (New Ways in Psychology and Educational Science). Like Roman Catholic psychiatrists,[38] he rejected Freud's theory because of its anti-moral nature.[39] He claimed that children's sexual feelings ought to be suppressed, not acknowledged. As a priest, he disliked the medical perspective of both psychoanalysis and individual psychology, but he agreed with Adler's positive message: always encourage, never discourage a child. Nonetheless, he also had serious objections to individual psychology. For Adler, personal happiness was the highest goal. This hedonism reminded the friar a little too much of Nietzsche's 'instincts'. He missed the Christian principle of ascesis: self-control instead of self-fulfilment, he explained, ought to be the final aim. Religion alone could compensate for feelings of inferiority.[40]

Nevertheless, at the end of the 1930s a young woman pedagogue and psychologist, Sis Heyster, cleared the way among Roman Catholics for the mental hygiene approach by accepting the principles of individual psychology without propagating it explicitly. She did not mention Adler but his Roman Catholic counterpart Rudolf Allers as a source of inspiration in one of her family advice manuals.[41] During the 1940s she became very popular among Roman Catholic mothers. A possible reason is that she did not content herself with sketching clinical cases; she continued to give positive advice on general goals and methods of child rearing. In a popular handbook on child psychology, for example, she did not forget to explain that all educational activity should be directed at helping a child to reach 'the deepest possible inner peace'. [42] Without avoiding the realities of parental authority altogether, she advocated a much gentler educational style than that still advocated by Catholic priests. This may explain why her public was not limited only to Catholics. She addressed all parents seeking experts' advice. Some of her books were even printed by non-Catholic publishers. Deliberately, she denied the boundaries of the Catholic sub-culture. In doing so, she contributed to the undermining of a separate Catholic identity, a process that gained momentum after World War II.

Orthodox Calvinists by contrast were involved relatively early in the medical discourse. One author of several volumes in a popular series on 'Biblical Education', a minister and superintendent of a Calvinist boarding school, was already using Adler's work in the 1920s. Without offering any form of critique, he applied Adlerian concepts and insights to the analysis of what was bothering 'difficult children'. Children's problems, mostly expressions of a 'sense of inferiority', were presented as the effects of incorrect treatment by parents. Often it was an authoritarian style of upbringing that made children fear their parents; less commonly it was spoiling which prevented the development of moral courage. He introduced Calvinist parents to dynamic-psychological concepts, like the 'unconscious', and at the same time he held onto the Bible as main point of reference.[43]

Other leading Calvinist pedagogues embraced individual psychology soon after 1930. The young educational psychologist Antoon Kuypers published an important study on the 'unconscious'. His comparison of psychoanalysis and individual psychology turned out to be a plea to use the latter in education, especially as a heuristic means of understanding the interaction between the individual and the community.[44] Discussing the same topic in a famous textbook, he praised individual psychology for conceiving the individual as responsible and autonomous. Unfortunately, however, this individual was too autonomous, as the theory left no room for God's will or for His ultimate moral law.[45] According to S.O. Los, a theologian and philosopher and the author of several pedagogical textbooks, Künkel's 'egotism' was nearly identical with Christian sin and the ideal of a 'realistic' education could be used to challenge 'the rebellion of youth against authority'.[46] Nevertheless, he missed God's Law as the ultimate criterion for morality. Though valuable, Künkels' concept of 'purification of the self' could not compete with scriptural lessons; only faith could cure the world, Los insisted.[47]

Most influential among orthodox Calvinists, however, was Jan Waterink, the Free University Professor of Pedagogy. In his 1934 textbook he praised individual psychology as 'a method to trace attitudes and reactions of the individual'. Despite these heuristic qualities, he criticised the theory for being too optimistic, too positive about the lower human instincts, too simple in its equation of 'lust for power' with 'assertiveness', and a dangerous weapon in the hands of those who wanted to oppose authority in general.[48] A few years later, in a profoundly revised edition of the textbook, Waterink admitted the importance of psychoanalytic concepts like the 'unconscious' and 'repression', but dismissed Freudianism because of the non-moral interpretation of the conscience and of feelings of guilt, as well as its pansexualism. As to individual psychology, Waterink repeated his objections but added an extensive discussion of the merits of Künkel's work.[49]

Waterink praised Künkel for his rich analysis of the complexities of an individual's unbalanced 'egotism'. Künkel's doctrine, he explained, offered a key to many everyday problems in child rearing. Unlike psychoanalysis, this theory pressed the individual to accept full responsibility for his own behaviour. Only a deep personality crisis, accompanied by remorse and feelings of guilt, could free the young adult from his extreme egotism. But there were drawbacks. According to this humanistic theory a well-balanced person could do without a conversion. Besides, a number of serious disorders, such as nervousness, could not be reduced to a simple 'lack of realism'. The worst thing, however, was that the theory left no room for sin, nor for God's grace. Therefore, it could not be matched with the Calvinist religion.[50]

Nevertheless, in the women's monthly *Moeder* (Mother), which Waterink edited personally between 1934 and 1961, he worked out a kind of synthesis between Christian morality and the humanistic medical discourse on child rearing. In the 1930s and 1940s the journal had more than ten thousand subscribers and many more women read it, as issues were passed on to neighbours. In his editorials, Waterink held on to the Calvinist anthropology of the child as a sinful creature and to the Bible as the source of morality. As to the desired educational style, he deviated considerably from the Calvinist tradition. Parental authority was limited and discipline had to be pursued so gently that it was better practised by women.

In his answers to 'Questions of Mothers' (fathers did not write and were apparently not expected to do so), however, Waterink joined the medical discourse. The readers themselves invited him to do so, as they presented their children's behavioural troubles in terms of mental health. Whereas his editorials continued to regularly deal with moral shortcomings, such as lying or stealing, the readers apparently were concerned above all else about the emotional disturbances of their children. The problems raised by Calvinist mothers were precisely the disorders discussed by psychiatrists in contemporary liberal family guidance manuals: nervousness, bed-wetting, fear, trouser-wetting, eating disorders, anger, sleeping disorders, and so on. Waterink interpreted them in terms of over-strung nerves, so-called 'neurasthenia'. It could easily happen to children with a hereditary predisposition to the disease. Quiet and calm treatment could defeat it even if it was hereditary. By contrast, vague aptitude, added to incorrect treatment, could bring about serious disturbances. Invariably, the emotional relationship between parents and children was held responsible.

Waterink's advice to letter-writing mothers was inspired by his interpretation of what was wrong with these children. In spite of his theoretical objections against individual psychology, the Calvinist professor used the popular theory to explain the nature and source of these children's 'illnesses'. Children might be suffering from neurasthenia because of a 'sense of inferiority' or jealousy caused by parental 'discouragement' or neglect. In those cases parents were recommended to show respect and understanding, to support and help their child to overcome the problem. Nervous symptoms could also be interpreted as unconscious protest against frustrated 'assertiveness'. Then parents were advised to ignore the child's behaviour and distract its attention. A 'sense of discrimination' or indeed spoiling could be the source of extreme 'assertiveness' in a child, manifesting itself as more or less conscious protest. These children had better learn to obey the rules. Punishment was only necessary, according to Waterink, when parents dealt with conscious wickedness, which fortunately was rarely the case.[51]

So, Waterink did not only use individual-psychological language; he also introduced a medical interpretation of children's problems. Sins turned into symptoms of mental illness. Therefore, we may conclude that in the 'Questions of Mothers' section of the journal Waterink lived up to his theoretical conviction: he used individual psychology as a heuristic means to understand individual children's disorders. Nevertheless, he never explicitly praised individual psychology, even as a method. He created a Calvinist version of the medical discourse on child rearing, in which he parted with both biblical education and patriarchal fatherhood.

Conclusion

In the Netherlands, the transition from a moral to a medical discourse on child rearing could be considered complete with the publication of the Dutch translation of Dr Benjamin Spock's *Commonsense Book of Baby and Child Care* in 1950.[52] Although formally addressing both parents, it also marks the return to an explicitly gendered child-rearing discourse. As in the nineteenth century, mothers were again to be responsible for the care of young children. The book immediately became very popular. The doctor's reassuring message of confidence, in yourself as a mother and in your child's potential for a healthy development, appears to have been very welcome among poverty-stricken post-war Dutch mothers. For the first time, the working class became part of the audience for this literature. Even more important, the American doctor was the first child-rearing expert who succeeded in pulling down the dividing lines between the religious communities or 'pillars'. His audience included not only liberals and social democrats, but also orthodox Calvinists and Roman Catholics. Therefore, Spock's work may be considered to have contributed to the post-war breakdown of the pillarized society that had prevailed throughout the first half of the century.[53] In one more respect his work marks a turning point. Implicitly, but no less successfully, the doctor introduced the concepts and interpretations of psychoanalysis into popular family guidance literature.

However, during the 1930s and 1940s, the ground had been prepared for Spock's popularity through the medicalisation of advice to parents. In the Netherlands, it was not Freud's own theory but Adler's individual psychology, which was responsible for introducing the psychiatric view of the child and its treatment into popular literature. Even denominational groups accepted the new perspective, probably because the concept of the child as a sinful creature was already under attack. Moreover, the mental hygiene approach, especially Künkel's theory, was not incompatible with the interpretation of growth as moral improvement and of growing up as submission to parental authority.

Unlike developments in Britain, medicalisation did not proceed at the expense of a behaviourist approach to child rearing. Dutch parental advice literature embraced mental hygiene as an alternative to a moral approach to the child. The healthy mind did not replace the child's body but his moral character as central issue in this literature. Attention was already directed at the mind as the seat of this character. As children's sins turned into symptoms of mental illness and child rearing became equivalent to the prevention and correction of mental disorders, parents' good example lost importance as a means of education. At the same time, children's behaviour did not matter so much any more; the underlying emotions became pre-eminent. Mental disorders were symbolic expressions of all kinds of feelings towards their parents. Experts had to explain to parents the real nature of what was upsetting these children. At the same time, the mental hygiene approach justified professional intervention in cases of abnormal development, a practice that extended rapidly after World War II.

As in Britain, parental responsibility was transformed from the authority and control of children's behaviour into the management of the emotional parent-child relationship. Dutch parents, not even the orthodox Calvinists or Roman Catholics, did not have to wait until Dr Spock sent out his message of self-confidence and emotional stability as the foremost aims of child raising. They did not even have to wait for Spock to learn that a healthy parent-child relationship was the nursery of national fitness in a secular society.

Nelleke Bakker

Notes

1 Siep Stuurman, *Verzuiling, kapitalisme en patriarchaat. Aspecten van de ontwikkeling van de moderne staat in Nederland* (Nijmegen: SUN, 1983).

2. Jeroen J.H. Dekker, *Straffen, redden en opvoeden. Het ontstaan en de ontwikkeling van de residentiële heropvoeding in West-Europa, 1814-1914, met bijzondere aandacht voor Nederlandsch Mettray* (Assen/Maastricht: Van Gorcum, 1985), 146–67.

3. For this concept, see Rima D. Apple, 'Constructing Mothers: Scientific Motherhood in the Nineteenth and Twentieth Centuries', *Social History of Medicine,* 8 (1995), 161–74.

4. Hilary Marland, 'The Medicalization of Motherhood: Doctors and Infant Welfare in the Netherlands, 1901-1930', in V. Fildes, L. Marks and H. Marland (eds), *Women and Children First. International Maternal and Infant Welfare, 1870-1945* (London/New York: Routledge, 1992), 74–96.

5. Dorien Graas, *Zorgenkinderen op school. Geschiedenis van het speciaal onderwijs in Nederland, 1900-1950* (Leuven/Apeldoorn: Garant, 1996), 145-55.

6. Cornelia de Lange, *De geestelijke en lichamelijke opvoeding van het kind* (Amsterdam: H. Meulenhoff, 1908, 2nd edn).

7. Nelleke Bakker, *Kind en karakter. Nederlandse pedagogen over opvoeding in het gezin 1845-1925* (Amsterdam: Het Spinhuis, 1995).

8. Nelleke Bakker, 'Child-rearing Literature and the Reception of Individual Psychology in the Netherlands, 1930-1950: The Case of a Calvinist Pedagogue', *Paedagogica Historica. International Journal of the History of Education,* Supplementary Series III (Gent: CSHP, 1998), 585–602.

9. Sol Cohen, 'The Mental Hygiene Movement, the Development of Personality and the School: The Medicalization of American Education', *History of Education Quarterly,* 23 (1983), 123–47, esp. 124.

10. Deborah Thom, 'Wishes, Anxieties, Play, and Gestures: Child Guidance in Inter-war England', in Roger Cooter (ed.), *In the Name of the Child: Health and Welfare, 1880-1940* (London/New York: Routledge, 1992), 200–19; Anneke van der Wurff, 'Aspecten van medicalisering en normalisering bij de opkomst van het medisch-opvoedkundig werk in Nederland in het begin van de twintigste eeuw', *Pedagogisch Tijdschrift* ,15 (1990), no. 2, 76–84.

11. Cathy Urwin and Elaine Sharland, 'From Bodies to Minds in Childcare Literature: Advice to Parents in Inter-war Britain', in

144

Cooter (ed.), *op. cit.* (note 10), 174–99.

12. Bakker, *op. cit.* (note 7), 105–32.

13. Ilse N. Bulhof, 'The Netherlands', in Thomas F. Glick, *A Comparative Analysis of the Reception of Darwinism* (Austin: University of Texas, 1974), 269–306; John R. Morss, *The Biologising of Childhood* (Hoeve, etc.: Erlbaum, 1990).

14. Marc Deapepe, *Zum Wohl des Kindes? Pädologie, pädagogische Psychologie und experimentelle Pädagogik in Europa und den U.S.A., 1890–1940* (Weinheim/Leuven: Deutscher Studien Verlag/Leuven University Press, 1993).

15. Peter Drewek, 'Educational Studies as an Academic Discipline in Germany at the Beginning of the 20th Century', *Paedagogica Historica. International Journal of the History of Education,* Supplementary Series III (Gent: CSHP, 1998), 175–94; Ernst Mulder, 'Patterns, Principles, and Profession: The Early Decades of Educational Science in the Netherlands', in *ibid.,* 231–46.

16. I.Kooistra, *Zedelijke opvoeding* (Groningen: J.B. Wolters, 1894), 104.

17. Bakker, *op. cit.* (note 7), 53–69, 105–52.

18. *Ibid.,* 133–52.

19. *Ibid.,* 177–96.

20. Nelleke Bakker, 'Opvoeden met de harde hand? Een historisch-kritische beschouwing van de neo-calvinistische opvoedingsmentaliteit 1880-1930', in B. Levering *et al.* (eds), *Thema's uit de wijsgerige en historische pedagogiek. Bijdragen aan de achtste landelijke pedagogendag* (Utrecht: SWP, 1998), 79–85.

21. Nelleke Bakker, 'A Head and a Heart: Calvinism and Gendered Ideals of Parenthood in Dutch Child-rearing Literature ca. 1845–1920', in Joyce Goodman and Jane Martin (eds), *Gender, Politics and the Experience of Education: An International Perspective* (London: Woburn Press, 2002, forthcoming).

22. Bakker, *op. cit.* (note 7), 197–213; Bakker, *op. cit.* (note 8), 589–90.

23. P.J. van Strien, *Nederlandse psychologen en hun publiek. Een contextuele geschiedenis,* (Assen: Van Gorcum), 148-50; *Nelleke Bakker,* The Lamp in the Living Room: Dutch Family Educationalists on Adolescence, 1915-1950', *Paedagogica Historica. International Journal of the History of Education,* 29 (1993) no. 1, 241–55.

24. Bakker, *op. cit.* (note 8).

25. R. Casimir, *Langs de lijnen van het leven* (Amsterdam: Becht, 1928, 2nd edn).

26. Outside psychiatry Freud's psychoanalysis was largely ignored until the 1940s: Ilse N. Bulhof, *Freud en Nederland. De interpretatie en*

invloed van zijn ideeën (Baarn: Ambo, 1983). Inside the profession denominational groups had serious criticisms: J.A. van Belzen, *Psychopathologie en religie. Ideeën, behandeling en verzorging in de gereformeerde psychiatrie, 1880-1940* (Kampen: Kok, 1989); R.H.J. ter Meulen, *Ziel en zaligheid. De receptie van de psychologie en van de psychoanalyse onder de katholieken in Nederland 1900-1965* (Nijmegen/Baarn: Ambo, 1988). Educationalists who took the trouble to discuss the theory were negative with the exception of F. van Raalte, who published two contributions to *Het Kind* in 1912 that were inspired by psychoanalysis. During the 1920s he preferred Adler, whereas during the 1930s he turned to spiritualism.

27. R. Jacoby, *Social Amnesia. A Critique of Conformist Psychology from. Adler to Laing* (Hassocks: The Harvester Press, 1975), 46–72.

28. Bakker, *op. cit.* (note 8).

29. P.E. Stepansky, *In Freud's Shadow: Adler in context* (Hillsdale N.J.: Analytic Press, 1983); H. Orgler, *Alfred Adler en zijn werk. Overwinning van het minderwaardigheidscomplex* (Utrecht: Bijleveld, 1940).

30. The first work to be translated into Dutch was *Menschenkenntnis* (Leipzig: Hirzel, 1927): A. Adler, *Mensenkennis* (Utrecht: Bijleveld, 1930).

31. A. Adler, *De psychologie van het individuele op school en in het gezin . Een serie lezingen* (Utrecht: Bijleveld, 1933); *idem et al., Het moeilijke kind* (Amsterdam/Antwerpen: Wereldbibliotheek, 1933); A. Adler, *Levensproblemen. Voordrachten en discussies* (Utrecht: Bijleveld, 1937); G. Adler, *Op verkenning in het onbewuste* (Hilversum: Rozenbeek en Venemans, 1934); R. Dreikurs, *Alfred Adler's Individualpsychologie* (Rotterdam: Bredée, 1934); P.H. Ronge, *Individualpsychologie. Een systematische uiteenzetting* (Utrecht: Bijleveld, 1934).

32. D.L. Daalder, 'Dr. Künkel spreekt in Amsterdam', *Het Kind,* 32 (1931), 619–20; *idem,* 'Tijdsignalen', *Het Kind,* 34 (1933), 272–4. A number of his books were translated immediately after the German edition had been published: F. Künkel, *Karaktervorming door zelfopvoeding* (Amsterdam: Wereldbibliotheek, 1930); *idem, Karakter, groei en opvoeding* (Amsterdam: Wereldbibliotheek, 1931); *idem, Individu en gemeenschap* (Den Haag: Servire, 1932).

33. F. Künkel and R. Künkel , *Opvoeding tot persoonlijkheid. Inleiding tot de Individualpychologie* (Amsterdam: Wereldbibliotheek, 1949, 9th edn).

34. R. Casimir, 'De ontwikkeling en verbreiding van de Individualpsychologie', *Mensch en Maatschappij,* 9 (1933), 198–233.

35. Ph.A. Kohnstamm, 'Boekbespreking', *Mensch en Maatschappij,* 7 (1932), 66.

36. D.L. Daalder, 'Boekbespreking', *Het Kind,* 36 (1935), 335–6, esp. 336.

37. Popular manuals showing these tendencies were: I.C. van Houte and G.J. Vos, *Moeilijke kinderen. Een boek voor ouders en opvoeders* (Utrecht: Kemink, 1929); F.H. Richardson, *Het nerveuze kind en zijn ouders* (Amsterdam: Van Holkema & Warendorf, 1929); J. Riemens-Reurslag, *Nieuwe zakelijkheid in de opvoeding* (Amsterdam: Van Holkema & Warendorf, 1932); R. Dreikurs, *Hoe voed ik mijn kind op?* (Utrecht: Bijleveld, 1936); H.J. Jordan, Jr., *Hoe opvoedingsfouten te vermijden?* (Zeist: Ploegsma, 1938).

38. Ter Meulen, *op. cit.* (note 26), 75–99.

39. Fr.S. Rombouts, *Nieuwste banen in psychologie en paedagogiek* (Tilburg: R.K. Jongensweeshuis, 1931), 44.

40. *Ibid.,* 72.

41. S. Heyster, *Opvoedingsmoeilijkheden van iederen dag. Een boek voor moeders en andere opvoedsters* (Amsterdam: Kosmos, 1938), 41; *idem, Opvoeden in de practijk. Het boek voor iederen opvoeder* (Den Haag/Gent: Populair Wetenschappelijke Bibliotheek, 1935).

42. S. Heyster, *Kinder- en jeugdpsychologie* (Leiden: Nederlandsche Uitgeversmaatschappij, 1946), 12.

43. G.W.C. Vunderink, *Van dieper leven. Bibliotheek voor Bijbelsche Opvoedkunde* VII (1924), no.6; *idem,* Conflicten, *Bibliotheek voor Bijbelsche Opvoedkunde* IX (1925), no. 2; *idem,* De gezinsopvoeding en hare gevaren, *Bibliotheek voor Bijbelsche Opvoedkunde* XI (1927), nos 4, 6.

44. A. Kuypers, *Het onbewuste in de nieuwere paedagogische psychologie* (Amsterdam: Paris, 1931), 116.

45. J.H. Bavinck and A. Kuypers, *Inleiding in de zielkunde* (Kampen: Kok, 1935, 2nd edn), 346.

46. S.O. Los, *Moderne paedagogen en richtingen* (Amsterdam: De Standaard, 1933), 117.

47. S.O. Los, *De individuaal-psychologie van Adler tot Künkel* (Amsterdam: Gereformeerde Psychologische Studievereeniging, 1937).

48. J. Waterink, *Hoofdlijnen der zielkunde* (Wageningen: Zoomer & Keuning, 1934), 211.

49. J. Waterink, *Ons zieleleven* (Wageningen: Zoomer & Keuning, 1946, 5th edn, 1st edn 1938, 176–92.

50. *Ibid.,* 192–202.

51. Bakker, *op. cit.* (note 8), 593–8.

52. Benjamin Spock, *Baby en kleuterverzorging* ('s-Graveland: De Driehoek, 1950).
53. Nelleke Bakker, 'Ouderadvisering in historisch perspectief. Over de geschiedenis van opvoedingsvoorlichting en opvoedingsonzekerheid', in Marga Akkerman-Zaalberg van Zelst , Harry van Leeuwen and Noëlle Pameijer (eds), *Ouderbegeleiding nader bekeken* (Lisse: Swets & Zeitlinger, 1998), 17–34.

7

'Grown-Up Children': Understandings of Health and Mental Deficiency in Edwardian England

Mark Jackson

> The child remains a child, whatever his age may be, he has a child's outlook, a child's pleasures and expectations. It rests with those responsible for him to decide whether he shall be a happy, good, pure child or a plague-spot upon the face of the earth.[1]

In 1892, the Metropolitan Association for Befriending Young Servants opened a small home for feeble-minded girls in Hitchin on the basis that young women 'on the borderland of imbecility' were 'liable to be the prey of vicious men or women, and to be dragged down into degradation'.[2] Two years later, an editorial in the *British Medical Journal* echoed such fears about the dangers of the feeble-minded by warning that those inhabiting 'the borderland of imbecility' were 'a greater danger to the State, than the absolutely idiotic', and by stressing the urgent need for institutional provisions designed 'to provide maintenance, protection, training, and employment for boys and youths who are mentally incapacitated from earning their own living and who are yet so far intelligent as not to be eligible for any asylum for the imbecile or insane'.[3] Such a scheme, the editorial suggested, was desirable 'not only from the point of view of philanthropy, but from that of social economy, for the segregation of those afflicted with feeble-mindedness in special homes would tend to diminish the evil in the next generation, while they would themselves earn something towards their support, and so be less of a burden to the community'.[4]

The naming of 'the borderland' in the 1890s marked the emergence of a distinct category of mental defectives, invested for the first time with positive, rather than merely negative, characteristics.[5] Since the introduction of the category of 'feeble-mindedness' to denote a mild degree of deficiency by P. Martin Duncan and William Millard in 1866,[6] feeble-mindedness had been characterised largely

149

by the mere absence of imbecility, on the one hand, and educational and social normality, on the other. Although both the Report of the Departmental Committee on Defective and Epileptic Children, published in 1898, and the subsequent Elementary Education (Defective and Epileptic Children) Act of 1899 continued to suspend the feeble-minded rather passively between the normal and the imbecilic,[7] it is clear that during the 1890s and 1900s the borderland was increasingly adorned with a distinctive set of topographical, biological, and historical characteristics. Fashioned within the context of anxieties about rising levels of insanity and deficiency, about the inherited and biological nature of educational and social ineptitude, and about the preservation of national and imperial strength, the feeble-minded (more than any other group of defectives) were perceived as a distinct and pathological 'class' in society, with constitutional tendencies to pauperism, criminality, bestiality, promiscuity, and excessive fertility.

By the first decade of the twentieth century, the problem of the feeble-minded had become, for some commentators, 'the most pressing of all the social problems of our time'.[8] Less overtly pathological than idiots and imbeciles, the feeble-minded constituted a covert source of physical, moral, and mental degeneration that was threatening to subvert the health and wealth of the nation. Critically, this rhetoric embodied a prominent belief that social pathology was clearly located in the biological nature of a distinct 'class' of the population rather than in socio-economic conditions. Although the productivity of the feeble-minded was understood to be determined in part by the environment in which they lived, the problems thought to be caused by those occupying the borderland of imbecility were inextricably linked to the constitutional and pathological nature of their condition.

During the late Victorian and Edwardian period, then, the feeble-minded occupied a critical social and cognitive space, a 'borderland' between the educationally and socially normal and the pathological. Use of 'the borderland' as an epithet for the feeble-minded was not coincidental. The term was regularly employed in this period either to describe phenomena that were ambiguously situated between the supposedly pathological and the normal,[9] or to depict conditions and behaviour that lay between, and sometimes served to connect, disparate clinical and social pathologies.[10] Significantly, the feeble-minded occupied borderlands that corresponded to both meanings of the term. In addition to bridging a gap between the mentally normal, on the one hand, and idiots and imbeciles, on the other, the feeble-minded also served to link contemporary conceptions of mental deficiency, criminality, poverty, and promiscuity.

The feeble-minded inhabited other borderlands during the early years of the twentieth century. They were situated, both literally and imaginatively, between childhood and adulthood, between charitable and state provisions, between the productive and non-productive, between educational, poor law, judicial, and asylum authorities, between the criminal and the law-abiding, and between the vulnerable and the dangerous. In this chapter, I want to concentrate on just one of these borderlands. In particular, I want to explore the manner in which the feeble-minded came to occupy an ambiguous space between childhood and adulthood. By exploring published medical and pedagogic texts, and by exploiting records from the Sandlebridge Boarding Schools and Colony which was founded in 1902, I shall argue that Edwardian attempts to regulate the borderland were forcefully framed by contemporary preoccupations with child development and, particularly, by the notion of arrested development. Significantly, such notions served not only to delineate the mental and physical characteristics of the borderland but also to provide a powerful metaphor for national and social decline. Inspired by fears of racial degeneration and by conceptions of the healthy child as an asset to the empire, contemporaries equated poorly developed children with a poorly developed nation. In spite of ambiguities in both rhetoric and practice, the construction of the feeble-minded as 'grown-up children'[11] provided a powerful rationale for repressive social policies that continued to dominate political and personal landscapes for much of the twentieth century.

Developmentalism and the feeble mind

By the end of the nineteenth century, it had become commonplace to explain a variety of social and natural processes (whether cosmic, geological, physical, psychological, national, or imperial) in terms of progressive development or evolution.[12] Childhood and the process of growing into adulthood were no exceptions. Childhood was routinely regarded as a period of profound anatomical, mental, and moral development.[13] And novel educational and medical approaches to children were designed ostensibly both to support and encourage the supposedly natural developmental processes whereby children evolved into adults, and to identify and overcome obstacles to normal development.

Significantly, as some historians have suggested,[14] the various

151

approaches to childhood that emerged in the nineteenth century were grounded in a physiological understanding of growth and development. Within the domains of medicine and education (and, more particularly, within the context of medico-pedagogic approaches to mental and physical deficiency),[15] physiological principles operated at several levels: firstly, they implied that maturation of the mind, the body, and the morals, was mediated through the physical body or the senses;[16] secondly, they emphasised the extent to which the education of both normal and defective children should emulate as closely as possible 'the mode in which nature herself proceeds in the development of the faculties of perfect children';[17] and, thirdly, they facilitated the emergence of the child as an object of scientific study, paving the way, as Lyubov Gurjeva has demonstrated, both for attempts to tabulate the normal stages of infancy and childhood and for the formation of the child study movement and the scientific management of children.[18]

Within this developmental discourse, childhood symbolised more than simply a stage in the life of an individual. Inspired by the notion of recapitulation, which assumed particular ideological significance in theories of evolution,[19] the child was historicised and both children and childhood were equated with the primitive.[20] As Dr Hastings Gilford insisted in the early twentieth century:

> It must never be forgotten that v. Baer's law that the racial ancestry is recapitulated in the development of the individual is not only true of pre-natal development, but is equally true of post-natal development. Hence defective growth or defective development shown during years of infancy, childhood, or youth may be no more than reminiscent of some corresponding backwardness during a past racial epoch, such as will be rectified when development has been carried on a little further.[21]

Within this context, the development of the child was not only analogous to, but a crucial constituent and exemplar of, the evolution of societies and races.[22] More pertinently, in the present context, child development embodied and symbolised human development.

The recognition, analysis, and tabulation of 'normal' child development was paralleled by growing interest in abnormal development, which was perceived increasingly as the disordered maturation of the physiological body.[23] In the middle decades of the twentieth century, the space opened up by this approach to childhood provided a site for the emergence of new clinical subspecialties, notably developmental medicine, developmental psychology, and developmental paediatrics.[24] In the last few years of the nineteenth and the early years of the twentieth century, however, developmentalism provided a clear theoretical basis for understanding the aetiology and pathogenesis of the defective mind.

Drawing on Henry Maudsley's bleak biological faith in the 'tyranny of organisation',[25] late Victorian and Edwardian doctors argued that feeble-mindedness was the product of a 'morbid inheritance' damaging the 'germ plasm' in such a way that normal development was impossible. Building explicitly on Seguin's physiological methods of education and training, for example, Dr George Shuttleworth, formerly medical superintendent at the Royal Albert Asylum in Lancaster, insisted in 1895 that 'with the idiot (and in less degree with the mentally feeble child) there is some hindrance to this normal evolution'.[26] Some years later, Dr Charles Paget Lapage and Dr Alfred Tredgold exploited both clinical and post-mortem findings to argue that all varieties of mental deficiency arose from 'imperfect or arrested development',[27] a phenomenon apparently generating not only inferior mental powers but also the bewildering array of physical anomalies (abnormal ears, eyes, palates, fingers, and so on) charted so meticulously by Dr Francis Warner in the 1880s and 1890s.[28] As the direct result of arrested development, the Edwardian feeble-minded were 'from their very nature feeble in all respects'.[29]

According to many commentators, this panoply of mental and physical defects rendered the feeble-minded child incapable of benefiting from an ordinary elementary education, and ensured that feeble-minded adults required permanent care and supervision. Although such accounts received powerful legitimation both from the Royal Commission on the Care and Control of the Feeble-Minded and from the terms of the Mental Deficiency Act of 1913 and the Elementary Education (Defective and Epileptic Children) Act of 1914,[30] for many alarmists definitions based entirely on educational capacity or the ability to earn a living failed adequately to capture the essence of the feeble mind. For example, for Mary Dendy, the most prominent advocate of institutional segregation of defectives, the defining feature of the feeble-minded was their lack of will-power, responsibility, and self-control.[31] Constitutional weaknesses of this nature not only apparently precipitated the feeble-minded into lives of crime, poverty, and prostitution but also ensured that the feeble-minded were never considered to have achieved adult maturity or, as Mathew Thomson has suggested, to deserve the rights of full citizenship.[32] Denied the capacity for normal development into adulthood, the feeble-minded were consigned to permanent childhood: as Alfred Tredgold insisted in 1910, 'children they always remain'.[33]   Routinely infantilised as 'grown-up children', feeble-minded people of all ages emerged from the authoritative rhetoric of developmentalism as a legitimate site for paternalistic intervention.

Edwardian arguments for intervention were closely shaped by preoccupations with class.   Although the *British Medical Journal* carried occasional appeals for more expansive institutional provisions for middle-class defectives, and although Mary Dendy and her colleagues claimed that feeble-mindedness was equally distributed across all social classes,[34] regular conflation of the borderland with the supposedly promiscuous, parasitic, and impoverished criminal classes guaranteed that both state and charitable interventions were almost exclusively directed at feeble-minded children and adults from the working classes.[35]

Crucially, the impact of developmentalism was evident not only in discussions of the aetiology and pathogenesis of deficiency, but also in the classification of defectives.   Edwardian doctors routinely divided feeble-mindedness into primary cases, which were the product of a morbid inheritance, and secondary or acquired cases, which occurred as the result of some external injury or infection. Although some medical authors referred to a separate class of primary 'developmental cases', in which neuropathic inheritance became manifest only at certain crises of development (such as dentition, puberty, and so on), in practice all primary, and many secondary, cases were regarded as the product of arrested development.[36]   In addition, developmental approaches also directed the treatment and management of the feeble-minded.   Drawing on Seguin's physiological principles, on the techniques of Froebel and Montessori, and on the practices of certain American and German institutions, the medico-pedagogic approach that dominated British special school, asylum, and colony regimes in the early twentieth century stressed the importance of educating the senses in order to develop both body and mind.[37]   Thus, in her domain at Sandlebridge, which was opened by the Lancashire and Cheshire Society for the Permanent Care of the Feeble-Minded in 1902, Mary Dendy incorporated a 'sense-room', which contained wooden models to train the senses and a variety of kindergarten materials designed to develop manual skills.[38]

However, there were clearly limits to the efficacy of such approaches.   Although Edwardian commentators certainly promoted means of developing the feeble mind, they nevertheless insisted that any development was necessarily restricted by the biological constraints of a feeble constitution. 'Feeblemindedness, just the same as idiocy', insisted Tredgold in 1911, 'is incurable, and no means can, or ever will, convert one of these persons into a normal citizen'.[39] From this perspective, the aim of education and training was primarily to prepare the feeble-minded for manual, productive work that would enable them to contribute 'something towards their own support'.[40] The potential benefits of this process were apparently profound, both for the feeble-minded and for society. 'There is much derelict land in England', asserted Mary Dendy imperiously, 'let us put our derelict humanity upon it and so reclaim both'.[41]

In the late nineteenth and early twentieth centuries, strategies to develop the feeble mind were generally construed as humanitarian and progressive. By identifying special educational needs and by devising pedagogic schemes to meet those needs, Shuttleworth, Dendy, Tredgold, Lapage, and others maintained that they were offering the feeble-minded opportunities to mature, to develop their abilities, and to work. In spite of such emancipatory rhetoric, however, it is clear that in the early twentieth century the impact of developmentalism was primarily despotic. The notion of arrested development clearly carried connotations of inferiority, an association evident particularly in discussions of 'mongolism' and in debates about the sexuality of feeble-minded women.

'Mongolian imbecility' was first perceived as a separate category of deficiency by Dr John Langdon Down in the 1860s. Apparently sharing characteristics with racial Mongols, 'mongolian imbeciles' provided Down with exemplary evidence both for his 'ethnic classification of idiots' and for the unity of human species.[42] Although Down's ethnic classification and his belief that 'mongolism' was the product of tuberculous degeneration were both discarded in the early decades of the twentieth century, the ethnological bias inherent in his approach clearly persisted. In particular, 'mongolian imbeciles' (like racial Mongols) were construed by Shuttleworth as 'unfinished children' whose 'peculiar appearance is really that of a phase of foetal life'.[43] Similarly, Dr D. Hunter revealed both the influence of developmentalism and the force of racial stereotypes by insisting that 'all the characteristics of the condition could be paralleled in the foetus, and that in short the Mongolian idiot was a grown-up foetus'.[44]

Insinuations of inferiority were also evident in Edwardian constructions of feeble-minded women. Possessing insufficient will-power to resist male sexual advances, 'even the best-behaved [feeble-minded women], and those of good parentage brought up amid every refinement' were, according to Tredgold, 'often so facile that it is utterly unsafe for them to be at large without protection'.[45] More disturbingly for contemporaries, feeble-minded women were thought to possess what Tredgold referred to as 'pronounced erotic tendencies' and to be 'utterly lacking in any sense of shame, modesty, or even ordinary decency'.[46] Echoing Mary Dendy's belief that 'when the higher faculties have dwindled the lower, or merely animal, take command',[47] Dr Joshua Cox painted a more evocative picture of the promiscuity and bestiality of feeble-minded women:

> The girls of this type have a much sadder fate. As they grow up into young women, they, being unfitted to retain any situation, drop lower and lower in the social scale, become the prey of ruffianly scoundrels unworthy of the name of men, and are under the grip of their more animal instincts, untramelled by any higher brain-power to keep them on a right line of life. They are often admitted to the wards of workhouses to await the birth of their illegitimate children - too often more feeble-minded than themselves.

> There is no sadder chapter in our social system than the lot of many of these half-witted girls in the poorest classes. They drift along the great river of life in our large towns, or perhaps in the smaller channels in the country, each week almost sinking lower and lower, physically and mentally, depraved through no real viciousness, but because they have no faculty of higher control, and debased by drink and vile associates.[48]

Manifestly shaped by concerns about lower-class sexuality and differential class fertility rates, the construction of feeble-minded women as 'animal' was reinforced by a range of prominent parallel conflations. In much late nineteenth- and early twentieth-century anthropological literature, women were readily equated with the primitive, the infantile, and the savage.[49] Constrained by the tyranny of their biological organisation, women, the feeble-minded, and certain racial types were collectively construed as undeveloped and incomplete. In this way, developmentalism provided a scientific rationale for constructing and maintaining social hierarchies and for reifying class and racial differences.

Child and empire

Clearly fashioned in the midst of rising middle-class anxieties about urban decay, racial degeneration, and declining national and imperial strength,[50] feeble-mindedness comprised not merely a single strand, but more usually the principal cause, of myriad social evils: the feeble-minded were the perpetrators of crime, the incubators of disease, the primary source of poverty, promiscuity, alcoholism, insanity and national deterioration, and the negligent parents of hordes of illegitimate children. As Tredgold cautioned an audience of the Manchester and Salford Sanitary Association in 1911:

> The feeble-minded, the insane and the epileptic have been allowed to mate to such an extent with healthy stocks that, although the full fruition of the morbid process may have been thereby delayed, the vigour and competence of many families has been undermined, and the aggregate capacity of the nation has been seriously reduced. The taint is, in fact, slowly contaminating the whole mass of the population.[51]

As Peter Bowler has suggested, the fear of degeneration that surfaced so forcibly in the late nineteenth and early twentieth centuries was not necessarily antithetical to Victorian notions of development and evolution. On the contrary, although opposed to the belief in progress that was adopted by many Victorians, concepts of degeneration and decline were implicit in contemporary theories of evolution.[52] What is crucial, in the present context, is that prospects of degeneration and aspirations to social progress together highlighted the need to safeguard the normal development of children into fit, healthy adults. With the child hailed as an asset of the empire,[53] child hygiene became a crucial tactic in the battle against race suicide.[54] As Dr Robert Rentoul warned in a characteristically plangent plea for the sterilisation of defectives in 1907, 'the hand that *wrecks* the cradle *wrecks* the nation'.[55]

In this context, the working-class feeble-minded child became a critical site for medical investigation and political intervention. Concerned about the proliferation of the borderland and about apparently declining numbers of healthy children,[56] contemporary commentators struggled to design strategies for limiting the birth of feeble-minded children, for maximising the development and productivity of those that were born, and for generating 'a nation of stalwarts'[57] rather than degenerates. Presuming that a poorly developed child was both analogous to, and constitutive of, a poorly developed nation, Dendy, Tredgold, Rentoul, and their associates situated themselves in the vanguard of efforts to revive national and imperial vigour.

The problem of the feeble-minded is intimately associated with the problem of insanity, epilepsy, alcoholism, and consumption. Again, such questions as the housing, feeding, and remuneration of the working classes, infantile mortality, teaching, employment, and pauperism are in urgent need of attention, but measures to deal with these matters cannot solve the problem of national degeneracy. National progress can only take place when means are taken to increase the fit and decrease the unfit. The establishment of suitable farm and industrial colonies is the only method whereby society can be protected from the feeble-minded. There they would be far happier than in the outside world and would contribute to their own support. Nothing is more wasteful than this army of degenerates who, when they are not living at the cost of the taxpayer in workhouses or prisons, are wandering at large, idling, pilfering, injuring property, and polluting the stream of national health by throwing into it human rubbish in the shape of lunatics, idiots, and criminals.[58]

For some Edwardian writers, the previous half century of welfare reforms had hindered efforts both to improve child health and to manufacture eugenic improvements in the race. According to Karl Pearson, for example, the cumulative effect of factory legislation and education acts in the late nineteenth century had been to reduce 'every possibility of a child being a pecuniary asset' to its parents.[59] Assuming that children constituted an economic commodity produced to meet demand, Pearson concluded that the principal effect of such legislation was that parents produced fewer children and failed to protect their health and welfare adequately.[60] From Pearson's perspective, legislative measures primarily intended to promote national progress had 'directly tended to enfeeble the race'.[61]

The error into which the legislature had fallen, according to Pearson and others, was that it had prioritised the environment over heredity. 'The whole trend of legislation and social action', insisted Pearson, 'has been to disregard parentage and to emphasise environment.'[62] Sir James Barr, consulting physician to Liverpool Royal Infirmary and President of the Liverpool Branch of the Eugenics Education Society, was more forceful. 'A good deal of the insane legislation and wasteful expenditure of recent years', he argued in 1911, 'has arisen from the teaching of sanitarians and some leading medical men, that everything depended on the environment, and heredity did not count'.[63] By improving the environment without due attention to biological laws, welfare and education reforms and indiscriminate charity had merely ensured the survival of the unfit: 'It is your miserable degenerate who is assisted by charity from the cradle to the grave that often survives the longest.'[64]

The solution to this dilemma, for Pearson, was not to repeal the Factory Acts, but to reverse their effects by espousing the principles of practical eugenics, which were committed both to encouraging 'sound parentage' and to making 'the well-born child' once again 'a valuable economic asset'.[65] While many Medical Officers of Health, School Medical Officers, and the Board of Education remained dedicated to environmental approaches to cultivating the physical and mental health of school children and stressed the role of the School Medical Service in improving 'the surroundings and physical life of the children',[66] most commentators on the problem of the feeble-minded in the early twentieth century preferred more intrusive solutions inspired by biological and hereditarian, rather than environmental, visions of the borderland. Adamant that 'national sanity and national well-being are of more importance than is the "liberty of the subject"',[67] Rentoul, Dendy, Tredgold, Barr, Pearson, and many others therefore advocated either the sterilisation of defectives or their permanent segregation in agricultural colonies.

Deceptive developments

In most contemporary professional accounts of the feeble mind, chronological growth failed to avert the consequences of arrested development. According to Alfred Tredgold, for example, the diverse mental and physical defects of the feeble-minded child ensured that 'bodily and mentally he is always in arrears, and with each advancing year his intellect is left farther and farther behind that of his more fortunate fellow'.[68] These deficiencies persisted into adult years. As Tredgold asserted, the 'child is father to the man, and in the main the physical and mental characteristics of the feeble-minded adult are similar to those of the mentally defective child'.[69]

Significantly, bodily growth could also generate new problems for the feeble-minded. In particular, the 'advent of puberty' (that is, 'the precise age . . . when the emotions and passions are under-going active development')[70] was thought to result in the 'evolution of habits and propensities which have the greatest effect upon the future life'.[71] The passage of time, therefore, could not only unleash dangerous sexual proclivities but also, in some cases, exacerbate emotional disturbances and reveal a 'strong predisposition to insanity and crime'.[72] In the absence of an appropriate environment or training, the innate intellectual problems of the feeble-minded

159

combined with their diminished power of self-control apparently ensured that educationally problematic children would become socially problematic adults.[73]

However, in spite of attempts to consign the feeble-minded to permanent childhood, it is evident that children on the borderland of imbecility did grow up and that those labelled as feeble-minded and their families vigorously endeavoured to resist efforts to classify and control them. Case records from Sandlebridge suggest that many of the children admitted to the Schools and Colony did possess (or develop) the ability to read and write and to work efficiently and productively on the farm and gardens or in the laundry and sewing rooms.[74] Indeed, the ability to work (an attribute more readily associated with normal rather than pathological development) may well have constituted a more decisive factor than educational ability or a particular diagnostic label in determining admission to, and retention in, the Schools. It is clear, for example, that although Sandlebridge was certified both by the Board of Education and, after 1914, by the Board of Control as an institution for the feeble-minded, a number of imbeciles and idiots were admitted on probation. Critically, those 'low-grade cases' that were retained were those specifically identified by Mary Dendy as good workers and useful to the Colony.[75]

The economic potential of defectives at Sandlebridge did not pass unnoticed by residents' families or poor law guardians responsible for their maintenance. In August 1907, Harry W.'s parents (whom Mary Dendy dismissed as 'unsatisfactory') attempted to remove him from the Colony so that he could 'work with horses under supervision'. The following year, they succeeded in taking Harry home and obtaining work for him.[76] Some years later, John M., whom Mary Dendy regarded as a 'hard-working lad' and who had apparently been dissatisfied with institutional life, was removed from Sandlebridge by the Salford Guardians to 'work on their own farm'.[77] Dendy was characteristically antagonistic to such efforts to normalise her 'children'. She not only struggled valiantly to retain productive residents in the Colony, but also openly criticised the manner in which parents were undermining her pioneering efforts to restore national efficiency: 'Were it not for the interference of bad parents, who, when they see the children grown into comparatively healthy boys and girls, try to remove them to make them earn money, we should be able to keep them all.'[78]

Significantly, several inmates from Sandlebridge managed successfully to reproduce their productivity outside the institution, thereby undermining Mary Dendy's insistence that the feeble-minded could only be productive and self-supporting in an appropriate institutional environment. In 1910, for example, Catherine P. was removed from Sandlebridge by her 'feeble-minded mother'. Two years later, Dendy noted that she had found 'a place' in domestic service.[79] In 1914, Harold M. was also removed by his mother after he had become 'very restless'. He immediately obtained a job as an under-gardener, before enlisting in the army. After the war, he worked as a tram-guard. Disturbed by her brother's removal, Harold's sister, Elsie, was also discharged from Sandlebridge in 1914 and obtained work as a servant.[80] Similarly, Andrew, Charles, and Robert W., admitted together from Harpurhey Hall Special School in Manchester in 1905, all succeeded in escaping from Sandlebridge to find work.[81] And in 1917, Harry H. was formally discharged after he had run away from the Colony and enlisted in the army. Some years later, Dendy noted that Harry was looking after animals as 'an attendant at Belle Vue'.[82]

Although Mary Dendy occasionally acknowledged the possibility that some of her 'little dullards'[83] might 'do fairly well'[84] beyond the boundaries of an institution, she generally regarded attempts to escape, efforts to remove defective children and adults from Sandlebridge, and employment outside the Colony not as evidence of successful development into competent adulthood but as proof of the troublesome, defective, and defiant nature of the feeble-minded and their families. Her private and public commitment to preventing the feeble-minded from leaving Sandlebridge, even (or perhaps particularly) if they had developed into productive adults, provided in part the inspiration for the Mental Deficiency Act of 1913, which authorised the certification of adults on the borderland of imbecility for the first time.[85]

Fashioned ostensibly in the name of humanity but manifestly opposed to notions of liberty, Edwardian constructions of the feeble-minded as permanent children and their compulsory segregation in rural colonies constituted a critical contribution to contemporary notions of health and deficiency. At one level, prominent perceptions of the feeble-minded child as a potential 'plague-spot upon the face of the earth'[86] facilitated the sacrifice of individual liberties in the interests of national health and imperial wealth. At a more intimate level, pessimistic assessments of the burden of arrested development, and conflation of the feeble-minded with criminals, paupers, and prostitutes ensured that many of the children admitted to Sandlebridge in the early decades of the twentieth century remained there for many years, trapped both literally and metaphorically in a borderland between childhood and adulthood, sometimes until they died.[87]

Acknowledgements

I would like to thank the Wellcome Trust for funding the research on which this chapter is based, and Hilary and Marijke for their comments on earlier drafts.

Notes

1. Mary Dendy, 'On the Training and Management of Feeble-Minded Children', in C. Paget Lapage, *Feeblemindedness in Children of School-Age* (Manchester: Manchester University Press, 1911), Appendix, 293.

2. *First Annual Report of Scott House* (1893), a copy of which is in the Local Studies Unit, Central Library, Manchester, M50/5/7/3, 2.

3. Anon., 'The Borderland of Imbecility', *British Medical Journal*, ii (1 December 1894), 1264.

4. *Ibid.*

5. References to 'the borderland' and to 'borderline' cases of deficiency appeared elsewhere around the turn of the century. See, for example: *Lancet*, i (18 June 1898), 1703; 'Dr Ashby's Report of the Manchester Special Schools', in *City of Manchester Education Committee Report, 1903-4*, Appendix 0, 122, located in the Local Studies Unit, Central Library, Manchester, classmark 379.1 M3; Mary Dendy, *Feeble-Minded Children* (Manchester, 1902), 4.

6. P. Martin Duncan and William Millard, *A Manual for the Classification, Training and Education of the Feeble-Minded, Imbecile, and Idiotic* (London: Longmans, Green, and Co., 1866), 12–13, 41–8.

7. *Report of the Departmental Committee on Defective and Epileptic Children* (C. 8746, London, 1898); Elementary Education (Defective and Epileptic Children) Act, 1899, 62 & 63 Vict. c. 32.

8. Mary Dendy, *The Problem of the Feeble-Minded* (Manchester, 1910), 6. Dendy was the most ardent advocate of permanent institutional care for the feeble-minded in the Edwardian period, and the driving force behind the establishment of the Sandlebridge Boarding Schools and Colony in Cheshire in 1902.

9. In 1874, in a chapter entitled 'The Borderland', the prominent physician Henry Maudsley referred to a miscellany of conditions (such as epilepsy, neuralgia, chorea, and dipsomania) that occupied 'a borderland between sanity and insanity': Henry Maudsley,

Responsibility in Mental Disease (London: Henry S. King and Co., 1874), 38–45. See also James H. Hyslop, *Borderland of Psychical Research* (London: G. P. Putnam's Sons, 1906); Sir William Richard Gowers, *The Border-Land of Epilepsy: Faints, Vagal Attacks, Vertigo, Migraine, Sleep Symptoms and Their Treatment* (London: J. and A. Churchill, 1907).

10. Maudsley, for example, referred to the 'borderland between crime and insanity': *idem, op. cit.* (note 9), 34. And J.B. Thomson, the resident surgeon at Perth prison in Scotland, described the criminal populations as lying on the 'borderland of Lunacy': J.B. Thomson, 'The Hereditary Nature of Crime', *Journal of Mental Science*, 15 (1870), 487–98: 487. Some years later, George Shuttleworth referred to the 'borderland class of mentally feeble deaf-mutes or deaf imbeciles': G.E. Shuttleworth, 'On the Treatment of Children Mentally Deficient', *Union of Teachers of the Deaf on the Pure Oral System: Transactions of the Society*, 2 (December 1895), 14. And in 1908, Alfred Tredgold, one of the leading Edwardian writers on mental deficiency, described 'insane aments' as occupying a 'borderland between this condition [mental deficiency] and insanity': A.F. Tredgold, *Mental Deficiency (Amentia)* (London: Baillière, Tindall and Cox, 1908), 312.

11. The phrase used by Dendy, *op. cit.* (note 1), 295.

12. For discussion of the history of evolutionism and notions of progress in the Victorian period, see Peter J. Bowler, *Evolution: The History of an Idea* (Berkeley: University of California Press, 1989); *idem, The Invention of Progress: The Victorians and the Past* (Oxford: Basil Blackwell, 1989).

13. See George F. Still, 'The Goulstonian Lectures on Some Abnormal Psychical Conditions in Children', *Lancet*, i (12 April 1902), 1008-12: 1008; Guy M. Campbell, 'Mental and Physical Development', *Journal of State Medicine*, 16 (1908), 617–22: 618. Significantly, surveys and discussions of abnormal development frequently started with an account of healthy infant growth. See Francis Warner, 'Abstract of the Milroy Lectures on an Inquiry as to the Physical and Mental Condition of School Children', *Lancet*, i (12 March 1892), 567–8; *idem*, 'Neural and Mental Disorder in Children', in William A. Edwards (ed.), *Cyclopaedia of the Diseases of Children Medical and Surgical* (London: Thomas Lewin and Co., 1899), 1304–16.

14. See, for example, Carolyn Steedman, *Strange Dislocations: Childhood and the Idea of Human Interiority 1780-1930* (London: Virago Press, 1995).

15. The term 'medico-pedagogic' was a frequent catch-phrase in late

Victorian and Edwardian school medicine and education circles. See
G.E. Shuttleworth, 'Mental Deficiency', in Chalmers Watson (ed.),
Encyclopaedia Medica (Edinburgh: William Green and Sons, 1901),
28–40: 39; John Arrowsmith, 'Medico-Pedagogical Methods in
Primary School Education', *Journal of State Medicine*, 22 (1914),
430–4.

16. See Arrowsmith, *op. cit.* (note 15); Campbell, *op. cit.* (note 13).

17. Shuttleworth, *op. cit.* (note 10), 6.

18. Lyubov Gennadyevna Gurjeva, 'Everyday Bourgeois Science: The
    Scientific Management of Children in Britain, 1880-1914'
    (unpublished PhD thesis, Cambridge, 1998), and Gurjeva's essay in
    this volume. See also William Ll. Parry-Jones, 'The History of Child
    and Adolescent Psychiatry: Its Present Day Relevance', *Journal of
    Child Psychology and Psychiatry*, 30 (1989), 3–11. The trend towards
    detailed scientific study of school children is exemplified by Dr
    Francis Warner's investigations during the 1880s and 1890s.
    Warner's studies were explicitly aimed at determining 'the average
    development and condition of brain-power among the children in
    primary schools': Francis Warner, 'Scientific Study of the Mental and
    Physical Conditions of Childhood', in Edwards (ed.), *Cyclopaedia of
    the Diseases of Children*, 122–34: 122.

19. See Peter J. Bowler, *The Non-Darwinian Revolution: Reinterpreting a
    Historical Myth* (Baltimore: Johns Hopkins University Press, 1988),
    6–13; Gurjeva, *op. cit.* (note 18), 189.

20. See Steedman, *op. cit.* (note 14), 12.

21. Hastings Gilford, 'Defective Growth and Development in Infancy,
    Childhood and Youth', in T.N. Kelynack (ed.), *Defective Children*
    (London: John Bale, Sons and Danielsson, 1915), 280–1. Gilford
    was medical officer to Leighton Park School, and Hunterian
    Professor at the Royal College of Surgeons.

22. These arguments were, of course, critical to the construction and
    maintenance of hierarchies according to race, class, and gender.

23. For an example of this dualistic approach to childhood diseases, see
    G.F. Still, *Common Disorders and Diseases of Childhood* (London:
    Hodder and Stoughton, 1909), which contains a discussion of
    normal development before turning to abnormalities and defects of
    development.

24. For a brief account of the history of developmental medicine, see
    Sheila J. Wallace, 'The Evolution of Developmental Medicine', in
    John Cule and Terry Turner (eds), *Child Care Through the Centuries*
    (Cardiff: British Society for the History of Medicine, 1986),
    80–107.

25. Maudsley, *op. cit.* (note 9), 31.

26. Shuttleworth, *op. cit.* (note 10), 7. In 1884, in his more general work on childhood diseases, Charles West had also quoted Seguin in his discussion of the delayed bodily and mental development of backward children: Charles West, *Lectures on the Diseases of Infancy and Childhood* (London: Longmans, Green, and Co., 1884), 288–9.

27. Tredgold, *op. cit.* (note 10), 56. See also: Lapage, *op. cit.* (note 1), 195; A.F. Tredgold, 'The Feeble-Minded', *Contemporary Review*, 97 (1910), 717–27: 718; *idem*, 'Mentally Defective Children', in T.N. Kelynack (ed.), *Medical Examinations of Schools and Scholars* (London: P. S. King and Son, 1910), 201–17: 205.

28. For further discussion, see Mark Jackson, 'Images of Deviance: Visual Representations of Mental Defectives in Early Twentieth-Century Medical Texts', *British Journal for the History of Science*, 28 (1995), 319–37.

29. W.A. Potts, 'The Problem of the Morally Defective', *Lancet*, ii (29 October 1904), 1210–11: 1210.

30. *Report of the Royal Commission on the Care and Control of the Feeble-Minded* (Cd. 4202, London, 1908); Mental Deficiency Act, 1913, 3 & 4 Geo. 5 c. 28; Elementary Education (Defective and Epileptic Children) Act, 1914, 4 & 5 Geo. 5 c. 45.

31. According to Dendy, 'the one defect most generally common to feeble-minded persons is great weakness of will power': Dendy, *op. cit.* (note 5), 2.

32. Mathew Thomson, *The Problem of Mental Deficiency: Eugenics, Democracy, and Social Policy in Britain, c.1870-1959* (Oxford: Clarendon Press, 1998).

33. Tredgold, *op. cit.* (note 27), 216. This rhetoric persisted on both sides of the Atlantic. Some years later, Mary Carpenter suggested that 'they are rightly termed "children" - and the majority of them forever remain so': Mary S. Carpenter, *A Study of the Occupations of 207 Subnormal Girls After Leaving Schoool* (Ann Arbor: University of Michigan School of Education, 1925), 9.

34. See, for example, the discussion in Manchester and Salford Sanitary Association, *Proceedings at a Conference on the Care of the Feeble-Minded* (London: Sherratt and Hughes, 1911).

35. For further discussion, see Mark Jackson, *The Borderland of Imbecility: Medicine, Society and the Fabrication of the Feeble Mind in Late Victorian and Edwardian England* (Manchester: Manchester University Press, 2000), 129–64.

36. See Shuttleworth, *op. cit.* (note 15), 29, 32–3; Tredgold, *op. cit.* (note 10), 72; G.E. Shuttleworth and W.A. Potts, *Mentally Deficient*

Children: Their Treatment and Training (London: H. K. Lewis and Co., 1916), 52, 64–5.

37. Fletcher Beach, 'Education of the Mind', in Watson (ed.), *op. cit.* (note 15), 110; Shuttleworth, *op. cit.* (note 15), 47; Shuttleworth and Potts, *op. cit.* (note 36), 186.

38. Dendy, *op. cit.* (note 1), 271–4. See also Jackson, *op. cit.* (note 35), 165–202.

39. A.F. Tredgold, 'The Problem of the Feeble-Minded', in Manchester and Salford Sanitary Association, *Proceedings at a Conference*, 6. See also Lapage, *op. cit.* (note 1), 154.

40. Mary Dendy, 'The Care of the Feeble-Minded', in Manchester and Salford Sanitary Association, *Proceedings at a Conference*, 44.

41. *Ibid.*, 55.

42. J.Langdon H. Down, 'Observations on an Ethnic Classification of Idiots', first published in *Lectures and Reports from the London Hospital for 1866*, reproduced in C. Thompson (ed.), *The Origins of Modern Psychiatry* (Chichester: John Wiley and Sons, 1987), 15–23.

43. G.E. Shuttleworth, 'Clinical Lecture on Idiocy and Imbecility', *British Medical Journal*, i (30 January 1886), 183–6: 185. See also Shuttleworth's comment that 'the whole bodily structure [of 'mongols'] points to a lack of finish', in a paper entitled 'On Mental Deficiency in Children', 14, handwritten notes for which are in the Western Manuscripts Department, Wellcome Institute for the History of Medicine, MS 4584.

44. *Lancet*, ii (20 November 1909), 1501. See also Gilford's assertion that 'mongolism' constituted 'a state of permanent infantilism': Gilford, *op. cit.* (note 21), 284.

45. Tredgold, *op. cit.* (note 10), 290.

46. *Ibid.*, 290.

47. Dendy made this point to Francis Galton in 1909 - see the letter dated 16/2/1909 in The Papers and Correspondence of Sir Francis Galton, UCL Library, 138/8. See also Dendy, *op. cit.* (note 8), 7.

48. J.J. Cox, 'Some Fundamental Points in Preventive Medicine Bearing upon the Question of Physical Deterioration in Children', *Journal of State Medicine*, 16 (1908), 641–54: 649. Cox was Dendy's co-secretary at the Lancashire and Cheshire Society for the Permanent Care of the Feeble-Minded.

49. See, for example Elizabeth Fee, 'Nineteenth-Century Craniology: The Study of the Female Skull', *Bulletin of the History of Medicine*, 53 (1979), 415–33; Nancy Leys Stepan, 'Race and Gender: The Role of Analogy in Science', *ISIS*, 77 (1986), 261–77.

50. For further discussion, see Jackson, *op. cit.* (note 35).

51. Tredgold, *op. cit.* (note 39), 17.

52. Bowler, *The Invention of Progress, op. cit.* (note 12), 192-201.

53. A.M. Paterson, 'The Child as an Asset of the Empire', *Liverpool Medico-Chirurgical Journal,* 31 (1911), 235–53.

54. See, for example, Sir John Byers, 'The Hygiene of Childhood', *Medical Magazine,* 20 (1911), 507–10.

55. Robert R. Rentoul, 'Proposed Sterilization of Certain Mental Degenerates', *American Journal of Sociology,* 12 (1906-7), 319–27: 327. Rentoul was a medical practitioner in Liverpool.

56. According to William Potts, investigators in Glasgow had been so disturbed at the level of physical and mental defect in school children that they had asked, 'Are there any healthy children left?': see W.A. Potts, 'Causation of Mental Defect in Children', *British Medical Journal,* ii (14 October 1905), 946–8: 948.

57. Sir James Barr, 'Address to the Section of Child Study and Eugenics at the Dublin Congress', *Journal of State Medicine,* 19 (1911), 705–19: 717. See also Barr's claim that 'there is still plenty of virility left in this country, and if we could only encourage its evolution and arrest the decadence which is seen on every hand, the nation might renew its youth': Sir James Barr, 'The Aim and Scope of Eugenics', *Liverpool Medico-Chirurgical Journal,* 31 (1911), 215–35: 229.

58. C.T. Ewart, 'Eugenics and Degeneracy', *Journal of Mental Science,* 56 (1910), 672–3.

59. Karl Pearson, *The Problem of Practical Eugenics* (London: Dulau and Co., 1909), 8–9.

60. *Ibid.,* 20–1.

61. *Ibid.,* 19.

62. *Ibid.,* 3.

63. Barr, 'The Aim and Scope of Eugenics', *op. cit.* (note 57), 230.

64. *Ibid.,* 222.

65. Pearson, *op. cit.* (note 59), 22–3.

66. *Annual Report of the Chief Medical Officer of the Board of Education, 1908* (Cd. 4986, London, 1910), 141.

67. Rentoul, *op. cit.* (note 55), 320.

68. Tredgold, *op. cit.* (note 10), 138.

69. *Ibid.,* 148.

70. Tredgold, 'The Feeble-Minded', *op. cit.* (note 27), 723.

71. Tredgold, *op. cit.* (note 10), 149.

72. *Ibid.,* 150. See also William C. Sullivan, 'Criminal Children', in Kelynack (ed.), *op. cit.* (note 21), 81–97: 84.

73. Tredgold, *op. cit.* (note 10), 149–50. See also Mary Dendy's comments on the necessary link between feeble-minded children and

subsequent pauperism and criminality: Mary Dendy, *Feebleness of Mind, Pauperism and Crime* (Glasgow: Glasgow Provisional Committee for the Permanent Care of the Feeble-Minded, 1901), 5.

74. Details are in the Sandlebridge Special Schools Album, in Cheshire Record Office, CRO NHM 11/3837/43. Sandlebridge was opened by the Lancashire and Cheshire Society for the Permanent Care of the Feeble-Minded in 1902.

75. Compare the cases of John E., Edith S., and George J. (who were all referred to as good workers and retained), with those of Edith W., Frank B., and Tom K. (who were released after a probationary period), in Sandlebridge Special Schools Album, CRO NHM 11/3837/43, 3, 18, 49, and 9, 11, 12. In 1914, Dendy proudly pointed out that although there were 'some very bad cases' at Sandlebridge, 'we have them all at work except one boy': Mary Dendy, 'Feeble-Minded Children', *Journal of State Medicine*, 22 (1914), 412–8: 417.

76. Sandlebridge Special Schools Album, CRO NHM 11/3837/43, 8. In 1908, Dendy noted, perhaps with some satisfaction, that Harry was '*not* [sic] at work'.

77. *Ibid.*, 7.

78. Dendy, *op. cit.* (note 75), 416.

79. Sandlebridge Special Schools Album, CRO NHM 11/3837/43, 10.

80. *Ibid.*, 45–6.

81. *Ibid.*, 55–6.

82. *Ibid.*, 66.

83. Dendy, *op. cit.* (note 5), 14.

84. Dendy's comment in Sandlebridge Special Schools Album, CRO NHM 11/3837/43, 59.

85. See Jackson, *op. cit.* (note 35); Thomson, *op. cit.* (note 32).

86. Dendy, *op. cit.* (note 1), 293.

87. See, for example, Lily F., who was admitted to Sandlebridge in 1902 and who was eventually discharged by order of the Board of Control only in 1947: Sandlebridge Special Schools Album, CRO NHM 11/3837/43, 19. For examples of people staying in the Colony until they died, see Day School Admission Register, CRO NHM 11/3837/42; Register of Admissions, CRO NHM 11/3837/48.

8

Mulock Houwer's 'Education for Responsibility': A Chapter from the Dutch History of Institutional Upbringing

Ido Weijers

D.Q.R. Mulock Houwer (1903-85) was for decades a key figure in child protection in the Netherlands, a demanding and critical public speaker. Although never identified with the child protection establishment - indeed he identified more with the rebels and avant-garde - his career presents a fascinating variation of the 'rags to riches' story. Mulock Houwer was born and grew up in Antwerp. His father died when he was only six years old. At eleven his mother placed him in an old-fashioned and very strict French-speaking boarding school. Three years later his mother died, after which he drifted from one distant relative to another. Eventually, his family on his father's side took him to *Maatschappij Zandbergen* in Amersfoort. He ran away from this institution twice, after which he stayed with several foster families. Nine years later, in 1926, on the invitation of his old headmaster, W.A. Ortt, he became a group leader at the same institution. After four years as deputy head and then head of the boys assessment centre (*Observatiehuis*) in Vosmaerstraat, Amsterdam, in 1933 Mulock Houwer succeeded Ortt as headmaster of *Zandbergen*. During the occupation, he spent three years in German concentration camps. After the war he became the first director of the newly formed National Child Protection Service and in 1957 he was appointed Secretary-General to the *Union Internationale de Protection de l'Enfance* in Geneva.

The first aim of this article will be to place Mulock Houwer's ideas on mental health and institutional upbringing into the context of debates surrounding the operation of the Children's Acts from the late 1920s to the late 1930s. Throughout this period, Houwer was formulating a number of ideas on education and upbringing as a critical response to contemporary practices in the world of re-education. These ideas, which stayed with him for the rest of his life, can be summarised in his own words, as *'verantwoordelijk-*

heidspedagogiek' (education for responsibility).

The second aim will be to concentrate on Houwer's ideas relating to the bringing up of children in institutions. These ideas were first expressed in papers submitted to the new journals on child protection and were later developed in his classic *Gestichtspaedagogische hoofdstukken* of 1938. In these pre-war years Houwer's main inspiration seems to have come from three very different intellectual movements, pragmatism, psychoanalysis and personalism. After reflecting on these three sources of inspiration, and analysing his most influential publications, I will show how Mulock Houwer linked these different insights in his own approach to institutional upbringing.

The introduction of the Children's Acts in 1905 is generally seen as the beginning of modern child protection. In fact, they were a result of philanthropic initiatives taken in the second half of the nineteenth century. These initiatives, particularily the creation of juvenile institutions,[1] signified the outcome of two major paradigmatic revolutions, in the field of law, especially criminal law, and in the field of social policy. The Children's Acts demonstrated both the power of the philanthropic movement and a victory for the Modernist School in criminal law. In turn this meant a victory for those who supported active state intervention in the social field.

'Improving the neglected child and the child offender' was the joint motto of these different movements. However, anyone who studies the many debates and the astonishing number of articles, dissertations, books, pamphlets and reports on this subject, hoping to find more precise educational ideas, soon comes up against the fact that hardly any practical ideas about how to tackle protecting and improving these children were developed. Everybody wanted to educate problem children, they wanted the children to learn discipline, while at the same time pushing back the prison-like approach, and they hoped that the pupils could learn a trade, but that was as far as it went. There was no clear picture drawn of the educational objectives or the educational conditions and resources needed for re-educating these children.[2]

The Children's Acts were based, purely and simply, on a 'needs' discourse in which neglected and delinquent children needed to be taken out of their family and placed in special care in institutions or foster families. In the 1930s, this needs discourse slowly became more sophisticated, paralleling the first steps in the direction of professionalisation of the work and the people working in this field. This change can be identified as a process of 'psychologisation' or 'individualisation' of the problem, the neglected and the delinquent child.

Apart from scattered initiatives elsewhere,[3] the *Observatiehuis* in Amsterdam, instituted in 1914, played a crucial role in this innovation process.[4] It was here, in the period of Mulock Houwer's (vice-) directorship, that pioneers like the child psychiatrist Frits Grewel, the psychologist Jan Koekebakker, and the first juvenile court judge of Amsterdam G. de Jong met and discussed new methods and international literature. Mulock Houwer developed his ideas in close co-operation with the first two of these men in particular. Grewel was head of the out-patient clinic of the *Wilhelmina Gasthuis* Psychiatric Hospital in Amsterdam. In 1955, he became a lecturer in child psychiatry and ten years later Professor in Special Education at the University of Amsterdam. Koekebakker was the first civil servant with an academic training in this field. In 1947, he became a lecturer and in 1950 Professor in Group Psychology at the University of Leiden. All three men published innovative and influential books between 1937 and 1941 (Grewel in 1937, Mulock in 1939 and again two years later, in 1941, Koekebakker) and to a large extent these publications resulted from the intensive exchange of their ideas.[5] They saw themselves as a kind of 'rebels club', seeking confrontation with the older establishment in child protection.[6] This 'rebels club' took the educational mission of the Children's Acts seriously. Their work has to be seen as both a sophisticated and psychological interpretation of the needs discourse. They focused on the individual child, whose personal needs were to stand at the centre of their attention.

It is fascinating that this same psychological and individualising discourse prepared the transition that took place at the beginning of the 1970s. At that time, a new stream of criticism emerged in the field of child protection and institutional re-education in particular. Far from being pushed aside by the new wave of radicalism, the psychological and individualising discourse of this older generation of rebels inspired the ideas and initiatives of the counter-movement. It was this individualising needs discourse that in turn brought forth or at least enhanced the new child rights discourse. Thus the counter-movement in Dutch child protection in the 1970s can be seen as another example of the 'legacy of a tolerant educative culture' in the post-war Netherlands.[7]

•

Criticism and alternatives

Around 1900, a 'world of re-education' began to develop in the Netherlands.[8] This world became visible in three ways. First, through the rapid proliferation of publicly-funded but privately-run institutions and their populations. There was a constantly growing need for places for children under 18. Since the Children's Acts, 1,500 to 3,000 children per annum required places either in an institution or a foster family. These were children whose parents had been divested of authority, or who were orphans or informally received children.[9] Whether responding to or creating this increasing need, in 1907 there were 60 private institutions, while ten years later there were already over 300, housing more than 20,000 children.[10] Secondly, a number of influential child protection societies emerged - *Pro Juventute* was founded in 1896, the *Nederlansche Bond van Kinderbescherming* (Dutch Association for Child Protection) was founded in 1899 and they were followed by their denominational counterparts and a guardianship system.[11] Thirdly, special forums for publications began to appear, the *Tijdschrift voor armenzorg en kinderbescherming* (Journal for poor relief and child protection, 1900) followed by the *Maandblad voor berechting en reclassering van volwassenen en kinderen* (Monthly Journal for the trial and rehabilitation of adults and children, 1922) alongside the authoritative and more general *Tijdschrift voor Strafrecht* (Journal of Penal Law, 1886).

Most of those involved saw their efforts as part of a triumphal march for the protection of neglected and criminal children, convinced as they were of the successes achieved since the introduction of the Children's Acts. In particular, those running the many private, denominational, but publicly-funded institutions, were convinced that what was needed was a steady expansion of re-education, since the fundamentals were in place. Nevertheless, dissenting voices, criticism, and doubts were to be heard centring on the lack of an adequate educational basis for the work being done with problem children.[12] Though several of the people who expressed criticisms knew the world of re-education from the inside, they had not been able to adjust the course plotted in 1901 and becoming operative four years later. In particular, they had not been able to initiate a thorough review of the educational theories behind re-education.

Mulock Houwer was among these critics of the late 1920s. His series of short articles on self-government prompted some of the most interesting discussions on the purpose and nature of re-education. From his institutional experience as pupil, group leader, member of staff and principal, he held up re-education practice against the light of its educational pretensions. In 1928, two years after he had become leader of a very diverse group of about 25 children at *Zandbergen*, Houwer described how, on a quiet winter evening, in response to a comment by one of the boys on 'our own laws', he suggested the idea of 'self-government'. The boys immediately took this seriously and responded with enthusiasm. Fascinated by their great alacrity and application, he outlined how they went about giving substance to this idea and developing it over the following days and weeks. He returned to this subject in a number of articles a year later. His underlying assumption was that neglected and offending adolescents needed some form of personal responsibility. Self-government offered the best opportunities for this and also had a positive effect on relationships and interaction within the group. At issue here, in his view, was 'education to take responsibility, demanding above all that the pupils exercise responsibility themselves... self-government is probably not a very good word, it should be called: education for co-responsibility'.[13]

He used self-government as a psychological experiment and as a vehicle with which he could voice positively his dissatisfaction with the way children in institutions were educated and brought up. He believed in the children in institutions and in their ability to change and develop, provided the people looking after them approached them with love, trust and adequate psychological knowledge and understanding. He contrasted these ideas with what he saw as unsatisfactory, short-sighted routines in re-education. This becomes clear in his handling of a number of issues familiar to institutions, namely, bed-wetting, the role of women in boys' institutions and the use of punishment.

The problem of bed-wetters, which all institutions continually faced, was completely misunderstood by the staff of institutions, according to Mulock Houwer. The usual approach was hard-handed: public washing of bed linen, making the child walk round with the wet sheets on his back, or making the child wear a sign. In his view, such actions were 'educational monstrosities'.[14] He argued that the underlying assumption of the carer should be that this problem caused distress to the child, distress that was made much worse by living in a group. Houwer suggested that the staff of the institution should first adopt the role of helper in order to win the child's trust. Neither punishment nor rewards were important, he argued, as at best they could only bring about a temporary improvement. Real improvement could only be achieved through a relationship of trust between pupil and carer and so institutional upbringing needed to offer explicit individual guidance. He wrote, 'A group must never be left to its own devices when it comes to expressing itself *vis-à-vis* an individual pupil. Without guidance in the background, the group can be inhumanly cruel.'[15]

From his views on the issues of women and punishment, an even stronger psychological perspective emerges. Regarding the issue of the role of women in boys' homes, Houwer again began by criticising the customary situation. He pointed out that, while the woman's role in bringing up children in the family was absolutely central, in institutional settings women had hardly any role at all.[16] Houwer felt that this situation was a consequence of the lack of educational considerations in existing forms of institution. In his opinion, the woman 'is better able to manage the inner structure of the child and the group ethos. The important question is whether the adolescent of all people... does not have all the more need of a woman's care, since she is better able to empathise with his feelings and difficulties than a man. To put it more succinctly: can a pupil in a home do without women in his life without being harmed.'[17]

This issue brought him to the theme of the bond between carer and pupil, which he considered crucial if re-education was to have any chance of success. He found the emphasis in boys' homes to be on speaking, preaching, and reprimands, whereas he believed that re-education was ultimately rooted in the emotional life and the personal relationship of trust between child and carer.[18] He felt that in this regard, institutional education and upbringing had generally made the mistake of learning hardly anything from psychoanalytical insights about the causes and treatment of problem behaviour. He argued that institutional upbringing was concerned with character development, moral education, education for responsibility and education to be a member of a community. It was clear 'that an uprooted child can only internalise norms and values if he can be brought to accept that they [can be made] better through a close relationship.'[19] The education for responsibility that he championed required feelings to be put at the heart of things and acted upon to benefit the emotional and moral development of the child. This could only happen by developing personal relationships

For Houwer, a close relationship along the lines of the psychoanalytical transference model was an important supplement and qualification to the concept of self-government. He elaborated on this in his discussion of the possible use of punishment, which he said was the 'most difficult' problem of institutional education and upbringing. 'Only where there is a close relationship can pain be suffered, which itself can lead to the desired improvement or rehabilitation.'[20] Against the idea of punishment as an instrument to break the stubborn will of a wicked child, that dominated all notions of education not oriented on the individual, he set the goal of appealing to the sense of guilt. He proposed that punishment should be used to appeal to the child's conscience and thus, he argued, the drive to self-control and restitution of guilt would be encouraged. He emphasised that the clear aim of punishment should always be to reinforce a sense of responsibility. 'The criterion must always be that the child will ultimately be able to acknowledge that the punishment given was justified.'[21] He asserted that punishment should never be meted out mechanically and that (lengthy) isolation punishments were completely wrong. In both cases, he pointed out, these methods were likely to be counter-productive because without intensive involvement and an appeal to the relationship that was at stake, they lacked the element that was so essential to punishment. Finally, from his critique of contemporary practice of frequent routine punishments in institutions, he concluded that punishment required the full input of the carer.

These educational insights illustrate the three most important sources of inspiration for Mulock Houwer. He developed the principle of self-government after long reflection on William George's approach. The idea that children in institutions primarily need love and a personal bond with their carer was inspired by the work of August Aichhorn, while the concept that (re-)education must ultimately come down to moral education had its origins in the ideas of Philip Kohnstamm. We will now analyse these sources of inspiration in more detail, after which the question of how and to what extent Mulock Houwer succeeded in linking these three important but different educational approaches will be addressed.

Self-government

At the beginning of the twentieth century, William 'Daddy' George and Fred Nelles pioneered the new style of re-education in the United States.[22] George founded his experimental Reform School based on a unique combination of modern ideas about education and upbringing and conservative economic principles. This earned him many admirers both in the United States and elsewhere in the Western world. The key to the organisational set-up of the Junior

Republic was inmate self-government. The pupils' daily lives were regulated in the main by their fellow pupils. Pupils were elected to posts such as president, senator and congressman. They sat on the management board, in 'parliament', and took up various other positions of responsibility in the school.

The young Mulock Houwer was very attracted by the idea of an institution being run as far as possible as a little society which had as much as possible in common with what went on outside. This could act as a copy of the outside world where people could learn and practise desirable behaviour. It also implied co-education, a principle that Houwer supported from the outset. William George's educational objectives were clearly derived from the concept of democratic education, as advanced from the end of the nineteenth century by the prophet of progressive education, John Dewey. Dewey, the philosopher of the pragmatic school, saw education and upbringing primarily as a social process. The key to this process was the child's practical experiences and constant reflection on those experiences. Experience was a fundamental concept of Dewey's philosophy of education. On the one hand, the child learned to know himself through his experiences in relation to his social surroundings whilst, on the other hand, he learned about the world in relation to himself. In Dewey's eyes, education was not so much about disseminating and transferring high moral ideas, norms and values, but about allowing the child to gain moral, practical experiences that related to his activities, abilities and interests. For Dewey, democratic living, in the family, at school and in various social groups was the starting point for educating children to become citizens in a democracy.[23] Through his involvement with Hull House, founded and run by Jane Addams, and as Professor of Philosophy, Psychology and Education at the University of Chicago, he set up the Laboratorium School in 1896. This gave him a concrete, practical outlet for his ideas.

George tried to apply Dewey's pragmatic line of reasoning directly in his Reform School, by setting it up as a democratic society in miniature. The intention was that practical experiences would prove to be a much more efficient way of educating juvenile delinquents to become good citizens than the route of social isolation, in which edifying lessons and admonitions were used to put the boys on the right track. Underlying the Junior Republic was the moral principle of 'nothing without labour', or 'earning your own keep'. In George's model of self-government, work and wages from work were seen as the basis of citizenship.

Tolerance

Mulock Houwer was fascinated by George's approach from the outset and at *Zandbergen* he had the opportunity to experiment with forms of self-government. However, he also had reservations about the model. One of the sources feeding his reservations was the re-education work of August Aichhorn. His practical and theoretical example was dominated by an entirely different way of thinking. An Austrian, Aichhorn had founded the *Oberhollabrun* children's home in 1918 with a number of like-minded people and had tried to apply psychoanalytical ideas to the work. Aichhorn came to international attention in 1925 with his collection of lectures *Verwahrloste Jugend* at exactly the time Mulock Houwer was starting work in the field and looking for inspirational examples.

Aichhorn's general diagnostic principle was that all maladjusted behaviour on the part of young people should be seen as a symptom of inadequate inner development, resulting from lack of love in early childhood. Maladjusted behaviour, varying from truancy and wandering the streets to stealing and burglary, were seen by him as symptoms of neglect. 'Neglect' was characterised by 'a limited capacity to suppress fits of anger and to divert the child from primitive purposes, and also the limited influence of moral standards prevailing in the community'. 'Problematic behaviour concealed a general problem', an unfulfilled longing for tenderness in the youth. We see a heightened need for gratification, primitive uninhibited release of anger, and a hidden, but all the greater for that, longing for affection.' Following on from this, Aichhorn formulated his general, radical, therapeutic principle. He wrote, 'If we want to abolish neglect, and not only suppress its symptoms, we must first respond to the needs of antisocial people, even when things are a bit wild at first and "sensible" people shake their heads in disapproval'.[24]

Mulock Houwer immediately discovered a kindred spirit in Aichhorn, whose criticism of the standard treatment in the average institution was exceptionally severe. In Aichhorn's view, standard education and upbringing completely ignored what should be at the heart of this work: 'They are educated not through words, exhortations, reprimands or punishment, but through what the pupils themselves experience.'[25] What was needed, therefore, was what he called 'a practical psychology of conciliation'. This chiefly involved two things: 'a pleasant environment for the pupils' and 'being rewarded with love'.[26] Aichhorn's approach applied three insights from psychoanalysis to the practice of re-education: 1) that the essence of neglect is a matter of 'the breakdown of love in early childhood'; 2) the application and translation to this field of what is known in analysis as 'transference'; and 3) the translation of Freud's insights regarding mass psychology into group-work. At the heart of this approach, was the idea that eradicating neglect was ultimately a libidinous problem, in which the emotional relationship between pupil and carer was the most important thing. 'Socialising the neglected child' was only possible if it was based on a strong attachment to someone from his environment.

Houwer was very impressed by Aichhorn's ideas and his interest only increased when in the early 1930s he became Principal at the Amsterdam assessment centre, where he came into contact with Grewel, Koekebakker and other pioneers in the field. One of the most important and forceful ideological weapons in their confrontation with the older establishment in child protection was their contribution to and dissemination of an unorthodox, man-in-the street's psychoanalytical view of difficult youth. They did this at the time mainly by adopting Aichhorn's basic assumptions regarding the general diagnosis - behaviour compensating for lack of love in early childhood - and his core therapeutic principle - understanding and tolerance, which would establish a re-education process by creating a strong, personal relationship based on trust.

Moral education

Immediately, upon beginning his work as group leader of 70 pupils at *Zandbergen* in 1926, Houwer felt the need to gain some relevant knowledge. It was a constant bugbear that most of the group leaders had a very low level of education. To gain an adequate education for himself, he went to Amsterdam each week to attend lectures given by Willem Bonger, the renowned criminologist, and social democrat. He also studied educational theory under Philip Kohnstamm. A prominent social liberal, physicist, theologian, and philosopher, Kohnstamm had been Professor of Educational Theory and Principal to the Amsterdam Public Seminary for Educational Theory since 1919, where many leading Dutch educationalists had been educated.[27] Kohnstamm, who was to guide Mulock Houwer for many years, had a very individual teaching style. All his students, without exception, were influenced by his philosophical world-view, known as personalism.[28] Mulock Houwer was also influenced, as is evident from his views on the use of punishment. Kohnstamm was his third source of inspiration and was entirely different from the two mentioned above. Where the work of both George and Aichhorn inspired Houwer largely at a practical level, the significance of Kohnstamm's educational theory lay in the way it inspired his thinking about the purpose of re-education.

Kohnstamm set his personalism against idealism;[29] his basic assumption was the idea of an I-Thou relationship between an individual and his own personal source of faith. Idealism hoped to persuade individuals to conform more or less to a generally prevailing ideal. Kohnstamm proposed that individuals should develop their diverse and unique personalities. In his inaugural speech, he summarised his personalism thus, 'Differentiation is the watchword'.[30] This led him to the educational principle of guarding against coercion and 'drumming things in' in either an intellectual or a moral sense. He wrote, 'Just leave the children to come to their own conclusions, the less people try to force "morality" upon them the better, so long as they have really lived through the personal side of the story'.[31] According to Kohnstamm, the issue, around which all education revolved, was the development of conscience. He postulated that no matter how a moral decision turns out, it is always taken with the engagement of the whole personality and is entirely concrete and individual. In his principal work on education, *Persoonlijkheid in wording*, he expressed it as '"Here I am, I cannot do otherwise" is what characterises all decisions of conscience. Anyone who "can also do otherwise", is acting arbitrarily, not following his conscience... That is what is so wonderful about this decision, that the individual personality is never so tied and never so free.'[32]

In Kohnstamm, Houwer immediately found another kindred spirit. He agreed with Kohnstamm that the role of the teacher was to develop, without pedantry, both the child's unique personality and a fully-developed conscience. Houwer also shared Kohnstamm's rejection of all forms of conformity. While Houwer was writing his dissertation on self-government for Kohnstamm, his teacher was working on his opus magnum, *Persoonlijkheid in wording* (The developing personality, 1929). In this work, the goal of educating children along typically Pestalozzian-personalist lines was identified as 'helping the growing person to find inner peace'.[33]

Clearly, this kind of educational objective in the re-education context was leading in an entirely different direction from that envisaged by reformers when the Children's Acts came into force. 'Inner peace', as a general aim of education in which the most important point is not to act against the voice of the individual conscience, was diametrically opposed to their basic assumption of protecting children and society. In this context, the problem child

179

was to be kept away from his family for as long as possible. In Kohnstamm's view of things, only minimal account was to be taken of the demands of the community in formulating educational goals. He said, 'Education is helping a developing person to find the deepest inner peace that he can find without being a burden or nuisance to others'.³⁴ In direct opposition to the views of those driving forces behind the Children's Acts, any form of determinism was taboo. On the contrary, notions of individual responsibility and personal moral development were at the core. Whilst at this time Mulock Houwer had already joined the child protection movement with independent, even rebellious but probably diffuse ideas, the educational theory of Kohnstamm at least reinforced a certain critical viewpoint and helped him to organise alternative ideas.

Education for responsibility in re-education

Self-government was the subject of Mulock Houwer's first publications, which were expressly grounded in the philosophy of pragmatism. However, as we have seen, there were two other sources of Mulock Houwer's thinking, personalism, represented by Kohnstamm, and the psychoanalytical approach championed by Aichhorn. How can we understand the relationship between these three very different educational approaches? None of the strong emphasis on individual moral development that characterised Kohnstamm's educational thinking is to be found in the pragmatism of Dewey or George, while the notion of moral development had hardly any role in Aichhorn's approach. Pragmatism for its part had no points of contact with the diagnostic and therapeutic insights that Aichhorn had borrowed from psychoanalysis. George's thinking left no room for the assumption about lack of love and where Aichhorn argued for large measures of tolerance from this perspective, George proposed strict discipline. George had no problem with group control and group pressure as controlling forces and Aichhorn wanted to use psychological processes within the group for therapeutic purposes, but both approaches were in opposition to the personalist goal of Kohnstamm. The traditional, liberal principle of productive virtue that underpinned George's approach was at odds with the modern, liberal, contemplative goal of 'inner peace' formulated by Kohnstamm. Finally, where care staff in George's system were in the background, operating merely as 'rule-givers', Aichhorn wanted group leaders to think up ways to intervene in order to develop a strong, personal relationship based on trust with each individual pupil.

Did Mulock Houwer create any relationship between these approaches, or did he simply allow these views to co-exist as partial sources of inspiration for a completely different picture of his own? In conclusion, I would like to show that from the outset Mulock Houwer tried to combine what for him were the most useful elements of these three approaches. This enabled him to formulate a theory of re-education in which, inspired by the ideas of Kohnstamm, the guiding principles were moral education and especially personal development. In Mulock Houwer's view the needs of the individual child should be geared to this.

These principles are relatively easy to demonstrate, as far as the idea of self-government is concerned. Mulock Houwer had always had reservations about the carer staying too much in the background. He felt that the pupils should voluntarily and totally involve the carer as a whole person and that he should be the key figure around which everything revolved. Above all, however, his relativisation of the concept of self-government is apparent from his criticism of self-government being operated as a system of laws, in the George Junior Republic. He believed it should rather be a way of experimenting with responsibility, offered in careful doses under guidance. For him the educational value of self-government lay in the attempt to make something of it, in thinking about it, discussing it and evaluating it together. He translated George's approach into an educational experiment, striving to achieve both positive effects for individual moral development and for the moral development of the group. From the very beginning, the theme of that experiment was moral development or what Houwer called responsibility-based education.

The integration of psychoanalytical ideas was more complicated. This was not so much a matter of explicit but rather implicit relativisation, reformulation and a tacit shift of emphasis. Typical of this, was his use of the neutral term 'relationship' where Aichhorn had deliberately spoken of 'transference'. This allowed for the maintenance of a certain distance from a too overt psychoanalytical inspiration in the area of therapy. It could be seen even more clearly in the field of diagnostics. Mulock Houwer was careful not to make pronouncements to the effect that all manifestations of neglect and problems of upbringing could ultimately be traced back to lack of love in early childhood. He also rejected Aichhorn's extreme tolerance. Control and discipline were not taboo for him, as they were for Aichhorn. For Mulock Houwer, the essential thing was that control and discipline were always guided by the motive of promoting the child's moral development and helping him in his search for 'inner peace'.

He defined his position most clearly in two articles in the early fifties. After explaining the crisis in which institutional education had found itself because of criticism from various quarters of its predominantly disciplinarian ethos, he argued that this 'down' period was merely apparent. In his view, the sense of crisis in the world of institutional education could be interpreted as an atmosphere of 'creative' or 'constructive uneasiness'. This, he believed, would lead to exciting comparison and open consideration of different approaches. He identified a number of approaches in theories of institutional education. The first was the 'disciplinarian system', which was no longer defended anywhere in the professional journals and which he, therefore, left out of the picture. Then he discerned the 'progressive step system', based on the pleasure-pain principle. Next, he examined the 'individual education system', for which the psychoanalytical approach was the model and then the system of 'social-educational upbringing', for which George's approach served as a model. Finally, he considered the 'eclectic education system', where the basic assumption was not a particular form of education and upbringing but the needs of the individual child.

He expressed without reservation his own preference for the eclectic system. It was non-dogmatic and gave priority to the problems of the individual child. He expressed its educational goal in typical Kohnstammian terms as, 'making the child as happy as possible, partly by helping him to achieve the best possible adaptation to normal life that he can'.[35] He acknowledged the strengths of both the individual and the social education system, and, where possible believed that they should be used in approaches to the institutional child, but under no circumstances should the system be determinist. In re-education, he argued, it was not possible to assume a specific, definite picture of the child, and one should not assume a particular ideal image to which all children must conform. For Mulock Houwer just as for Kohnstamm, differentiation was the watchword of education. As for Pestalozzi the choice of education system should be geared to the child, rather than choosing the child to fit in with the education system.

Lifelong critic

By the end of the Second World War, residential child care in the Netherlands had been completely disrupted. Institutions had been taken over by the occupier or destroyed by bombs and at the same time there was an enormous increase in the number of children for whom care needed to be organised as a matter of urgency. There were 4,000 Jewish war orphans and close on 20,000 children of Dutch National Socialists whose parents had been interned and who had been left to their fate. Mulock Houwer and his friends were among the first to point out the pressing problems in the field of child care.[36] This emergency spurred the government into becoming more involved in residential care. Government funding increased tenfold over 20 years, more places were created and more staff taken on.[37] Nevertheless, the local, denominational organisations remained unchanged for a long time and, against that background, planning and the professionalisation of workers was very slow to get off the ground.[38] A major enquiry was set up in 1950 to take stock of the situation in the institutions and its report was ready two years later. The conclusions were devastating, which is probably why the report was not published until 1957.[39]

Mulock Houwer was one of the key figures in this research team, which was led by his friend, the psychologist Koekebakker, and he was one of the authors of the report. The report's main criticism voiced his typical view that there was a fundamental lack of recognition of the needs of the individual child. An analysis of the daily routine in the homes made it clear that at many times of the day it was simply not possible to take account of the fundamental bio-social needs of the individual child. In the view of Mulock Houwer and his co-authors, this meant that there was no caring foundation on which to base any responsible educational approach. There were no educational diagnoses or treatment plans and no account was taken of the children's past, their individual problems or their age. The few specialists that were attached to some of the institutions were working in a vacuum. The whole environment failed to provide any basis for therapeutic intervention and the majority of the staff were untrained.[40]

This report seems to have set the ball rolling, towards further professionalisation in the 1960s. A more individual approach to the children and more homely design and organisation of children's homes was initiated. From 1946 internal training started, organised by Middeloo (neutral), followed by De Kopse Hof (Roman Catholic) and De Jelburg (Protestant). 1952 saw the beginning of a new academic study, Special Education or *Orthopedagogiek*.[41]

In 1967 Mulock Houwer became an associate professor at the University of Amsterdam, joining his old comrade Frits Grewel, the child psychiatrist, who had become Professor of Special Education in 1965. Just as Houwer had criticised the state of institutions in the

1950s, as witnessed by his contributions to the report of the Overwater Commission (1951),[42] he continued to vent his critical views in the 1960s and 1970s as a mouthpiece of the broadly-based action movement being established in this sector. In the extremely influential report of the Wiarda Commission (1971)[43] and various articles published around 1970, he made it clear that he had developed very strong reservations about the readiness with which children were removed from their homes.[44] The protests that began to be heard from young people and parents in the 1960s had made him aware of the dangers and problems of this practice. It would be far better, he argued, to listen to the children themselves and look for solutions in the family's immediate home environment. He pointed out that there was a need to develop greater variety of provision in the form of day-care centres for example. In this he was not only giving voice to the existing trend towards exercising greater caution in the imposition of child protection measures, he was also offering alternative perspectives which formed a focal point for the newly-created interest groups of parents and young people to rally round.

Above all, Houwer focused on the differentiation principle. By always adopting an eclectic position with the aim of helping the child to find inner happiness, he remained sensitive to the fundamental defects of institutional education. The point that he had raised in the mid-fifties - the strength of the individual educational approach - and his new focus on the bond between parents and child[45] was now extended to the bond between the child and his whole environment. He gave increasing weight to this aspect. Whereas, in his early work, he had focused on specific problems that could face some children in the institution, such as isolation and being cast out from the group, the general problem of the bond between parents and child now became central to his thoughts.

Finally, after almost half a century of involvement with re-education institutions, and attempting to improve mental health care for neglected children from within the institutions, Mulock Houwer came to the conclusion that this form of educational work had very limited potential.[46] He believed that the institutional rationale and its general needs discourse, based as it was on the idea that anything was better than leaving the children in their familiar, damaging environment, had turned out to be flawed. Houwer was able to make this final drastic about turn because he held fast to the principle that the starting point should not be a particular type of education and a traditional, general needs discourse, but the strictly individual needs of the child relating to its concrete individual situation and its own story. Holding to this principle he was among the first in the 1960s and 1970s to place a new emphasis on autonomy, self-determination and the rights of children, and to recognise their implications for child protection and juvenile justice.[47] He can be seen as trying to articulate a new balance between the needs discourse and the new rights discourse in child protection. Mulock Houwer can also be seen, through his and his rebellious comrades' psychological and individualising interpretation of the needs discourse, as having inspired the emergence of the counter-movement with its typical mix of individual children's needs and rights.

Notes

1. Jeroen Dekker, *Straffen, redden en opvoeden. Het ontstaan en de ontwikkeling van de residentiële heropvoeding in West-Europa, 1814-1914, met bijzondere aandacht voor 'Nederlandsch Mettray'* (Assen: Van Gorcum, 1985) and Carol van Nijnatten, *Moeder Justitia en haar kinderen. De ontwikkeling van het psychojuridisch complex in de kinderbescherming* (Lisse: Swets & Zeitlinger, 1986).

2. See, for the debate on punishing and re-educating juvenile offenders, Ido Weijers, 'Het pedagogisch tekort van de strafrechtelijke kinderwet', *Comenius*, 18 (1998), 12–27; *idem*, 'The Debate on Juvenile Justice in the Netherlands, 1891-1901', *European Journal of Crime, Criminal Law and Criminal Justice*, 7 (1999), 63–78; and *idem*, 'The Double Paradox of Juvenile Justice', *European Journal on Criminal Policy and Research*, 7 (1999), 329–51.

3. See, for instance, E.A.D.E. Carp, *Het misdadige kind in psychologisch opzicht* (Amsterdam: Scheltema & Holkema, 1932).

4. Irene van der Linde, *Stoute jongens: van boefjes tot pupillen. Een geschiedenis van het observatiehuis van de vereniging 'Hulp voor onbehuisden' 1914-1970* (Amsterdam: Stadsuitgeverij, 1993).

5. F. Grewel, *Paedagogische verwaarlozing en opvoedingsfouten* (Purmerend: Muusses, 1937); D.Q.R. Mulock Houwer, *Gestichtspaedagogische hoofdstukken* (Eibergen: Heinen, 1939); J. Koekebakker, *Kinderen onder toezicht: psycho-pedagogische beschouwingen over patronaat en gezinsvoogdij* (Purmerend: Muusses, 1941).

6. See Peter Hoefnagels, 'Een halve eeuw kinderbescherming. Portret van D.Q.R. Mulock Houwer; 1903–1979', *Tijdschrift voor familie- en jeugdrecht*, 1 (1979/80), 193–7; 15–23. See also W. Hellinckx and J. Pauwels, *Orthopedagogische ontwikkelingen in de kinderbescherming. Leven en werk van dr.D.Q.R. Mulock Houwer* (Leuven: Acco, 1984).

7. See Ido Weijers, 'The Dennendal Experiment, 1969-1974: The

Ido Weijers

Legacy of a Tolerant Educative Culture', in M. Gijswijt-Hofstra and R. Porter (eds), *Cultures of Psychiatry and Mental Health Care in Postwar Britain and The Netherlands* (Amsterdam: Rodopi, 1998), 169–83.

8. See Dekker, *op. cit.* (note 1).
9. Centraal Bureau voor de Statistiek, *Vijfennegentig jaren statistiek in tijdreeksen* (Voorburg & Heerlen: CBS, 1995).
10. Piet de Rooy, 'De beschutte kooi. Gezins- en gestichtsverpleging, 1870-1940', in B. Kruithof, T. Mars and P.E. Veerman (eds), *Internaat of pleeggezin, 200 jaar discussie* (Utrecht: WIJN, 1981), 90–110: 98; Thom Willemse, 'De 20e eeuw, 1905-1988. Van opvoedingsgesticht tot behandelingstehuis', in S. Groenveld, J.J.H. Dekker and Th.R.M. Willemse (eds), *Wezen en boefjes. Zes eeuwenzorg in wees- en kinderhuizen* (Hilversum: Verloren 1997), 339–400: 359.
11. Jan-Paul Verkaik, *Voor de jeugd van tegenwoordig. Kinderbescherming en jeugdhulpverlening door Pro Juventute in Amsterdam 1896-1994* (Utrecht: SWP, 1996).
12. For instance K. Andriesse, 'Kindergebreken', in C.F.A. Zernike (ed.) *Paedagogisch Woordenboek*, (Groningen, 1905), 597–612; S. van Mesdag, 'Opleiding van personen, die met de berechting en met de opvoeding in gesticht en maatschappij van het tot misdrijf vervallen kind belast zijn', in *Verslag van het eerste Nederlandsch Paedagogisch Congres* (Groningen: J.B. Wolters, 1926), 449–64; G.H. Honing, 'Straf en opvoeding (in de praktijk)', in *ibid.*, 480–509.
13. D.Q.R. Mulock Houwer, 'Zelfbestuur in opvoedingsgestichten', *Tijdschrift voor armwezen, maatschappelijke hulp en kinderbescherming*, 30 (1929) 2268, 2273; see also *idem* 'Het moeilijke kind als helper in ons werk', *Tijdschrift voor ervaringsopvoedkunde*,7 (1928), 190–4; *idem*, 'Rechtspraak door kinderen', *Tijdschrift voor ervaringsopvoedkunde*, 7 (1928), 327–31; *idem*, 'Zelfbestuurtoepassing als gestichtspaedagogiek', *Maandblad voor berechting en reclassering van volwassenen en kinderen*, 8 (1929), 225-8; *idem*, 'Zelfbestuur', *Tijdschrift voor armwezen, maatschappelijke hulp en kinderbescherming*, 30 (1929), 2063–4.
14. D.Q.R. Mulock Houwer, 'De behandeling van enige bedwateraars en de resultaten', *Tijdschrift voor ervaringsopvoedkunde*, 8 (1929), 220–3.
15. D.Q.R. Mulock Houwer, *op. cit.* (note 5), 79.
16. D.Q.R. Mulock Houwer, 'De vrouw in het jongensgesticht', *Het kind*, 4 (1930), 157-9.
17. D.Q.R. Mulock Houwer, *op. cit.* (note 5), 162–3.

18. D.Q.R. Mulock Houwer, *Het tuchtprobleem in opvoedingsinrichtingen en tehuizen* ('s-Gravenhage: De Nederlandse bond tot kinderbescherming, 1948), 41–6.
19. D.Q.R. Mulock Houwer, *op. cit.* (note 5), 163.
20. *Ibid.*, 166.
21. *Ibid.*, 107.
22. S. Schlossman, *Love and the American Delinquent: The Theory and Practice of 'Progressive' Juvenile Justice, 1825-1920* (Chicago: University of Chicago Press, 1977).
23. G.J.J. Biesta, *John Dewey. Theorie en praktijk* (Delft: Eburon, 1992).
24. August Aichhorn, *Verwaarloosde jeugd. De psychoanalyse in de heropvoeding* (Utrecht: Bijleveld, 1952), 119.
25. *Ibid.*, 129.
26. *Ibid.*, 120.
27. Nathan Deen, *Een halve eeuw onderwijsresearch in Nederland* (Groningen: Wolters, 1969).
28. See Ernst Mulder, *Beginsel en beroep. Pedagogiek aan de Universiteit in Nederland, 1900-1940* (Amsterdam: Dissertation University of Amsterdam, 1989).
29. See Ido Weijers, 'Philip Kohnstamm: universeel intellectueel, vrijzinnig', *Comenius*, 8 (1988), 259–73.
30. Philip A. Kohnstamm, 'Staatspedagogiek of persoonlijkheidspedagogiek' (1919), reprinted in Philip A. Kohnstamm, *Persoon en samenleving. Opstellen over opvoeding en democratie* (Amsterdam: Boom, 1981), 89–120: 100.
31. Philip A. Kohnstamm, *Bijbel en jeugd* (Haarlem: Erven Bohn, 1923), 125.
32. Philip A. Kohnstamm, *Persoonlijkheid in wording* (Haarlem: Tjeenk Willink, 1929), 67.
33. There is a fascinating consensus between Mulock Houwer's two mentors, Kohnstamm and Ortt, about the crucial place of Pestalozzi in their educational orientation: see Jhr.W.A. Ortt, 'Pestalozzi leeft nog voor ons', *Tijdschrift voor armwezen, maatschappelijke hulp en kinderbescherming*, 28 (1927) 1398–1400.
34. Kohnstamm, *op. cit.* (note 32), 136.
35. *Ibid.*, 65.
36. D.Q.R. Mulock Houwer, F. Grewel and R. Friedman-Van der Heide, *Vijftigduizend kinderen roepen om hulp!* (Amsterdam: De Arbeiderspers, 1946).
37. C.P.G. Tilanus, *Jeugdzorg: historie en wetgeving* (Utrecht: SWP, 1998), 35.
38. K. de Bloois, *Veertig jaar 'Zoekt het verlorene'. Een onderzoek naar het*

maatschappelijk geslaagd zijn van oud-verpleegden (Rotterdam, 1951); see also D.Q.R. Mulock Houwer, *Gestichts- en gezinsverpleging 1899-1949* ('s-Gravenhage: Nederlandse Bond tot Kinderbescherming, 1949).

39. Werkgroep Gestichtsdifferentiatie, *Verzorging en opvoeding in kindertehuizen* (Utrecht: Nationale Federatie voor Kinderbescherming, 1957).

40. *Ibid.*, 446–8.

41. Willemse, *op. cit.* (note 10), 386–91.

42. Commissie Overwater, *Rapport van de commissie ingesteld met het doel van advies te dienen over de vraag in welke richting het Rijkstucht- en Opvoedingswezen en in verband daarmede het kinderstrafrecht zich zullen moeten ontwikkelen* ('s-Gravenhage: SDU, 1951).

43. Commissie-Wiarda, *Jeugdbeschermingsrecht* ('s-Gravenhage: SDU, 1971); see also Ido Weijers, *Schuld en schaamte. Een pedagogisch perspectief op het jeugdstrafrecht* (Houten: Bohn Stafleu Van Loghum, 2000), 88–91.

44. D.Q.R. Mulock Houwer, 'Een "missing link" in het welzijnsbeleid en de justitiële kinderbescherming', *De Koepel* (1970) 50; *idem*, 'Inrichtingen', in G.P. Hoefnagels, D.Q.R. Mulock Houwer and A. Peper, *Een nieuw plan voor de kinderbescherming* (Meppel: Boom, 1970), 37–45.

45. D.Q.R. Mulock Houwer, 'Aspecten van (gestichts) groepspaedagogiek', *De Koepel* (1952), 61–5; *idem*, 'Gestichts- en gezinsverpleging. Over de doorbraak en de constructieve onbehaaglijkheid', in *Straffen en helpen. Opstellen over berechting en reclassering aangeboden aan Mr.dr. N. Muller* (Amsterdam: Wereldvenster, 1954), 75–91.

46. D.Q.R. Mulock Houwer, 'Noodzaak van een anders georiënteerd inrichtingswezen', in G.P. Hoefnagels, D.Q.R. Mulock Houwer and J. Keizer, *Kinderbescherming, jeugdbescherming of welzijnszorg* (Meppel: Boom, 1971), 36–56.

47. A. van Montfoort, *Het topje van de ijsberg. Kinderbescherming en de bestrijding van kindermishandeling in sociaal juridisch perspectief* (Utrecht: SWP, 1994).

9

The Healthy Citizen of Empire or Juvenile Delinquent?: Beating and Mental Health in the UK

Deborah Thom

The relation between the child and its parent is 'the last irrevocable, unexchangeable primary relationship', the one thing that late modernity has left fundamentally unaltered, writes Ulrich Beck in his account of the *Risk Society*.[1] Di Gittins points out that parents still have absolute control over their children's bodies.[2] Both commentators see the relationship between the child and its parents as altered by a changing distribution of power within the family in which women have acquired more power over their children's lives at the expense of fathers. A third argument comes from the changing contribution of the modern state and welfare agencies, both public and private.[3] The parental relationship is radically affected by the state's intervention through schooling and, to a lesser extent, the juvenile justice system. Yet, the child's mental and physical health is not in this instance to the forefront of the state's concerns. There remains a separation between health and justice; nor does health supersede questions of social order.

This paper presents corporal punishment in twentieth-century Britain as an example of the ways in which state, civil society and the family interact. It also questions why the infliction of physical pain remains so important in discussions about the control of the delinquent child, despite the development and general acceptance among professionals of psychological discourses recommending its abolition. Hegel argued that, 'the family is the ethical root [basis?] of the state' and that the family remains the location of ethical life for children'. Yet the family remained the place where a healthy British child could 'reasonably' expect no protection from beating until a very recent decision of the courts attacked the concept of parental right to punish on the basis of the human rights of the child not to endure cruel and unreasonable punishment. There is clearly something about the resistance of parents to psychological discourses, and the way in which the state fails to support the professionals, that needs examination.[4]

Children were beaten in twentieth-century Britain as a matter of course in the home, the school and under summary jurisdiction in the magistrates' court. Whenever the topic is debated in public life in the first half of the twentieth century beating is seen by many as a creator of psychologically healthy children, not as a health problem but a cause of good health. The idea that the twentieth century sees the dominance of ideas of mental hygiene in the construction of the healthy citizen is also called into question by the concepts used to describe and treat criminal or anti-social children, as is the argument put forward by Jacques Donzelot and some feminists about feminist politics leading to greater humanitarianism in child-rearing practices. The dangerous child becomes the child in danger.[5] Until the end of the Second World War, professionals in the field of child health were ignored and their arguments rejected when punishing the delinquent child was raised as an issue, and ideas deriving from psycho-dynamic theory of child development were less influential than an older discourse based upon the concept of the child as a bundle of instincts; a social dynamic based on the idea of energy which could both incorporate physical chastisement and be used to reject it, but certainly had little time for the unconscious.

Debates about corporal punishment remained astonishingly consistent despite the expansion of mental health services until the Second World War. The practice of corporal punishment fluctuated in magistrates' courts where it first began to be questioned and subsided more slowly in the school and the home. It is identified as one of the key components of national character and this account starts with these links.

A 'virile training':
The debate on corporal punishment before the
First World War

In 1908 the new Children's Act, which codified and reformed the criminal justice system for juveniles, raised the question of flogging as a punishment in the juvenile justice system, the school and the home. There were several debates on the issue, which set the scene for an account of social and psychological health which have continued almost until the present day. The fullest was in the journal *Outlook* which echoed those of the nineteenth century, and which could have been written at almost any time up until 1948 when magistrates' power to inflict the birch was finally removed. The arguments were used consistently until the late 1930s when the rhetoric of citizenship replaces the rhetoric of Empire, nation and race.

> Some form of physical correction is essential to the training of the young. This does not imply cruelty. Are we to spend our money on training an enfeebled, soft and effeminate generation of boys and girls who are afraid of the pain of a well-deserved whipping? If so what is to become of that dogged pluck and endurance, that prompt response to the call of duty, grit and determination that have so long distinguished our nation?[6]

Beating was thus seen as a major determinant of British national character, explicitly so in the argument of this contributor to the journal who said that French delinquents were worse that the British because they were 'youthful, unflogged apaches'. Others argued that beating was a class privilege which the children of the poor should enjoy as much as 'children educated at public schools'.[7] The emphasis on national character is reiterated by several correspondents. One writes of the upper and middle classes, 'Who can say whatever other faults they may have had that they failed in courage, fortitude and endurance or any of the robust virtues which go to make a nation great?'[8] Another linked it specifically to the Imperial mission:

> If we would maintain our position in the world as an imperial race, we must insist upon a virile training both in the home and the school, which shall raise up a people hardy, bold, accustomed to concentration of thought, firm of purpose and not afraid of struggle and difficulty. Such a people cannot be raised without discipline.[9]

It is not accidental that the word virile was used to describe the desired type of young person. Assumptions about gender variation and sexual difference lay at the heart of this debate, and many commentators shared the view of scientists investigating the subject of gender at a time when boys were more various than girls.[10] This theory went through discussions about education in relation to intelligence and criminality alike. The power of a social theory of gender, which assumed male energy as the root cause of misbehaviour, can be seen in Stanley Hall's *Adolescence* published in Britain in 1907. Hall famously wrote that, 'the young man is fighting the hottest battles of his life with the Devil'.[11] Psychology was beginning to assert that normal male adolescents were slightly disturbed by the fluctuations in their energies and the vigour of their growth into adulthood. A gendered notion of psychological development meant that the treatment of the delinquent children maintained a double standard of male violence and female victimhood. August Aichhorn described delinquents thus in 1936 in the title of his book as *Aggressive Youth and Wayward Girls* and this differentiation ran through psychology, criminology and social work. As a result, the two sexes faced different structures of regulation in youth. Women and girls were governed *informally* by auxiliaries to the state or local, minor state functionaries; men and boys far more at the formal level of law and punishment, directly by the state.

War 1914-18

The limits of the psychologisation of young people were, in part, sustained by the persistence of theories of gender, theories which wartime was to make far more acute.[12] Military mobilisation created grave anxieties about militarism and the creation of an aggressive and brutal juvenile underclass. There was also a moral panic about girls falling into sexual delinquency, the rise of illegitimacy and the so-called 'war babies'. The discussion on civilisation under attack fell on ears already sensitive to the concern for psychological health and discipline. Victor Bailey described the development of the Borstal system and juvenile institutions designed to create healthy boys in his account of the juvenile criminal justice system *Delinquency and Citizenship*.[13]   In this account, the social health of the young delinquent is primarily attributed to the penal system but the book looks more to institutions than discourses. It is the pervasive discourse of male energy, its repression and inhibition that punishment discourse addresses and thus creates a very different notion of health and normalcy than either the psychological or medical model provides.

Ian Gibson's excellent account of the persistence of corporal punishment in British culture and society, *The English Vice,* records some of the rhetoric which returns each time this subject is raised in Parliament, a rhetoric of masculinity and discipline which claims the public school as the ideal.[14] The debate in *Outlook* provides powerful examples of the model of children's moral nature that lies behind a belief in whipping, flogging, birching or caning of children, seen as particularly suitable objects for the practice. The argument gives to beating a role in socialisation which can still be heard in discussions of child punishment. The action of violent chastisement affects the child's character and nature operating through the body onto its psyche. It instils national character, the argument runs; it encourages good relations with adults, teachers in this case, as one anonymous correspondent wrote, 'In nine times out of ten a caning has been the beginning of an intimate relationship between master and boy'.[15]

Another saw it as working directly through the body, 'It hardens the body and the mind... town upbringing and town life undoubtedly tend to softness'.[16] Some pointed out the problems with this argument - why should the working class not have the privileges of the public school, if it was so productive why not beat girls, and, since summary beatings were used for offences which involved committing cruelty, did they not simply repeat the painful experience on the body of the offender?

The debate also shows the muddle in the public mind between judicial beating and punishment by teachers and parents. This debate demonstrated at great length and very clearly how far ideas of nation, state and socialisation were tied to theories of discipline, a tie which the outbreak of war in 1914 made more emphatic. Juvenile delinquency rates registered in crime statistics and social commentary soared during the First World War. The sociologist Hermann Mannheim saw this as partly a result of declining emigration and expanding juvenile labour, but also the diminishing effect of domestic control.[17] Others argued that juvenile delinquency was a result of changes in the economy. The Departmental Committee on Juvenile Employment after the War suggested that we must, 'replace the conception of the juvenile as primarily a little wage earner by the conception of the juvenile as primarily the workman and citizen in training', that is, the citizen is still usually seen as a boy, and yet he is an economic agent.[18] Secondary schools, which took about 10 per cent of the age group at 11 from the elementary schools (for an elite education under state auspices) had never been fuller, numbers rising in wartime by more than 50 per cent, up from 51,141 to 81,056 under the 1907 special places regulations. War increased formal educational provision for the few, the minority of academic children, and reduced it for the mass in elementary schools, whose buildings were used by the military and whose hours of study were cut.

Criminal children created a particular anxiety about the effects of war, far more significant really than the rising number of adolescent wage-earners. There was an increase in children charged with punishable offences in the first year of war which Cecil Leeson in his pamphlet *The Child and the War,* published in 1916, concluded, 'represents an actual increase in wrong-doing, and not an increase in prosecutions only'. Leeson's concern reflected a demographic concept of society, expressed (as so often in this period) by the use of the term 'population': 'With a population decimated by war, it is the concern of everyone to prevent the waste of human material... the country will require to make each human unit go farther than before'.[19] Thus each child was described as a unit of production and of socialisation. 'The great thing the war has taught us to be is less selfish', wrote Charles Russell, Chief Inspector of Reformatory and Industrial Schools, in *The Problem of Juvenile Crime* in 1917. Certainly, many contemporaries claimed that the war had created a wider concern with society, in which criminal children became less a problem in themselves since dealing with them was quite easy, but more a problem as a symptom of the possibility of degeneration among the mass of children, a portent of the malign effects of war . In what sense did the war actually encourage criminality, or, at any rate, be seen as encouraging deviance among the young?

The Home Office circular on criminal statistics of 1916 records an increase in offences in one year of 34 per cent from 2,500 to nearly 4,000. As Russell pointed out, there was nothing mysterious in the decrease in adult crime during war-time:

> What has really happened is that very large numbers of potential criminals, and of those whose irregular ways of living had from time to time brought them within prison walls, have found in naval or military service a healthy outlet for energies frequently misdirected before the war.[20]

But the increase in juvenile crime was also, he said, explicable, and effectively for the same reasons. The model used was the same as the authors of letters to *Outlook*. It was based on an assumption of animal spirits, instinctual dynamics analogous to other natural forces like water or electricity. Their energy was not given an healthy outlet, children were more physically vigorous, many schools were used half-time by military authorities, so schooling was also half-time. He denied the influence of cinema, arguing that the real cause of social dislocation and a failure of moral values is 'the national disgrace of the slum and over-crowding'. Leeson saw the causes of crime not in the nature of the child but in the social circumstances of military mobilisation and war-work; thus it is an absence which is causing crime, an absence which he characterises as 'the withdrawal from child-life of adult personal influence'.[21] Leeson was Secretary for the Howard Association for Penal Reform, and while he did not see it as causing criminality, he did criticise the influence of the cinema, seeing the 'fascination of the cinema as more an indictment of the child's dull home conditions'.[22] At best, Leeson comments, the case for any direct influence by the new medium is unproven. The pamphlet speaks strongly against the remedy still available to the juvenile court magistrate, flogging. Here Leeson demonstrates the general tendency to psychologise, so characteristic of reformist comments about delinquency, that marks the discussions of reformers. Here he offers a clear demonstration of the theory of child mind and development in the period, which attributes the norms of child development to all children so that the delinquent is simply behaving along a spectrum of normalcy responding to abnormal social conditions.

> It is said that corporal punishment arrests the child's imagination, debases his character, destroys his initiative. We would not advocate anything tending to dwarf imagination or initiative - for we all require more of both; nor do we think the instances are numerous in which thrashing is the proper remedy. It should be remembered however that there is such a thing as an unhealthy imagination, and that initiative itself is not everything: initiative in a wrong direction is certainly better than none at all; but initiative rightly directed is what we need in the child, and in some rare cases the change of direction is to be achieved only at the expense of a disagreeable experience. Punishment by itself , however, whatever shape it takes, is no real remedy. The remedy is found only when we recognize in the child a centre of deeply rooted instincts needing diversion and guidance, of an unbounded vitality which simply must be released. Our business is not to repress but wholesomely to direct...[23]

Psychology and delinquency 1918-38

After the war the reformers dominated in the public discussion of what to do about juvenile delinquency. The language of treatment not punishment, based on the same model of the dynamics of normal development and natural youthful energy became general. However, the task of the criminal justice system remained one of control rather than treatment and this contradicted the assumptions of mental health practitioners. Children's lack of citizenship, their openness to surveillance, is very evident in the statistics on juvenile crime in the inter-war period, as psychological explanations began to become more significant to those associated with juvenile delinquency. A survey of over a 1,000 inhabitants of the new institution to punish juveniles separately from adults and to redeem through educational re-adjustment - the Borstal - was carried out for Hermann Mannheim, who taught at the London School of Economics. The survey demonstrated the social basis of much delinquency in the mind of an advanced criminologist. Of 606 boys and 411 girls currently in Borstal, 'home conditions or lack of home' was identified as the main cause of criminality in 133 and 75 respectively.[24] The years of economic depression and the flowering of the Borstal system added some theoretical insights to the debate about how far delinquent children were normal children with contingent problems, or how far they were irretrievably or innately different. Psychology became a way of describing, diagnosing and treating delinquent children with strong claims to be taken seriously as the most effective way of analysing a general social problem. British psychology was eclectic, under-theorised and self-consciously sociological rather than medical. The 'new psychology' supported the ideals of a society freed from repression in which frustration or deformation of otherwise healthy instincts was the driving developmental determinant of anti-social behaviour. It was *not* the same discourse as that of the individual therapy known as psychoanalysis, but they had in common ideas of inhibition, repression, fantasy and the significance of sexuality and the body in the life of the adolescent. The long debate over the new institution, the child guidance clinic, reflected the divisions in thinking about behaviour as a problem of psychic development rather than as evidence of the innately anti-social.[25] Unlike the rest of Europe, particularly German-speaking Europe, British theorists were relatively untroubled by the acute theoretical divides between those who believed in a single unconscious (Freudians), a collective unconscious (Jungians), or a socially determined notion of development which did not acknowledge the unconscious at all (Adler). There was also in Britain a more systematic relationship between hereditarians and psychologists in which the psyche was seen as one of the key areas for the identification of inherited qualities.[26]

Volume 1 in the series *The Sub-Normal School Child* by Cyril Burt was *The Young Delinquent*,[27] published in 1925, the most popular and most cited of all his books. In this volume Burt staked a claim for the new psychology as the single most important discourse to explain educational malfunction, social disorder and the nature of the future which children embodied. Through the psychological case study which investigated the 'past, the present and the future' the adjustment of the child could be fine-tuned, a mass system for psychological health could be created, by placing this mass of individual cases into an institutional setting, the child psychological clinic. Society played a contributory role.

> If the majority of delinquents are needy, the majority of the needy
> do not become delinquents... Poverty can only engender crime by its
> ultimate action, through ways more often circuitous than plain,
> upon the inner, mental life of the potential offender.[28]

Burt asked questions about the cinema as other commentators had
done, and, as they had argued earlier, he concluded that its influence
was slight. He suggested that the cinema's general moral tone was
significant. Films had, of course, developed since Russell's dismissal
of the argument in 1917.

> Throughout the usual picture palace programme, the moral
> atmosphere presented is an atmosphere of thoughtless frivolity and
> fun, relieved only by some sudden storm of passion with occasional
> splashes of sentiment. Deceit, flirtation and jealousy, unscrupulous
> intrigue and reckless assault, a round of unceasing excitement and
> the extremes of wild emotionalism, are depicted as the normal
> characteristics of the every day conduct of adults. The child with no
> background of experience by which to correct the picture, frames a
> notion altogether distorted, of social life and manners.[29]

He went on to explain the effect by the most direct account of the
way in which these attitudes and feelings become physically
influential. They 'stir the curiosity, heat the imagination, and work
upon the fantasies, of boys and girls of every age'. Psychic forces still
manifested themselves through the body at puberty, although Burt
followed Freud's follower, Ernest Jones, and the psychologist William
McDougall as seeing these changes as primarily and simply physical;
rejecting Stanley Hall's theory of radical character change, a kind of
temporary madness for all boys at adolescence. Burt saw puberty as
a problem of body out of step with mind or moral sense which is, he
argued, particularly likely for girls, who menstruate and become
fertile before they are morally informed or socialised into adult
sexuality. Burt's solution was primarily to psychologise deviancy and
therefore to argue for psychological remedies. Children were to be
observed in psychological clinics and treated elsewhere according to
this idea of a mixture of the physical and the psychological causes of
delinquency; treatment involving the expenditure of energy and
psychological therapy in Borstals for some, self-governing 'colonies'
for others. The Borstals were new, set up under the provisions of the
Children's Act of 1908, and when Burt wrote in the early 1920s there
were five for boys, each holding about 1,000 youths aged between 16
and 21, and only one for girls with 125 places. In 1920 the Juvenile

197

Organisation Committee of the Board of Education had recommended that all children coming before a court be medically examined because they found doctors would often support the child's defence that this was illness, not wickedness: 'the child was suffering from some disease which tended to make the offender irritable, passionate, and at times perhaps hysterical, or even temporarily insane'.[30]

Burt's account reaches its climax in the account of the regulatory grid he proposed to pass over all delinquents and all disturbed children and in which he makes most explicit the programme of loading all these manifestations into the psyche.

> The study of the criminal thus becomes a distinct department of this new science - a branch of individual psychology; and the handling of the juvenile offender is, or should be, a practical application of known psychological principles. To whip a boy, to fine him, to shut him up in a penal institution, because he has infringed the law is like sending a patient, on the first appearance of fever, out under the open sky to cool his skin and save others from infection.[31]

Burt was making a strong claim for the utility of psychological enquiry, but it is not accidental that he uses physical and medical analogies in making his case. The science of psychology was to heal minds as medicine healed bodies, but children were still being described through bodily symptoms. He failed to win the supremacy for psychology of the analysis and treatment of problems of juvenile misbehaviour for which he had hoped. One of the reasons for this was the way in which psychological explanations were now more general, more acceptable and more persuasive, so that the special insights of psychologists became seen merely as so much common sense. In other words, the ideology of child development was extraordinarily successful in changing the reaction to the idea of a delinquent child from fear to pity, in the general population, but it did not advance the professional claims of psychological professionals where delinquency was concerned.

The Young Delinquent was published at exactly the same time that the London magistrate Mrs St Loe Strachey was investigating the possibilities of establishing an English system of child guidance clinics along the American model.[32] This new institution was to spread rapidly in England, sponsored by Rockefeller money from the Commonwealth Trust, and creating a network of clinics and a professional training for psychiatrists, psychologists and psychiatric social workers to staff the clinics. Many of these newly-trained professionals were women, many of them had been volunteers, previously working unpaid, but increasingly they were young, unmarried women who needed wages to survive. Burt had been one of the main protagonists of the 'psychological clinic' as the pressure point where suasion could be exerted on the child, the family and society. He was to be disappointed in the subsequent structure of clinics in that they were, mostly, headed by medical men rather than psychologists and the key personnel were in fact women, who made up the majority of the psychiatric social workers, rather than professional men. They were responsible for investigating home conditions, the relations between clinic and school and for the preliminary diagnostic interviews with parents and child. They also carried out the interviews with new schools, foster parents and the child itself - in other words they were mainly responsible for the treatment as well as the framing of the diagnosis. They represented, then, a group of philanthropic workers whose behaviour and professional practice was neither punitive nor empowered legally or customarily, but whose jurisdiction extended widely as far as children were concerned. Their powers were actually slight in theory, but in practice their recommendations could affect the future of a child radically. In this sense, they were a prime example both of the penetration of new therapies but also of the limits of regulation, as informal enforcement hardly touched the criminal justice system it had been designed to reform.

The first research commissioned by the Child Guidance Council investigated bedwetting. This seems insignificant now perhaps, but it was the single largest presenting problem at most early clinics and parents, children themselves and social workers all found it a serious problem. The other main problem was also nothing that could be described as delinquency, but what is variously described as 'nerves' or 'nervousness'. The outcome was that early clinics were full of male children between 9 and 11 years old who wet their beds, slept uneasily at night, had strange dreams, walked in their sleep or cried for no reason, not with the 13- to 16-year-olds whose delinquency was the motive for the scheme in the first place. Those who were seen as delinquents were still quite likely to find themselves passing through the criminal justice system, untouched by the more humane concerns of clinic staff and much more severely treated both in institutional care and after they had served their sentences in civil society. The clinics too had more middle-class children than their initiators had expected, more than in the population at large, and far fewer of the minority ethnic groups who predominated in the children's courts, particularly Irish migrants. Both groups were however overwhelmingly male.

The persistence of punishment:
The Cadogan Committee on corporal punishment

By 1938 the professions were beginning to acquire secure status, the institutions of professional life were in place and the notion of psychic disturbance as a cause of delinquency and maladjustment was clearly entrenched, substituting earlier eugenic models or ideas of punishment. But this progress was not unresisted. The shift from body to mind in modern societies as identified by Michel Foucault in *Discipline and Punish* was strikingly slow in Britain.[33]   The Departmental Committee on Corporal Punishment of 1938 met to discuss the repeated demands of the Howard League for Penal Reform, doctors and educators that children should no longer be beaten as a judicial punishment. As their appendix points out, apart from in several American States and supervised parental punishment in Sweden and Denmark, Britain and its Dominions were the only industrialised nations where beating was regularly, if infrequently, passed as a sentence on children and young people. The report describes in full detail the nature of the punishment and the instrument used to inflict it. Successive changes in the criminal law had left the only male adults being beaten for mutiny or gross assault on an officer in prison or the Armed Services, while male young persons of 14 to18 and male children of 7 to14 could be beaten for a range of offences, including deer poaching, malicious damage and offences under the White Slave Act of 1912 of procuring and soliciting. This demonstrates the inhibition on developing modernity in an additive legal system which still drew upon the 1824 Vagrancy Act, which had allowed whipping for being a 'rogue' or a 'vagabond', and overlaid on that the new terms of the White Slave Act, which assumed that youth prostitution was a result of corruption by adult men.

Youths sentenced to summary corporal punishment were beaten, in England and Wales, not with a rod or cane, but with a birch broom made of twigs bound together about 6 inches across. In Scotland the tawse, a strap made of leather, was also used. Ironically, these instruments were made by prisoners in prison workshops. Children under 14 could be given six strokes if beaten summarily in a magistrate's court, aged over 14 they got twelve; if beaten in a superior court the maximum was 25 strokes. In Scotland the

Table 9.1
The Incidence of Corporal Punishment in Magistrates Courts

1910	1702	1919	1689	1928	188
1911	1727	1920	1380	1929	186
1912	2164	1921	661	1930	135
1913	2219	1922	556	1931	147
1914	2415	1923	561	1932	160
1915	3514	1924	633	1933	162
1916	4864	1925	474	1934	146
1917	5210	1926	365	1935	218
1918	3759	1927	247	1936	166

Source: Report of the Departmental Service Committee on Corporal Punishment: Statistical Appendix.

number of strokes was not fixed, but was designed to be 'sufficiently severe to cause the repetition of it to be dreaded'. The report even describes the posture in which this punishment was carried out, and the variants in local practice, in what sounds like horrified detail: 'The birch is applied across the buttocks on the bare flesh, bent over a table, with the hands and, sometimes, the feet, held by police officers.[34]

This practice of judicial beating had been attacked in the past. In 1932, the entire Children's Act had been held up while members of the House of Lords reinstated beating for those aged under 14. It was also falling to some extent into disuse as probation and Borstal or industrial schools were seen as perfectly adequate punishments for most offences. The rise in juvenile crime and the absence of many auxiliary professionals on military service, as well, perhaps, as the emergence from retirement of many emergency magistrates, meant that beatings rose in wartime (in both wars) along with the male juvenile crime wave. Although they did not go on rising during the Depression's comparable growth in adolescent crime, they were to rise again slightly in a similar but much smaller epidemic of wartime delinquency between 1939 and 1945. The boys who were being beaten ranged from the incorrigibles to male prostitutes, and tended *not* to be the largest or most brutal boys but those whose parents refused to take responsibility for them.

The figures were recorded for the 1938 Committee up until the year 1936. These figures do not simply reflect changes in criminal offences. In 1932 there had been 8,449 offences dealt with summarily in magistrate's courts in this age group (at 404 per 100,000). In 1936, when the number beaten was almost the same, there had been 13,707 (or 717 per 100,000) offences. The Committee concluded that the general tendency in the juvenile penal system argued against beating: 'Changes in our general methods have been aimed at subordinating the retributive element to other elements of deterrence and reform'.[35]

The committee's report concluded that professional evidence from England and Wales (though not from Scotland,) had overwhelmingly rejected beating, caning or other physical punishments as well as rejecting custodial care for young offenders. Evidence from psychologically informed witnesses entirely supported this general conclusion. Yet the committee's rejection of beating was based far more on the evidence of magistrates that it was *ineffective.* They showed that boys who were beaten were more than twice as likely to re-offend as those punished in other ways, most of them within six months of being beaten. The exigencies of cutbacks in government spending were used to reject Cyril Burt's evidence that an extensive, lengthy assessment of each child in a psychological clinic was necessary for any punishment process.

> His proposals could not be carried out unless every juvenile court could call upon the services of a fully equipped psychological clinic. We find it impossible to relate these proposals to the practical realities of the existing situation.[36]

Burt's proposals were rejected as too expensive and impractical. However, Freudian theory was rejected because it undermined the basis of the whole system of punishment itself. The British Psychoanalytic Association argued that the main problem of corporal punishment was the development of sadistic pleasure in the mind of the beater. The state was thus seen to be encouraging perversity of a most damaging and sexual kind.

> Conscious sadism is recognised as a form of sexual perversion, and a system of judicial corporal punishment may pander to unconscious impulses which, in essence, are sadistic and sexual. The full implications of this view would extend far beyond our terms of reference. We do not think its [psychoanalytic theory] development has yet reached the stage at which its hypothesis can safely be made the basis for a drastic and far-reaching reconstruction of our penal code.[37]

So, although it was recognised that this sort of description, with its attribution of powerful unconscious motives of a sexual kind, might one day provide a basis for change, the Committee members were not yet convinced. It is, however, interesting that the lengthy exposition of the damage to the individual child, and to other children looking on, of corporal punishment provided by the Child Guidance Council does not merit anything like the same careful public attention. This may be of course because it was so solidly congruent with the views of doctors, magistrates, policemen and probation officers as to occasion no particular remark. Indeed, the discussion was never of great general public interest, but it is evidence of the slowness of change in relation to delinquency and psychological explanations that the case against beating still had to be made then and later. The psychologisation of the discourse of bodily punishment in the penal system was not as significant as the empirical justifications of criminologists.

Discussion on corporal punishment in the *British Medical Journal* reflected the diversity of professional opinion and the dominance of the energy model of the psyche within popular and professional thinking about criminality in boys. The editorial of 20 March, 1937, ended, 'To tie him hand and foot to a tripod and flog him with a brine soaked birch seems the best way to make a boy of eight years look upon society as his enemy'.[38] Most of the letters responding to this editorial which helped set up the Departmental Committee were entirely in agreement. They cited the magistrate Clarke Hall, who had conclusively demonstrated the statistical relationship between flogging as a punishment and speed of re-offending as evidence of the complete inefficacy of corporal punishment. One defended beating on the grounds that though it was painful, the boy 'accepts it as part of the game'. This prison doctor feared far more the introduction of psychoanalysis, which is how he described psychological medicine.

> Psychoanalysis is a double-edged weapon and should only be applied in certain cases; applied haphazardly it can do the most incalculable harm, and turn healthy young people into hypochondriacs and incurable neurotics.[39]

This comment was challenged by Lindsey Neustatter who asked for evidence of this harm, which was not forthcoming. Indeed, in the very next year two of the Tavistock Clinic's workers, Sturge and Maberley, produced a survey of 500 children treated at the Tavistock to assess the impact of psychotherapy. They contacted 1,330 and found 500 who could confidently be described as having a known outcome. Their questionnaire, they concluded, showed 36 cured, 87 improved and 37 not improved, that is a 78 per cent improvement. A survey of visits to another subset of patients gave comparable proportions of 40 cured, 81 improved and 39 not: that is, a total of 76 per cent relieved of their symptoms. 'Symptoms are by definition what the patient complains of but in children they are much more often what the adult complains of in the child'. The cases included 87 who were stealing, 53 who were 'difficult to manage', truancy in 13, and enuresis in 45. Symptoms which were more internal to the child included 44 cases of anxiety, 23 of fears, 31 of tics, and 33 with physical symptoms. It is unclear who would have complained about masturbation or sex difficulties, but only 17 cases were recorded in this survey. Sturge and Maberley explained the much larger number of boys in the clinic's client population and thus in the sample:

> their psychoneurotic symptoms tend to take a more spectacular and socially difficult form than those of girls. The present form of social organisation gives a better chance for boys who show neurotic symptoms to adjust as they grow up, whereas girls who may possess only a latent tendency to neurosis in childhood develop more definite symptoms in every day life later.[40]

The committee's report of 1936 demonstrated very clearly that beating was being seen as characteristic of national character but that this was now a cause of embarrassment rather than the pride it had reflected in 1908. Appendix V listed practice in 15 foreign countries. In 12 of these beating was not used: Austria, Belgium, Czechoslovakia, Denmark, France, Germany, Holland, Hungary, Italy, Portugal, and Switzerland. In Finland and Norway a parent might administer punishment beatings, in Sweden prisoners could be beaten but had not been since 1926, and in the USA, some, mainly Southern, states used it on offenders in prison. In the Dominions, although it was clearly falling into disuse, the punishment was still available in some Australian provinces, New Zealand, South Africa, Eire and Newfoundland for juveniles. Only Southern Rhodesia used the punishment extensively as an adjunct to labour discipline and mostly on what the report called 'natives'. In 1932-36, they recorded that 43 'European' juveniles were whipped, 1,656 'natives'. All were, as far as I can tell, male.

•

War 1939-45

The report concluded that much delinquency was a result of 'a misdirection of the spirit of adventure which should be the natural characteristic of any normal adolescent boy'.[41] History and the theory of the child's mental nature both militated against the retention of this punishment which could only legitimately be retained if it was a deterrent not a retributive act. The committee recommended its abolition. Interestingly, there is no discussion of girls who did not in theory or in law get beaten at all, and might thus demonstrate alternative ways of thinking about punishment. But there were very few girls classified as delinquents, The lack of theory to explain clearly the gender imbalance of twentieth-century adolescent crime rates is echoed in the 1941 survey of juvenile delinquency published jointly by the Home Office and Board of Education. The first page includes the pious hope that the needs of girls must not be overlooked but then does not mention these needs again. Obviously, this is partly because this multiplication of criminal offences in young people is almost entirely among boys at the peak age of 13.

> Many of them (the offences) are due to high spirits or a desire for adventure or indicate the absence of discipline in the home life... it would be unwise to ignore the effect of the excitement and unsettlement of war on adolescent boys... boys are stirred by stories of deeds at sea, on the field or in the air... the spirit of adventure finds outlet in ways readily open to them and this type frequently works in gangs.[42]

The policy solution for these young men was to establish the Service for Youth scheme in 1940 which attempted to spread the benign influence of the youth club onto a national stage, using healthy, physical outdoor exercise to challenge youthful exuberance to interest itself in sport and social service. The government circular on juvenile delinquency did recognise the possibility of war making visible serious existing psychological problems, it applauded the 'invaluable' help of the few child guidance clinics in existence, and commended them to all local education authorities for 'the treatment of maladjusted children'.[43] Yet their main solution of vigorous team sports and the encouragement of group identity helped to maintain gangs, while competition tended to help violence. The Service for Youth did address the body rather than the mind of young people; hence it was not to some contemporary observers a solution to the problem of delinquent male youth but an evasion of it.

The effect of general acceptance of a notion of psychic economy deriving from physical energies, manifested in the body, was to normalise the war and the energy associated with it rather than to pathologise concepts of violence. The only professionals who were able to expand on pre-war ideas of the loss of love as the most influential social danger for young people were those who dealt with the most disturbed children of all, children who could not be evacuated to someone's home because it was thought no normal billet could take them. A Ministry of Health survey noted in the discussion of the Hostels for Difficult Children, 'that violence or anti-social behaviour is often a symptom of emotional disturbance and that what is needed is, in the first place, sympathy and understanding'.[44]

Here is the authentic voice of familial privatised health, human sympathy and a location of disturbance and its solution in the intimate life of the family or its substitute which has been rightly observed by Rose, Denise Riley,[45] and others. However, why did the Chief Medical Officer of the Board of Education *not* comment in his annual reports on the statistics of child death which showed that more children aged 10 to15 regularly died from violence of all forms than from any other single cause, and that, apart from years of whooping cough epidemics, so too did those aged 5 to10.[46] The anti-social behaviour and violence of parents upon their children is probably the cause of these deaths, far more directly damaging to public health than most other causes of death, yet until the spectacular and brutal murder of Dennis O'Neill in 1946 and the Curtis Committee on children without homes, violence *against* children was much less an object of concern than the violence or misbehaviour *of* a very few.

Schools and homes

Corporal punishment in schools reflected similar assumptions about child regulation to those of the system dealing with delinquency. In 1967, the Plowden Committee's report showed that 80-90 per cent of teachers were opposed to any abolition of their power to punish. The report, in an odd formulation, summarised the evidence: 'Psychologists are agreed that the advantages of corporal punishment are far outweighed by its disadvantages'. They pointed out that no other European countries allowed it, but that 'a lack of corporal punishment will often contrast sharply with what goes on in a child's home'.[47] In both cases the argument is expressed negatively. This reforming body was then offering psychological expertise against cultural norms and insisting that in the end the experts should be heeded. Earlier, in 1961, the education officer of West Riding of Yorkshire had demonstrated convincingly that secondary schools which caned vigorously were probably increasing their disciplinary problems; 'The higher the caning, the heavier the delinquency rate and the worse the behaviour'.[48] He also pointed out that in fact the schools with the best disciplinary records were among those with the lowest rateable value for housing, in other words that economic affluence was not a direct determinant of child behaviour, nor poverty a direct cause of misbehaviour.

If the school in Britain gradually became a place in which corporal punishment was first tightly monitored and then abolished in 1982 after lengthy campaigning, what of the home? Oral history shows that the culture of parental power and responsibility for general social regulation went hand in hand. Steve Humphries records a stepmother who slapped and pinched her stepchildren and hid their books to keep them away from school in the 1930s.[49] Elizabeth Roberts, in a more generally enthusiastic account of parent-child relationships, records few strict parents including one who himself said that he was very strict but 'never laid a finger on them'.[50] Paul Thompson's comparative account of child-rearing practices has been the most systematic effort to consider whether there is a national culture of child discipline and records the difference in parental punishment as one of the key determinants of variation within British culture[51]. Punitive cultures encourage early leaving of home and discourage creativity. All these accounts based on oral evidence record the same phenomenon as Willmott and Young's classic sociology of the family did - that the bad old days of child brutality are safely historicised, a thing of the past: 'I whack mine now but not the beatings we used to have.'[52]

The question of how far there had been change is difficult to unravel when so many people across time believe that things were better now, but record a quite substantial use of corporal punishment in the recent past whether it be the 1920s or the 1970s. One change that may be older than is often thought is in the balance between parents administering punishment. Ellen Ross, writing about London life between the wars, saw daily discipline as actually practised by mothers but attributed to fathers in theory.[53] Ross sees neighbourhood sanctions as the major check on excess violence. Others have noted the significant gap as being not between working-class families but between the family and state agencies, particularly policemen who, as shown in many oral histories, often used informal corporal punishment to reinforce their authority in the streets. However, such sanctions should not be contrasted. In many examples, the same children may appear at any site of punishment, because parents often 'smacked children who had been smacked at school'.[54] Donzelot argues that there is no private, separate realm of the family: 'psychoanalysis made the family amenable to social requirements and a good conductor of relational norms,'[55] but this seems a long way from the experience recorded by these oral historians of different periods of the twentieth century. Hermann Mannheim reported in the 1960s that since the grounds for admission to the 'approved school' (where delinquent children were sent in the 1940s) *included* poor quality home conditions, the assumption that 'the experience of approved school' and 'poor home conditions' were in any sense separate or distinct measures of delinquency seemed inappropriate. The health of society was not being measured differently in different sites. These sites referred *to each other* to define the delinquent, a process which might involve psychological or medical intervention in a clinic, but more often passed by these institutions into others more punitive in style where the child's health was measured by his acceptance of discipline, not his mental state. Donald Winnicott, the psychologist, added a new factor to the debate. He saw delinquency as created in part by the child's own desires, when he argued in the 1950s that actually delinquency could indicate the wish of the child for 'control by strong, loving confident people'.[56]

Psychological and sociological explanations alike retained the stronger recognition of the autonomy of the child in relation to both family and civil society that is characteristic of the descriptions found in oral history. Family members do not adopt the language of the state agencies that impinge upon the parental task, nor do they necessarily accept recommendations for change in deep-rooted cultural practices. The child's independence from punishment appears to be closely related to its economic independence, so that the structure of family, civil society and state seems to resemble most closely Hegel's version, the family as the primary site for different models of love rather than justice which leaves us some room to consider how far the family remains profoundly constructed by contemporary notions of love and its role in regulation, and profoundly resistant to the attempts by psychology and psychiatry to alter its practices. Secondly, institutions' powers to punish is often used in relation to a model of a 'healthy child' representing the nation's moral character which goes back to the nineteenth century and ideas of energy, drive and instincts. This set of ideas is also resistant to professional argument and advice for a long time after the change in professional discourse which rejects corporal punishment as an unhealthy way to discipline a child.

Notes

1. Ulrich Beck, *Risk Society: Towards a New Modernity* (London: Sage, 1992), 118.

2. D.Gittins, *The Family in Question: Changing Households and Familiar Ideologies* (Basingstoke: Macmillan,1985), 179.

3. J. Donzelot, *The Policing of Families* (London: Hutchinson, 1980) expounds this change most elaborately, seeing the family as a site of discursive negotiation rather than an object of social construction. See also Nikolas Rose, *The Psychological Complex: Psychology, Politics and Society in England, 1869-1939* (London: Routledge and Kegan Paul, 1985), who describes a pattern of governmentality which calls into question interventions by a 'state' acting on 'the family'. In his later books *Governing the Soul: The Shaping of the Private Self* (London: Routledge, 1990) and *Inventing Ourselves: Psychology, Power and Personhood* (Cambridge: Cambridge University Press,1996), Rose has developed an analysis of self-invention to explain the construction of subjectivity While he has extended his account of the play between different forms of power, the account has lost some of the distinction between one sort of discursive practice and another in which social institutions are insufficiently distinguished from each other. I am arguing here that social practices are different from professional discourses and indeed often undermine them.

4. G.W.F. Hegel *Elements of the Philosophy of Right,* trans. H.B. Nisbet (Cambridge: Cambridge University Press, 1991), 272, cited by P. Ginsborg, 'Family Civil Society and State in Contemporary European History', *Contemporary European History,* 4 (1998), 249-74: 259.

5. On feminism's contribution to ideas about the family, see Carol Dyhouse, *Feminism and the Family in England, 1880-1939* (Oxford: Blackwell,1989).

6. *Outlook,* 5 September 1908, 306, letter from DM.

7. *Outlook,* 12 September 1908, 338, letter from ER.

8. *Outlook,* 10 October 1908, 513, letter from HEP.

9. *Outlook,* 19 September 1908, 369, letter from 'A Lover of my Country'.

10. Cynthia Eagle Russett, *Sexual Science: The Victorian Construction of*

Womanhood (Cambridge, Mass: Harvard University Press, 1989) provides an elegant account of the debates between Havelock Ellis and Karl Pearson on this subject.

11. G. Stanley Hall, *Adolescence: Its Psychology and its Relations to Physiology, Anthropology, Sociology, Sex, Crime, Religion and Education* (New York: D. Appleton & Co., 1904), 2 vols, vol. 1, 458, cited by S. Humphries, *Hooligans or Rebels: An Oral History of Working Class Childhood* (Oxford: Basil Blackwell, 1981), 18.

12. Pam Cox, *Bad Girls: Gender Justice and Welfare* (London: Macmillan, 2001), on theories about delinquency among girls and the respective roles of theft and sexuality in its construction.

13 Victor Bailey, *Delinquency and Citizenship: Reclaiming the Young Offender 1914-1948* (Oxford: Clarendon Press, 1987).

14. Ian Gibson, *The English Vice: Beating, Sex and Shame in Victorian England and After* (London: Duckworth, 1978).

15. *Outlook*, 17 October 1908, 512, letter from XYZ.

16. *Outlook*, 31 October, 1908, 584, letter from MMcL.

17. H. Mannheim, *Social Aspects of Crime in England between the Wars* (London: George Allen & Unwin, 1940), chapters 9 and 10, on juvenile delinquency, 233–333.

18. *Final Report of the Departmental Committee on Juvenile Employment after the War*, vol. 1, cd. 8512, 1917, 8.

19. Cecil Leeson, *The Child and the War* (London: Howard League for Penal Reform, 1917), 22.

20. C.E.B. Russell, *The Problem of Juvenile Crime* (Oxford: Oxford University Press, 1917).

21. Leeson, *op. cit.* (note 19), 22.

22. *Ibid.*, 44.

23. *Ibid.*, 60.

24. Mannheim, *op. cit.* (note 17), 262–3.

25. D.Thom, 'Wishes, Anxieties, Play, and Gestures: Child Guidance in Inter-War England', in R. Cooter (ed.), *In the Name of the Child: Health and Welfare 1880-1940* (London: Routledge,1992), 200–19.

26. See Mathew Thomson, *The Problem of Mental Deficiency: Eugenics, Democracy and Social Policy in Britain c.1870-1940* (Oxford: Clarendon Press, 1998); Adrian Woolridge *Measuring the Mind: Education and Psychology in England* (Cambridge: Cambridge University Press, 1994) for a full account of the debates on the influence of eugenics on psychology, as well as the pioneering account of Gillian Sutherland, *Ability, Merit and Measurement: Mental Testing and English Education, 1880-1940* (Oxford: Clarendon Press, 1984).

27. One other volume was published in the series, *The Backward Child* (London: London University Press, 1937), but, sadly, the projected third volume *The Neurotic Child* never appeared.

28. Cyril Burt, *The Young Delinquent* (London: London University Press, 1925, revised 3rd edn 1938), 92.

29. *Ibid.,*148.

30. Board of Education, Juvenile Organisation Committee, *Report on Juvenile Delinquency* (London: HMSO, 1920), 12.

31. Burt, *op. cit.* (note 28), 5.

32. See Thom, *op. cit.* (note 25), and, for the American clinics, Margo Horn, *Before It's Too Late: The Child Guidance Movement in the United States, 1922-1945* (Philadelphia: Temple University Press, 1989).

33. Michel Foucault, *Discipline and Punish: The Birth of the Prison,* translated by Alan Sheridan (Harmondsworth: Penguin, 1991).

34. *Report of the Departmental Committee on Corporal Punishment* (the Cadogan Committee, henceforth CCP), Cmd 5684 (London: HMSO, 1938),16–19.

35. CCP, 22.

36. CCP, 32.

37. CCP, 33.

38. *British Medical Journal,* i (20 March 1937), 618.

39. Letter from HM Prison, Jersey, Dr P.G. Bentlif, prison medical superintendent.

40. *British Medical Journal,* i (3 June, 1939), 1132.

41. CCP, 46.

42. Board of Education circular 1504/Home Office circular 807624, *Juvenile Offences* (London: HMSO, 1941), 4.

43. *Ibid.,*11.

44. Ministry of Health, *Hostels for Difficult Children. A Survey of Experience under the Evacuation Scheme* (written by Claire Britton) (London,HMSO, 1943), 13.

45. Denise Riley, *War in the Nursery* (London:Virago, 1983).

46. *Annual Report of the Chief Medical Officer to the Board of Education:* Table of causes of death among school-children, for the years 1939-45 (London: HMSO, 1945), 72–5. These list deaths due to the war separately, and violence is 'other' violent deaths.

47. Department of Education and Science, *Children and their Primary School. A Report of the Central Advisory Council for Education* (London: HMSO,1967), 270–1.

48. D.H. Stott, *Studies of Troublesome Children* (London: Tavistock Publications, 1966) 80–2, citing Alec Clegg's unpublished paper

prepared for the Local Education Authority, 'Caning, behaviour and delinquency in secondary schools' (West Riding, 1961). The report also appears in *Education 1904-64*, West Riding Education Committee, 178–80.

49. S. Humphries and P. Gordon, *A Labour of Love: The Experience of Parenthood in Britain* (London: Sidgwick & Jackson), 184–5.

50. E. Roberts, *Women and Families: An Oral History, 1940-1970* (Oxford: Blackwell, 1995), 160–4.

51. Paul Thompson, *The Edwardians* (St Albans: Paladin, 1975), 62–7.

52. M.Willmott and M.Young, *Family and Kinship in East London* (London: Routledge and Kegan Paul, 1957), 27.

53. E.Ross, *Love and Toil* (Oxford: Oxford University Press, 1993), 150–2.

54. Lynn Jamieson,'The Experience of Being Brought Up', in Michael Drake (ed.), *Time, Family and Community* (Oxford: Blackwell, 1994), 106–28.

55. Donzelot, *op. cit.* (note 3), 209.

56. D.Winnicott, *The Child, the Family and the Outside World* (Rickmansworth: Penguin, 1957), 229.

10

Children's Emotional Well-being and Mental Health in Early Post-Second World War Britain: The Case of Unrestricted Hospital Visiting

Harry Hendrick

This chapter is intended to be a study in emotionology, which has been defined as 'the attitudes or standards that a society, or a definable group within a society, maintains towards basic emotions and their appropriate expression'.[1] The argument presented here is that between the late-1940s and the late-1950s something of a cultural shift began to occur (and the emphasis is on the early stages of what would be a long, drawn-out process) in the prevailing emotional standard by which the medical profession acknowledged and judged the emotions of hospitalised young children, in particular that known as 'separation anxiety'. No attempt is made, however, to examine the nature (psychological, physiological and philosophical) of emotions themselves; nor is the chapter concerned with the politics and day-to-day practices of what by the early 1960s had become an organised pressure group campaign. Instead, the intention is to show why and how the distress of pre-school patients at being separated from their parents, especially their mothers, came to be regarded as a legitimate emotion, deserving of 'entitlement', meaning ameliorative action on the part of those adults attending to their care.

After some introductory remarks, the chapter is divided into three parts, the first of which sets the scene for post-Second World War developments by outlining what will be a familiar trajectory of trends and influences involving the emotional welfare of children during the period circa 1918 to 1948. The purpose is to illustrate (albeit somewhat schematically) the different degrees of continuity and discontinuity in the making of a particular emotional standard, and also to show that sick children were the last group to have their 'feelings' included in the glossary of emotions. Part one, then, provides a brief overview of the following: the influence of the 'New Psychology' on child care and child guidance; the impact of

American psycho-medical research and the related appearance of liberal child-rearing literature during the 1940s; the significance of war-time evacuation schemes; and the changed perception of institutionalised children brought about by the Report of the government appointed Care of Children Committee (1946). The core of the chapter lies in part two, which examines of the role of John Bowlby, the child psychiatrist and psychoanalyst, and founder of the Separation Research Unit at the Tavistock Clinic, and that of James Robertson, his principal research officer and director of the seminal documentary film, 'A Two Year Old Goes to Hospital'. Bowlby and Robertson, it is argued, working within the environment of the 'Tavistock Programme', made a decisive contribution towards both a scientific and a popular understanding of the significance of 'separation anxiety' and, therefore, were instrumental in changing the attitude of society towards this emotion and its expression. In the concluding section, the focus switches to the sociology of emotions in order to draw attention to questions of power and authority in the making of emotional standards, and to identify children as sentient beings in possession of their own emotional perspectives.

Introduction

The developing awareness of and interest in children's emotions can best be understood if we appreciate the multi-faceted concern with the condition of national mental health in the early years of the new welfare state – a state, it should be remembered, that was marked by a sharp social democratic turn towards collectivism, and by the need to find its place in the emerging new world order which, as every political commentator understood, would be dominated by the Soviet Union and the United States on the one hand, and, on the other, would witness the birth of a new Europe. Influential persons within medicine, social science and party politics were coming to argue that in such a social and geopolitical climate, British social democracy required citizens who were not only willing and creative participants in groups, but also well-adjusted individuals in their own right. Consequently, within the context of a comprehensive concern for children's psychological welfare, the specific issue of hospital visiting became one of the areas where 'separation anxiety', as a psycho-analytic condition in young children, was held to constitute a direct threat to national fitness on three levels. Firstly, emotional deprivation in childhood could inhibit healthy character formation, thereby risking the emergence of a delinquent lifestyle; secondly, as the disturbed child grew into adulthood, it might be unable to develop effective parenting skills and so threaten the future of the normal family; thirdly, mental distress might easily frustrate the individual's ability to reach an equilibrium between fulfilling the demands of the self and those of society. This raised more than just the spectre of ill health; there was also the possibility of social and political conflict.

Prior to the 1940s there does not appear to have been any public suggestion that it was desirable for young children in hospital to be visited on either a daily or an unrestricted basis by their parents. Visiting times were usually once a week, once a month, or not at all. Sometimes no physical contact was allowed, with parents having to view their child through a window. It was well known that many children were upset on entering hospital, that they cried on being separated from their parents and that there were often distressful scenes when visiting time was over. Although this was regrettable, it was regarded as the inevitable consequence of being hospitalised. Many reasons were advanced to justify restricted visiting: parents could spread infections; their visits 'unsettled' the child; they disturbed hospital routines; some mothers were 'difficult'; there was no guarantee that all children would be regularly visited and, therefore, it would be unfair on those whose homes were far away, or whose parents were too busy with home commitments, to see other children having daily visits; and, anyway, only a minority of mothers asked for either longer visiting hours or to stay overnight.

In 1943, however, Harry Edelston, a Leeds psychiatrist, in a series of case histories, tried to draw attention to the risk of psychological damage caused by 'hospitalisation trauma', but the concept met with fierce resistance from his colleagues. A few years later, L.A. Parry, a consultant surgeon, supported by an editorial in *Nursing Times*, also called for urgent reform. A further sign of growing disquiet came in 1949, perhaps in response to the new interest in hospitals as a result of the establishment of the National Health Service in 1948 (NHS), when the *Spectator*, a weekly magazine, published the results of a survey of visiting hours in London hospitals, showing that the majority allowed visiting at best for one or two hours a week, and that at two hospitals no visiting of any description was allowed for children under three. This was followed by the first of several circulars, issued by the Ministry of Health (MOH), asking hospitals to liberalise their visiting regimes, but to no avail.[2] Within the year, the matter assumed the full glare of press publicity when the annual conference of the National Federation of Women's Institutes (NFWI) passed a motion deploring visiting restrictions and called upon

Hospital Management Committees to make the necessary changes: 'Cruel to keep us away, plead 438,000 women' (*Daily Mirror*).[3] The issue was of increasing importance given the large number of children involved: on census night 1951, 46,856 children aged 4 weeks to 14 years were hospitalised, and the annual figure was approximately 685,000.[4] Moreover, as a government report later noted, in the years before the NHS, hospital patients were often from poverty-stricken backgrounds, 'while children of better families were nursed at home or in private nursing homes. Today… (the) NHS (has) widened the hospitals' sphere to cover the whole community… Hence new attitudes to patients of all ages are demanded.'[5] Thus, by the early-1950s a debate was under way.

**Psycho-medicine,
child-rearing and social policy 1920s-40s**

The 'New Psychology' and its Influence

Inter-war and wartime developments were crucial in promoting what were relatively new attitudes towards children as psychological persons, especially in respect of beliefs about the nature and role of their emotions vis-à-vis their intellectual, social and emotional growth. A number of accounts have shown that as the inter-war years progressed, the realm of child-rearing advice mutated from an emphasis on habit formation to a recognition and understanding of the emotions – from 'problems of management to problems of meaning'.[6] This is not to say that there was a comprehensive rebuttal of the former in favour of the latter for throughout the period the dominant voices were those of J.B.Watson, the American behaviourist, whose theories of baby care had little time for wishes, sentiment or tenderness, and F. Truby King, the New Zealand doctor, who was a popular advocate of strict regularity in all areas of infant feeding and management. Nevertheless,the 'New Psychology', which emerged in the aftermath of the First World War, and slowly gained influence, viewed the experiences of a child in its family as being integral to proper emotional and mental development. The importance of the family lay in its ability to channel and organise the child's impulses in such a way as to produce a harmoniously balanced individual. In part this was done through habit training, but also through personal relationships between parents and children. And it was integral to this process that parents should respect the child's 'self regard', for this was responsible for the direction of the will. This way of conceptualising the child emphasised two distinct insights:

216

children might be in conflict with their nurturing environment, and the significance of the natural, biological family[7] - both of which highlighted the role of emotions, which were now coming to be seen as guides to the course of mental health.

Among the more influential authors propounding such views was Susan Isaacs, educationalist and psychoanalyst, who, through her books, especially the much reprinted *The Nursery Years* (1929) and her advice column in *Nursery World* (1929-36), advised parents to be liberal and tolerant towards their children and to understand that they had their own perspectives. Isaacs was by no means a solitary figure: what was in effect a psychodynamic approach to child-rearing was also clearly advocated in John Rickman (ed.), *On the Upbringing of Children* (1935), a series of lectures given by child analysts. Other well-known studies included a number of articles by Margaret Lowenfeld, director of the Clinic for Nervous and Difficult Children, which were intended to explain the reasons for children's antisocial behaviour.[8] The emphasis on understanding was reiterated through the publications of the Home and Schools Council, where it was stressed that while children should be brought up to make a contribution to the community, they had to 'be ready and glad to make it'. The child must not only be a good citizen, 'but, if possible, a happy one'.[9] The message of all these texts was that besides the regulation of habits and morals, sympathetic consideration should be given to anxieties, fears, wishes and aspirations. If any of these were ignored, the result might be either troubled or troublesome children.

Many, if not the majority, of the new authorities on child care came from the child guidance movement as it developed from the 1920s onwards. Although the clinics, of which there were more than 40 by 1939, represented many different analytic persuasions, they were all committed 'to understanding children's problems, from acute anxiety, phobias and nightmares, to bed-wetting, truancy, stealing and aggressiveness – problems now to be understood in terms of deeper aspects of mentality and emotion'.[10] The child guidance movement acted 'to integrate a range of diverse concerns and orientations into a coherent framework of argument and advice'.[11] This meant that the clinics were intended to be co-ordinating centres for research, investigation, analysis and treatment of disturbed children. To this end, the movement was important in spreading the vision of the child as a person with a mental and emotional interiority, requiring careful and sensitive management if it were to grow into a mature and healthy adult.

•

The influence of American psycho-medical research and the coming of liberal child care

In many respects the post-war literature on hospital visiting was a continuation of work begun in the 1930s, though not published by and large until the 1940s, much of it originating in America. The research fell into five categories: the emotional significance of illness; the effects of long-term hospitalisation; programmes of ward management in pursuit of children's 'mental well-being'; accounts of institutional practices; and the role of the ward nurse in relation to patients and parents.[12] Several of the specific observations focussed on the effects on personality development of prolonged institutional care/or lack of a permanent mother-figure during the child's early years. Among the best-known and most authoritative authors, whose work would be further publicised by Bowlby in his famous World Health Organisation (WHO) Report (1951), were Levy (1937), Bender and Yarnell (1941, 1947), Spitz (1945, 1946, and 1947), and Goldfarb (1943). The work of Goldfarb and Spitz, for example, was widely cited with reference to the claim that maternal deprivation could result in lasting emotional damage and that it risked impairing an individual's ability to make stable and co-operative relationships with other people.[13]

The other American influence on the prevailing emotional standard was the new philosophy being advocated in the child-rearing literature which, prompted by war and fear of the consequences of authoritarian regimes, such as fascism and communism, promoted liberal parent-child relations and, in so doing, added to the significance being attached to maternal care and the family environment. The swing against Watsonian behaviourism began in the late-1930s with the publication of Anderson and Mary Aldrich's *Babies are Human Beings*, which was followed by two ground-breaking anti-authoritarian texts: Dorothy Barauch, *Your Children and War* and C.Madelaine Dixon, *Keep Them Human*. The outcome of the trend was Benjamin Spock's *The Common Sense Book of Baby and Child Care*.[14]

It is worth pausing a moment to look in a little more detail at Spock since he represents what is perhaps the best-known example (apart from Bowlby) of a 'popular' social scientist who consciously responds to what are said to be the social and political issues of his time, through seeking to influence them. In order to appreciate the significance of Spock, and how he connects with the British debate on child care in general, the historical fixture of his book has to be recognised. Spock was part of a generation which was deeply affected by the Depression, the rise of totalitarian regimes, and the war itself.[15] In such an unstable, threatened and threatening world, Spock felt that it was necessary to create a society that was 'more cooperative, more consensus-orientated, more group conscious…'; thus he was led to develop 'a "democratic" model of child-rearing, featuring the family as a small group, the parent as group leader, and the child as an occasional participant in the group-making process'.[16] This model was not Spock's alone. It was the product of American social science, in particular the writings of Kurt Lewin, the social psychologist , who was well-known for his experiments into the workings of democracy and group leadership, and whose ideas would figure in Bowlby's political thinking, while resonating throughout the post-war 'social psychiatric' practices at the Tavistock Institute of Human relations.[17] Spock, then, embraced, and gave expression to, a particular social scientific ethic, which contemporaries expounded in pursuit of a stable environment for liberal democracy.

Evacuation and the Curtis Report on the care of children

The foregoing suggests that for a decade or more prior to the emergence of the hospital reform debate of the 1950s, there was a growing literature devoted to the psychological effects of separation on personality development, the importance of democratic child-rearing and the propriety of the mother-child relationship. However, as historians of social policy know so well, what finally shaped the diverse concerns of child care workers, from psychiatric as well as social welfare backgrounds, was the social and political reaction to evacuation and the appointment of the Curtis Committee to enquire into the care of children deprived of a normal home life. In that they opened up a number of welfare topics for discussion, popularised more humane attitudes to child care, and made specific recommendations relating to children's mental health and physical well-being, both are crucial to any understanding of the evolution of the emotional standard pertaining to the distress experienced by young hospital patients.

In the realm of research into children's emotional disturbance, a particularly important context was provided by the various wartime evacuation schemes. Among many child psychiatrists evacuation was always a controversial process, being described by one of them as 'a cruel psychological experiment on a large scale'.[18] Once in progress, the schemes offered doctors, educationalists, social workers, and psychologists and psychiatrists unique opportunities to study several hundred thousand children - in the first wave 826,959 were sent to reception areas. One important study, the *Cambridge Evacuation Survey*, under the editorship of Susan Isaacs, stressed the central theme of much of the research, namely the significance 'of family ties and of feelings of parents and children towards one another'. Unfortunately, those responsible for the schemes were said to be unaware of the 'strength of the family tie ... and the need for skilled understanding of the individual child'.[19] And the point, with respect to pre-school children, was reiterated in Burlingham and Freud's influential accounts of their wartime residential nursery.[20] It was well known, they wrote, that food and vitamins were essential for proper bodily development in early childhood. Less widely recognised was that in the absence of the fulfilment of essential psychological needs – 'personal attachment', 'emotional stability', and 'permanency of educational influence' – 'lasting psychological malformations will be the consequence'.[21] As Nikolas Rose has observed, the distinguishing feature of these studies was that they showed how fragile was the life of *normal* children, unlike others which had dealt with those already suffering from emotional disturbance.[22] This was the critical consideration where young hospitalised children were concerned: though they were 'normal' on entering hospital, many reformers claimed that their personality development risked being fractured through enforced and prolonged separation from their parents.

Hardly had discussion of the consequences of evacuation subsided, when a new debate arose over the direction of post-war social policy for neglected children. In 1945 the government somewhat reluctantly appointed the Curtis Committee to inquire into the care of children who were deprived of 'a normal home life with their own parents or relatives'.[23] The Committee's Report and the subsequent Children Act (1948) are too familiar to require detailed consideration here,[24] though the psycho-analytic presence among the committee's key witnesses should be noted.[25] The central message of the Report was the recognition that in many local authority and charitable Homes, 'The child... was not regarded as an individual with his rights and possessions, his own life to live and his own contributions to offer... Still more important, he was without the feeling that there was someone to whom he could turn who was vitally interested in his welfare or who cared for him as a person.'[26]

In the light of the hospital visiting debate, the importance of Curtis was twofold. First, the emphasis on the nurturing role of the family and the attention given to 'separation' confirmed the growing view among social workers that the latter, in certain circumstances, could be emotionally damaging. Second, in recognising the significance of the 'self', the Report highlighted the role of psychological health in a child's development: children were to be treated as individuals whose experiences could mark them for life, especially in their personal relationships. As was noted years later, the establishment of a comprehensive child care service, under the Children Act, 1948, meant that 'New understandings of the *emotional* (emphasis added) needs of children began to seep through';[27] they did not, however, reach as far as the hospital service. Nevertheless, both the Report and the Act, through their focus on children's emotionality, made important contributions towards the change in emotional standards and certainly helped to prepare the way for the debate on hospital visiting regimes.

The 'Tavistock Programme', John Bowlby's Separation Research Unit and James Robertson's film, 'A Two Year Old Goes to Hospital'

The 'Tavistock Programme'

The politics of mental health raised a number of concerns among contemporaries during and after the Second World War. On the one hand, the war appeared to illuminate several sources of anxiety: for example, anti-social behaviour, moral uncertainties, the effects of bereavement and, not least, the condition of the evacuees and their families. On the other hand, there was the global context to consider: the emergence of the Soviet empire, the growth of nationalism and communism within the British empire, the stirrings of a New Europe, and the political and economic supremacy of the USA. In Britain, the election of a left-wing government, accompanied by aspirations to social justice, collectivism and democratic citizenship, posed several potential difficulties for the place of the individual in the community. At the same time, the post-war 'consensus' around the government's commitment to full employment, the erection of a comprehensive, universal and free social services system, and the creation of a National Health Service made it seem as if all social problems deriving from lack of income and ill health were well on their way to being solved. Even so, many social and medical scientists feared that psychological ailments, and estimates suggested than one third of all illnesses were psychological in nature,[28] were in danger of being ignored or of passing unnoticed, owing to difficulties inherent in recognising symptoms. Psychological science, however, they argued, working in common with sociology, could not only identify and attend to mental illness, but also could help to structure human relationships in such a way as to promote health, harmony, productivity, happiness and stability – all through the development of an individual's emotional maturity.

The programme for the theory and practice of preventive mental health strategies was most clearly articulated at the Tavistock Clinic and the newly established Tavistock Institute of Human Relations (TIHR). Having been founded in 1920, the Tavistock was revitalised after the war, in large part by what was known as the 'army group': psychiatrists and psychologists who had worked together under J.R.Rees, at the time director of the Tavistock and consultant psychiatrist to the army.[29] The war was important in encouraging a particular kind of psycho-medical approach for it illustrated the links between minor mental problems and major pathologies, as well as the extent of minor disturbances, and, therefore, the potential danger of debilitating consequences. Thus, after the war, the group began practising 'social psychiatry', which involved associating psychiatry (as a 'therapeutic agency') with social psychology and social medicine.[30] This approach soon attracted the financial attention of the Rockefeller Foundation with a donation of £20,000 in 1946 for the establishment of the TIHR. The plan was for the TIHR to focus on social psychiatric activities while the Clinic, which had been absorbed into the NHS, would concentrate on patient care and training programmes.[31] In this way, the clinical and the sociological would be linked together so as to enable staff to devise programmes for what Miller and Rose have termed 'the government of subjectivity and social life' - involving families, communities, institutions and industrial organisations - the purpose of which was 'the transformation of the conception of citizenship in the post-war era'.[32]

At the centre of the desire to create a form of citizenship suitable for the new democracies lay 'group relations' theory. The concept of 'the group' owed much to the development of armed-service psychological selection procedures during the war,[33] and to the influence of Kurt Lewin.[34] (Until Lewin's death in 1948, there was a close connection between the TIHR and his Research Center for Group Dynamics at MIT, and together the two institutions established the journal *Human Relations* as an outlet for their ideas.) For those who were concerned to create a balanced and efficient relationship between the individual and the collective, the group concept was of primary relevance. Many social scientists saw such a relationship as an essential prerequisite for the emergence of a 'humanist morality',[35] one that was intended to reflect the superiority of western democracies over authoritarian regimes. The danger lurked in the alienation of the individual from the group as, for example, in the post-war demobilisation period when it was feared there would be 'a loosening of bonds of mutual support of the larger group loyalties... The social conscience of the individual... will be weakened and there will be a return of personal ambition and self-centredness...'.[36] As Wilfrid Bion, one of the principal advocates of social psychiatry, wrote 'the failure arises when it comes to producing any method for dealing with underlying emotional tensions in human relationships. And yet it is precisely these primitive unconscious tensions which present the fundamental problem in all human relationships.'[37] This emphasis on 'human relationships' operated at two levels: that of individuals in one-to-one contact and that of the individual and the group. Much of the concern for children's mental and physical welfare, certainly from the 1930s onwards, was motivated by the expressed need to produce 'citizens' who would be able to function harmoniously in both respects. As we shall see, this objective was at the heart of Bowlby's Separation Research Unit, and it fed directly into his interest in the hospital visiting issue.

John Bowlby and the Tavistock Separation Research Unit

In the post-war reorganisation of the Tavistock Clinic, Bowlby, who had worked at the London Child Guidance Clinic before the war, was appointed head of the Children's Department in 1946 (renamed the Parents' and Children's Department in 1950), and by 1947 he was also Deputy Director of the Clinic. In the initial grant application to the Rockefeller Foundation for the establishment of the TIHR, it was stated that there would be more emphasis placed on collaboration with paediatricians, obstetricians, local authority child-care workers and education authorities. This was regarded as essential given the recognition of 'the growing awareness of the significance of childhood in individual and social development'.[38] Bowlby, of course, had long been aware of this significance. He was interested in the idea of 'separation' because he wanted to emphasise the importance of the environment and the interaction between it and the child (in opposition to the Kleinians who saw the child 'almost as a closed system').[39] After securing a couple of small grants, Bowlby established his Separation Research Unit in 1948 which, from the outset, cooperated with the TIHR, and was financially supported during the next decade by the WHO, the International Children's Centre in Paris and, most generously, by the Rockefeller, Ford and Joseph Macy, Jr., Foundations.[40] There is no doubt, then, that Bowlby was closely associated with the political and medical objectives of the 'Tavistock Programme', the American Foundations (which were deeply involved in sustaining the 'American way of life' in a period of rabid anti-communism), and the growing international interest in mental health as an ethical and political goal.[41]

This raises the question: what was the nature of Bowlby's political position and how did it relate to his research and his interest in hospital visiting? Important insights into his political thinking are evident in a paper he delivered in 1947 to a Fabian conference on 'The Psychological and Sociological Problems of Modern Socialism', in which his theme was 'liberty and democracy'.[42] It is perhaps easy now to forget the urgency of the notion of 'willing co-operation' in the post-war era - a period of widespread economic and social reconstruction. As Bowlby said: 'The necessity of humanity learning to live together peacefully and co-operatively has never been greater'. One of the principal problems was how to overcome the psychological difficulties in persistent cooperative behaviour; such a society would be 'historically rare' and would require a balance of psychological and social forces 'not easily attained'. The problem of ensuring co-operative behaviour stemmed fundamentally from the fact that it required from the individual some degree of denial or frustration. This could be enforced through fear and compulsion, but in a democracy it has to be voluntarily accepted. Here Bowlby cited the example of the Tennessee Valley Authority scheme which, through a model of grass-roots democracy, was said to have created 'a remarkable degree of willing co-operation and in so doing released undreamed of reserves of social energy'. In the same vein, he referred to the work of Kurt Lewin, in particular his experiments in boys' clubs where it was found that those run on democratic lines produced 'a marked feeling of "we'ness" rather than "I'ness"'. Although willing co-operation demanded a commonly accepted objective, it also required libidinalisation of group aims, which could be best facilitated if the individual's earliest libidinal relationship – with the mother – was undisturbed. Failing this, the child would experience frustration and hostility, which could have long-term consequences for its emotional development. It was on the basis of the simple, loving, sympathetic and tolerant family pattern 'that all later personal relationships rest'. And properly functioning personal relationships were a political necessity as post-war Britain required 'an understanding and acceptance of the need for inevitable controls required for… full employment, a maximising of production… or a maximising of personal efficiency'. Such collective goals required the sacrifice of private goals. In his closing remarks, Bowlby referred to the Labour government's commitment to a 'high degree of internal and external co-operation', made even more important with the 'advent of the atomic bomb'. Such a weapon could not be controlled either by moral exhortation or fear of punishment. 'The hope for the future lies in a far more profound understanding of the nature of emotional forces involved and the development of scientific techniques for studying them.'

It seems reasonable to assume that Bowlby brought these concerns to his research. However, the Research Unit was little more than a year into its first project on 'The Effects on Personality Development of Separation from the Mother in Early Childhood'[43] when Bowlby was asked by the WHO to report on the mental health aspects of the problem of homeless children in their native countries. He proceeded to travel throughout Europe and America, talking to researchers and practitioners while familiarising himself with the literature. The resulting volume, *Maternal Care and Mental Health* (1951), propelled him into international fame, and, where the changing attitude towards children's emotions was concerned, besides emphasising the psychological nature of social distress, it promoted both the idea of 'maternal deprivation' and its relationship to 'some origins of mental ill-health':

> what is believed to be essential for mental health is that the infant and young child should experience a warm, intimate, and continuous relationship with his mother (or permanent mother substitute) in which both find satisfaction and enjoyment. Given this relationship, the emotions of anxiety and guilt, which in excess characterise mental ill-health, will develop in a moderate and organised way... The outstanding disability of persons suffering from mental illness... is their inability to make and sustain confident, friendly, and co-operative relations with others... The growth of this ability... is determined to a very high degree by the quality of the child's relation to his parents in his early years.[44]

Bowlby made clear the social and political implications of neglect when he concluded that the proper care of deprived children:

> can now be seen to be not merely an act of common humanity, but to be essential for the mental and social welfare of a community ... (such children) are a source of social infection as real and serious as are the carriers of diptheria and typhoid. And just as preventive measures have reduced these diseases... so can determined action

greatly reduce the number of deprived children… and the growth of adults liable to produce them.[45]

The influence of this message can perhaps be gauged from the fact that the Report was reprinted in 1953 in an abridged form as *Mother Care and the Growth of Love*, eventually selling over 400,000 copies in the English edition alone, and was translated into fourteen languages.[46] Unsurprisingly, as one reviewer noted, the Report marked 'a turning point in the study of the mental hygiene of childhood'.[47] The power of the image of 'maternal deprivation' was derived from the real experiences of millions of neglected children throughout post-war Europe: orphaned, deserted, neurotic, delinquent, angry, frightened and often hungry. Besides being an affront to the humanist principles enunciated by democratic societies, these children were also a threat to such societies – both in their present condition and as citizens of tomorrow.

There is little doubt that when the Separation Research Unit turned its attention towards hospitalised children, it did so under the auspice of the 'Tavistock Programme' and in particular Bowlby's growing international reputation. Bowlby, however, does not appear to have been responsible for initiating what came to be called 'Hospital Visiting Project No.1'. According to his own account of events, the London Advisory Committee, associated with the Research Unit from its inception, consisting of representatives from paediatrics, nursing, child psychiatry, psychology and social work, 'pressed for operational research into the problems associated with the visiting of children in hospital'.[48] Work began on the Project in April 1951 when James Robertson, principal research officer at the Unit, made a reconnaissance of the problem. At the time, the Unit's research emphasis was on separation among school children, rather than those of a pre-school age and, therefore, only limited resources were put into the Project between 1950 and 1953. Bowlby later admitted that this had been a mistake 'since, as experience deepened, it became increasingly clear that here was a particularly fruitful field of enquiry'. Indeed, as it turned out, 'this has been the unit's most useful endeavour'.[49]

If Bowlby was relatively slow to grasp the significance of the visiting issue for his own research, he also seems to have been a little anxious about the fact that 'public sensitivity… and… pressures… spring largely from humanism'. 'Our role', he wrote, 'is to keep clear of partisan involvement'.[50] Thus he was careful to specify that the research concern was not simply with unrestricted visiting as 'a form of social amenity', but with the extent to which nursing and visiting 'can safeguard the mental health of the child'.[51] The relevance of 'separation anxiety', however, was vehemently disputed in hospitals where, as Bowlby reported, resistance is 'high... for many reasons' and as a result 'we find that the progress of our concepts... is much slower than in the child care field'.[52] Notwithstanding medical opposition, by the early-1950s the reform of hospital visiting practices was publicly associated with both Bowlby (and Robertson) and the work of the Tavistock's Separation Research Unit.

James Robertson and his film: 'A Two Year Old Goes to Hospital'

In 1948, Robertson, who was the sole field worker in the Unit, began to visit London hospitals in search of samples of children who would be suitable for Bowlby's research project.[53] During these and other visits over the next three years (including those for the 'Hospital Visiting Project'), Robertson came face to face with what he saw as the trauma of separation as it affected young children. He felt that older children could cope with the situation: they were used to going to school; they had a sense of time; they could match explanations with their own experience; and they had some understanding that the medical staff were there to help them to get well. But where younger children were concerned, especially those aged three and under, Robertson observed them as quiet, tearful, desolate and overwhelmed: 'If a nurse stopped beside a silent toddler, he would usually burst into tears at the human contact and the nurse would be rebuked for "making him unhappy". A quiet ward was prized above all, so nurses kept away from recently admitted young patients except to feed and clean them.'[54] When Robertson mentioned his unease at the situations he was observing to hospital staff, he met with almost universal opposition: 'there was an enormous meshing of defences against acknowledging the distress and psychological deterioration in young patients. I saw defences so powerful that the kindest of staff could be wholly unaware of the emotional abuse they were practising and colluding in.'[55] And even with colleagues at the Tavistock, he had 'a sense of the inadequacy of words to convey what I saw and how I understood it'. The typical response was to say that the distress he witnessed was 'usual and inevitable and that because it was commonplace there was no cause for concern'. All young children were unhappy and tearful at first, but within a few hours or days they 'settled down', in time they would 'forget' their mothers. Parental visiting was generally frowned upon since it was said to 'upset' children. In every hospital Robertson visited, he found the same situation: 'staff inattention to distress in young patients because it was thought unimportant and would soon pass'. When he did follow-up research with selected children back in their own homes, it was often found that the 'settled' child of the ward developed behavioural problems where none had previously existed, such as 'clinging to the mother, temper tantrums, disturbed sleep, bed-wetting, regression and aggression particularly against the mother as if blaming her'.[56] Robertson's frustration stemmed from his inability to show the continuum of the young patient's emotional states. Within the hospital ward children were seen as '"content" or "cheerful" or "friendly" or "tearful" or whatever'. While the child's physical changes were noted on a day-by-day basis, behavioural patterns were not.[57] During the course of his work, Robertson had read about the power of visual communication and, with the intention of educating both his colleagues and paediatricians, he decided to make a film record of a child's short stay in hospital in order to examine and re-examine what was shown and to avoid mis-understandings that could arise from either the written or purely verbal form.[58]

The resulting silent film, 'A Two Year Old Goes to Hospital' (1952) premiered at the Royal Society of Medicine and immediately became controversial, but also influential. At the initial showing and after there were bitter denunciations and calls for it to be withdrawn. Robertson explained the abusive attacks as 'a desperate attempt to maintain the myth that had sustained the hospital professions for generations – the myth that children's wards were happy places, that young patients "settled" and became content in the absence of their parents'. The visual record 'had pierced the defences and compelled attention to the problem'.[59] Bowlby, however, decided that the film should not be given a general release outside the medical profession for fear that it would encourage public protests against hospital procedures and, therefore harden resistance to reform. Consequently, it was not widely shown until 1957.[60] Even so, the British Film Institute declared the film a work of 'national and historic importance', the WHO bought many copies for international distribution, it was discussed at international conferences, and became a standard text in schools of psychiatry, psychology, social work and nursing. Robertson embarked on a lecture tour of Britain and North America and, together with Bowlby, wrote several articles. Robertson became the acknowledged expert on the matter, so much so that it was he who submitted the official Tavistock (TIHR) memorandum to the government inquiry into the welfare of hospitalised children.[61]

The importance of Robertson's observations and of the film were two-fold: where previously parental visiting was said to 'upset' young children, he showed that it was merely *revealing* the distress which had been 'hidden by the quiet exterior of the "settled" child'. Similarly, when the child cried to a friendly, sympathetic nurse, she was not causing the distress, but *discovering* it. Secondly, three phases of 'separation anxiety' were identified (according to JR he formulated them): Protest, Despair and Denial (later changed by Bowlby to Detachment). Protest was the initial phase, involving crying, shaking, throwing about, and eager looks towards any sight or sound that suggested the arrival of parents. This was followed by Despair, characterised by a 'continuing conscious need of the mother coupled with an increasing hopelessness'. The physical movements have diminished or ended and crying has become quietly monotonous and intermittent. The child is withdrawn, undemanding of the environment and in a state of 'deep mourning'. Denial gradually succeeds Despair and appears to suggest that the child is settling in. In reality, this is a device for coping with distress. The child finds the distress intolerable and, therefore, begins to repress feelings for the mother. Also, in addition to the need for the mother, the child needs food and comfort, and these are pursued in the third phase.[62]

It has been said that the film let in a 'shaft of light' on the subject of visiting, but that it was only one influence among many.[63] Another contemporary described it as the single most influential event in the campaign for reform.[64] Of course, in some respects, both opinions may be true. On the one hand, the film cannot be separated from the social psychiatric role of the Tavistock in the community and that of Bowlby who, by the 1950s, was an internationally respected figure. Bowlby clearly provided the fundamental scientific substance for the arguments that the film was said to illustrate.[65] On the other hand, aside from Spitz's American film, 'Grief – A Peril in Infancy' (1946), this was the first time that film had been used to document a child's emotional journey during a period of anxiety and in a frightening environment. Robertson identified the power of visual representation and its ability to portray emotion through moving images. The audible silence of the images (in its original form, the film was also without a commentary) reinforced the spectacle of 'the body', which was both the messenger and the expression of the distress. The former made known the condition, while the latter staked out an identity. Bearing in mind how little is known about children as patients, it is useful to think sociologically here: to see the body not simply as a material form, but as an experiential subjective experience.[66] In sum, the cinematic narrative inclined the viewer to think of the child as a human being in and for itself.

Furthermore, the film was unique in that it provided not only a longitudinal record, which could be examined over and over again - every facial expression, every bodily movement (many of which were easily missed amid the preoccupations of a busy ward), but also it compelled the viewer to *look* and to *see* in new ways (indeed, it connected 'looking' to 'seeing'- it made viewers active rather than passive): for example, to look at what the child was *not* doing – not crying or calling for its mother; not throwing itself about in the cot – this, it warned, was the danger sign: doctors and nurses should not be deceived by the apparently 'settled' child. Similarly, hospital staff should *see* the crying child as *distressed*, not as 'demanding', or 'naughty' or 'spoilt'. Instead of dismissing the distress as 'natural', meaning temporary and, therefore, unimportant, it was to be seen as meaningful and, therefore, of significance. The point was well made by Ronald MacKeith, a sympathetic paediatrician. 'The film,' he remarked, 'opens our eyes to the quiet unhappiness that a young child in hospital may suffer much of the day, almost unnoticed by the nurses and doctors. We do not want to see the grief and we see only a "good" quiet child. If a child is crying, we may equate this... to the crying of a small child who is hungry or has fallen. We tend to dismiss all crying as unimportant.' And, he added, 'doctors, nurses, and parents all do well to give a child, however small, credit for understanding - or feeling – what is said or felt'.[67]

None of this is to deny that there were other influences, besides that of the film. From 1948 onwards the general medical, nursing and child welfare press, drawing upon the research and practice of a number of psycho-medics, began the long process of educating their readers in the importance of children's mental and emotional health. The picture emerging from the articles and editorials (many of which referred to Bowlby and Robertson) was one that showed the child in several different contexts: as a citizen, as a fragile participant in family relationships, as vulnerable to trauma, and as a person, and while not all of these were new in themselves, together they presented the child as a psychological individual with a developing sense of self.[68] In so doing, this literature implicitly questioned the prevailing emotional standard and proposed a number of critical revisions.

Where the film, together with Robertson's writings and those of Bowlby, can certainly be said to have been a significant influence, was as evidence given before the government appointed Committee on the Welfare of Children in Hospital, under the chairmanship of Sir Harry Platt, the distinguished orthopaedic surgeon. Robertson was invited to show both his films (in 1958 he had made another: 'Going to Hospital with Mother') and, as previously mentioned, he also authored the official memorandum from the Tavistock and the TIHR. In its Report (1959), the committee acknowledged the role of the TIHR in educating public opinion and concluded:

> We are unanimous in our opinion that the emotional needs of the child in hospital require constant consideration. Changes of environment and separation from familiar people are upsetting and frequently lead to emotional disturbances which vary in degree and may sometimes last well into adult life.[69]

Among the 55 recommendations were two that would be central to the reform movement as it developed from the 1960s onwards: unrestricted visiting and the provision of overnight accommodation for mothers of under fives. Despite government acceptance of the recommendations, the majority of hospitals continued to resist liberalising their visiting hours.

By this time Robertson was no longer merely a member of Bowlby's research unit, he was an active campaigner. His submission to the Platt Committee was published in 1958 and was quickly translated into eight European languages and Japanese. *The Guardian* (particularly through the Women's Page under the editorship of Mary Stott) and *The Observer* newspapers were increasingly committed to unrestricted visiting and in January 1961 Robertson wrote an article for the former and three for the latter.[70] A month or so later excerpts from his films were shown on BBC television where, at the end of a discussion with sympathetic paediatricians, Robertson (apparently ignoring direction from the producer) spoke directly to the camera and appealed to parents to tell him about the experiences of their children in paediatric wards.[71] The programme and *The Observer* articles drew over four hundred letters, which were published in book form. Among the viewers of the television programme was Jane Thomas, a young mother living in Battersea who, after seeking Robertson's advice, contacted several of her neighbours and together they launched Mother Care for Children in Hospital (MCCH) in order to campaign for the implementation of the Platt Report. In 1965, in recognition of the broad membership of the reform movement, MCCH changed its name to the National Association for the Welfare of Children in Hospital.[72]

Children and emotional standards

This chapter has sought to argue that during the 1950s the prevailing emotional standard with respect to the treatment of young hospitalised children began to undergo change and development. Contemporary participants in the debate, whatever their position, were in no doubt that 'emotions' in relation to emotional growth lay at the core of mental health. The contested issue was the relative importance of different forms of childhood distress. But, it may be asked, why are emotions important, and what is an emotional standard, and how does it arise? Furthermore, given that the standard was eventually moderated with greater sensitivity towards children, in what way did they benefit from the changes, and how was the child-adult relationship affected? By way of a brief answer to these questions, it will be helpful to consider them from the sociology of emotions perspective – as 'a way of seeing'. This will enable us to focus on the 'sociocultural *determinants* of feeling' as well as the 'sociocultural bases' through which emotions and feelings are defined, appraised and managed.[73]

First, what is 'emotion'? There is no clear answer since differences of opinion abound within academic study. At a basic level, emotions cover a wide range of phenomena: knee-jerk responses to fright, loyalty, feelings of hunger and thirst, moods of contentment or depression, and so on. The search for an exact definition, though, is bound to be elusive since both the definition and the experience are always known within particular sociocultural meanings: 'The very mutability, ephemerality and intangible nature of "the emotions", as well as their inextricable interlinking with and emergence from constantly changing social, cultural and historical contexts, means that they are not amenable to precise categorisation.'[74] And yet, however difficult they are to define, they remain a constant source of grounding for our lives. Why is this? In general, because 'emotionality lies at the intersection of the personal and society'. We are all joined to our societies 'through self-feelings and emotions' which we 'feel and experience on a daily basis'. Thus, 'to be human is to be emotional'.[75] In other words, emotions are essential for the integrity of the self; thinking about emotions draws attention to feelings and the manner in which they help us to constitute our subjectivity. Emotions, in effect, are 'ways of experiencing relationships between embodied selfhood and existence. Along with being hungry, thirsty, wide-awake, tired... being emotional is a fundamental mode of being.'[76] These considerations are of special importance for the historical study of children, since it is so easy to overlook the legitimacy of their emotions; to dismiss them, as was done with respect to 'separation anxiety', as being 'childish' (natural) and, therefore, of no significance. In this way the cries of the young patients were silenced by an adult-centric form of logic that explained their 'experience' by reference to their age, while simultanenously drawing upon an equally adultist perception of their age (one that underplays reason and feeling) to describe their experience.

Turning to ask what is an emotional standard and how it arises (and how is it maintained), at the outset it is worthwhile reminding ourselves that there is indeed such a standard. Emotions do not free-float, willy-nilly, in an all-embracing egalitarian universe. In her influential sociological study, *The Managed Heart*, Arlie Russell Hochschild refers to the 'emotional dictionary' and to concepts of 'emotion management', 'feeling rules', and 'status shields'.[77] The 'emotional dictionary' – 'a giant cultural entity' – is a particularly useful idea where adult-child relations are involved, given the degree to which these are governed through adult power and authority, for by definition it includes only those feelings which are held to be 'feelable'.[78] The dictionary, as Hochschild says, reflects 'agreement among the authorities of a given time and place':[79] in the case of the welfare of sick children, it represented the collective view of the hospital profession (and, broadly speaking, of the wider society). Clearly, however, during the 1950s new and critical voices (from within and outside of medical science) began to challenge the composition of the existing conceptual vocabulary, so that gradually (over many years) the 'separation anxiety' became 'legitimate' and, therefore, began to be included in the list of references. However, it should not be overlooked that the vast majority of these voices were stimulated by international and national political interests far removed from a simple concern with the contentment of children. Only when a sufficient number of influential adults deemed the *consequences* of children's distress (not the distress itself) to be a danger to mental health and the long-term social stability of society did attitudes began to change – the dictionary, that 'giant cultural entity', was amended. Occasionally, the 'humanism' of the issue was mentioned, as when Dermod MacCarthy, a paediatric reformer, proclaimed: 'Our primary concern is to prevent the unhappiness that is caused to young patients by separation from the mother. The possibility of after-effects or lasting harm has always been a secondary consideration.'[80] The prevention of such unhappiness was undoubtedly the concern of a minority of hospital staff, several Ministry officials, and of Robertson himself. On balance, though, it is hard to conclude that it was ever anything other than a 'secondary consideration' for the medical scientists with their social-psychiatric agendas.

If an emotion is not in the dictionary, how, then, does the individual child deal with it? Prior to the acceptance of 'separation anxiety' as a proper emotion, the young patients were distressed by virtue of their situation, and many were led into despair brought on by having their anxieties ignored. And to have one's feeling invalidated in this way is a profoundly wounding experience, for 'feelings as a form of information are experienced as the deeply, existential ground of who we are'.[81] In part this was due to children's lack of a 'status shield' – no social, legal, economic protection – their distress carried no 'entitlement'. Thus they were compelled to do 'emotion work', to engage in 'emotion management', that is, they had to adjust ('work on') their emotions to the predicament in which they found themselves.[82] This is what they were doing when Robertson observed them manifesting the three phases of Protest, Despair and Detachment. It was not just that their feelings were at odds with a set of 'feeling rules' such as those governing a wedding or a funeral, but that they were deemed to be 'unfeelable': they were in a similar position to homosexuals in China where, according to Hochschild, homosexual love is not 'bad'; it is held not to exist.[83] The hospitalised children shared this state of non-being – they had 'an extremely powerless social status', which increased the likelihood of experiencing an unpleasant sense of emotional being.[84] Young children were vulnerable in three respects: their relative powerlessness as children *per se*; their lack of verbal dexterity; and their low status as 'patients' in a profoundly hierarchical environment. Hence they had no way of protecting 'the boundaries of their self';[85] except by turning inwards: through Detachment. And this, it began to be argued throughout the 1950s, posed a variety of risks to society. The vulnerability of young children, it was realised, had to be protected if the art of social psychiatry was to be effectively practised among individuals and throughout the community.

Did children benefit from the newly developing emotional standard? It has been shown that the standard by which children's emotions was judged had been changing in quite specific ways since the advent of the 'new psychology' after 1918, and had reached something of a high point, at least in theory and among professionals, with the passing of the Children's Act (1948) which, in common with the Curtis Report (1946) gave expression to psychodynamic principles of child care. Nevertheless, as Bowlby belatedly realised, the welfare of children in hospital was more or less completely ignored. Not until 'separation anxiety' began to be acknowledged as 'real', were these children brought within the ambit of a changing culture of emotions. Once this occurred, it would seem to be undeniable that having a more extensive range of their emotions recognised as legitimate, as requiring an entitlement, was of enormous advantage to them. Broadly speaking, it bestowed upon them a greater sense of personal security in that their feelings were seen to be 'true'. Consequently, their selfhood was enhanced. More specifically, as a result of the entitlement, it seems reasonable to suggest that individual children cried less, suffered less upset, experienced less anxiety and, therefore, were made happier during what was for many of them already a traumatic time in hospital. Lessening suffering and unhappiness, even in these postmodernist days, is surely an unconditional good.

As for the ways in which it affected the child-adult relationship (for the better), this can best be explained if emotion is seen as 'relational' – as involving a 'deep sociality'[86] – in that it mediates the workings of our interactions as we make contact with others: we are compelled to admit that they, too, have a self. Through a recognition of 'separation anxiety', groups of adults came to see and to understand children's emotions (at least this particular emotion) as manifestations of what (in a different context) has been described as 'the personal and private apprehensions (they, the children) have made of the world... (their) emotions are emblematic of...(their) understanding of self, others and the social milieu'.[87] Put simply, these adults began – very slowly, and in limited circumstances – to acknowledge a new level of emotional interiority in children, which hitherto had been denied, disregarded, and ridiculed. This new entitlement implicitly saw children as agents participating in the creation of their own being and, in so doing, it went further along the path towards including them in a shared humanity.[88]

Harry Hendrick

Acknowledgements

It is a pleasure to record my thanks for interviews to Peg Belson, Sir George Godber, Dr Mary Lindsay, Joyce Robertson and Mary Stott. Kay Hardwick, librarian at Action for Sick Children, was unfailingly helpful, and the Wellcome Trust was generous with its financial assistance. I'm also pleased to acknowledge Bernard Harris and John Stewart, both of whom made constructive suggestions for the restructuring of earlier drafts.

Notes

1. Quoted in Peter N. Stearns and Carol Z. Stearns, 'Emotionology: Clarifying the History of Emotions and Emotional Standards', *American Historical Review*, 90, 4 (1985), 813–36.

2. The growing interest in visiting hours is chronicled in James and Joyce Robertson, *Separation and the Very Young* (London: Free Association Books, 1989), 7-8.

3. NFWI, Verbatim Report of AGM, June 1950, London; *Daily Mirror*, 15 June 1950; see also 'Press Cuttings 1945' and 'Articles, 1941-73' in Action for Sick Children (ASC) Archive, London.

4. Ministry of Health, *The Welfare of Children in Hospital. Report of the Committee* (London: HMSO, 1959), 1. Hereafter the Platt Report.

5. *Ibid.*, 2.

6. Cathy Urwin and Elaine Sharland, 'From Bodies to Minds in Childcare Literature: Advice to Parents in Inter-war Britain', in Roger Cooter (ed.), *In the Name of the Child: Health and Welfare, 1880-1940* (London: Routledge, 1992), 186. For useful accounts of child-rearing literature, see Christina Hardyment, *Perfect Parents: Baby-Care Advice. Past and Present* (Oxford: Oxford University Press, 1985) and Daniel Beekman, *The Mechanical Baby: A Popular History of the Theory and Practice of Child Raising* (London: Dobson, 1977).

7. Nikolas Rose, *The Psychological Complex* (London: Routledge and Kegan Paul, 1985), 185–90.

8. *The New Era*, November 1930, 137–9; May 1933, 82–4, 93–6.

9. Home and Schools Council, *Advances in Understanding the Child* (London: Home and Schools Council of Great Britain, n.d. 1935?), 5.

10. Urwin and Sharland, *op. cit.* (note 6), 184; also Rose, *op. cit.* (note 7), 200–5; D.Thom, 'Wishes, Anxieties, Play and Gestures: Child Guidance in Inter-War England', in Cooter (ed.), *op. cit.* (note 6), 200–19.

11. Rose, *op. cit.* (note 7), 200–5.

12. Dane E. Prugh, *et al.*, 'A Study of the Emotional Reactions of

Children and Families to Hospitalisation and Illness', *American Journal of Orthopsychiatry,* 23 (1953), 70–105.

13. For full bibliographical details, see Prugh, *ibid.* and John Bowlby, *Maternal Care and Mental Health* (Geneva: WHO, 1951).

14. Charles Anderson and Mary M. Aldrich, *Babies are Human Brings* (New York: Macmillan, 1938); Dorothy Baruch, *You, Your Children and War* (New York: Appleton,1942); C. Madelaine Dixon, *Keep Them Human* (New York: John Daly, 1942); and Benjamin Spock, *The Common Sense Book of Baby and Child Care* (New York: Duell Sloan, 1946).

15. William Graebner, 'The Unstable World of Benjamin Spock: Social Engineering in a Democratic Culture, 1917-1950', *The Journal of American History,* 67, 3 (1980), 612-29: 613. I am indebted to this excellent article for the rest of this paragraph. See also Michael Zuckerman, 'Dr Spock: The Confidence Man', in Charles Rosenberg (ed.), *The Family in History* (Philadelphia: University of Penn Press, 1975), 179–207.

16. Graebner, *op. cit.* (note 15), 612–13.

17. *Ibid.,* 624.

18. K.M.Wolf, 'Evacuation of Children in Wartime', *The Psychoanalytic Study of the Child,* 1 (1945), 389–405: 389. See this for a review of the literature.

19. Susan Isaacs (ed.), *The Cambridge Evacuation Survey* (London: Methuen, 1941), 9.

20. D. Burlingham and A. Freud, *Young Children in War-Time* (London: George Allen and Unwin for the New Era, 1942) and *Infants without Families: The Case for and Against Residential Nurseries* (London: George Allen and Unwin, 1943).

21. Burlingham and Freud, *ibid., passim.*

22. Nikolas Rose, *Governing the Soul: The Shaping of the Private Self* (London: Routledge, 1990), 159–60.

23. MOH/Ministry of Education, *Report of the Care of Children Committee* (London: HMSO, 1946). Hereafter the Curtis Report, 5.

24. Jean Packman, *The Child's Generation: Child Care Policy from Curtis to Houghton* (Oxford: Blackwell, 1981); Jean Heywood, *Children in Care* (London: Routledge and Kegan Paul, 1959); Harry Hendrick, *Child Welfare. England. 1872-1989* (London: Routledge, 1994).

25. Among its members were Lucy Fildes, a child guidance psychologist and Sybil Clement Brown, a leading exponent of psychiatric social work; the witnesses included Bowlby, D.W. Winnicott and Clare Britton, a psychiatric social worker.

26. The Curtis Report (1946), para 148.

27. Eileen Younghusband, *Social Work in Britain, 1950-1975* (London: Allen and Unwin, 1978).

28. Contemporary Medical Archive Centre (CMAC), Wellcome Institute for the History of Medicine, PP/BOW/C/6.1, Paddington Group Hospital Management Committee, *The Tavistock Clinic*, n.d. [1960?]; Henry V. Dicks, *Fifty Years of the Tavistock Clinic* (London: Routledge and Kegan Paul, 1970), 112.

29. CMAC, PP/BOW/A.5/2 Milton Senn, Interview with John Bowlby, October 1977 (Hereafter Senn Interview); Dicks, *op. cit.* (note 28), 112.

30. Lawrence K. Frank, 'Social Order and Psychiatry', *American Journal of Orthopsychiatry*, 11 (1941), 620–7; Edward Glover, 'The Birth of Social Psychiatry', *Lancet*, 24 August 1940, 239.

31. Senn Interview, *op. cit.* (note 29), 10; PP/BOW/C.6/1; *The Tavistock Clinic, op. cit.* (note 28).

32. CMAC, PP/BOW/C.6/1, Eric Trist, *The Tavistock Institute of Human Relations in Retrospect and Prospect* (1957), 6-7; Peter Miller and Nikolas Rose, 'The Tavistock Programme: The Government of Subjectivity and Social Life', *Sociology*, 22, 2 (1988), 171-92:187. I am indebted to this article for a number of references.

33. Rose, *op. cit.* (note 22), 40-52.

34. Alfred J. Marrow, *The Practical Theorist: The Life and Work of Kurt Lewin* (New York: Basic Books, 1969); Gertrud Weiss Lewin (ed.), *Kurt Lewin. Resolving Social Conflicts: Selected Papers on Group Dynamics* (New York: Harper and Brothers, 1948), 711-83. His work was promoted within the 'army group' and in the post-war Tavistock by Eric Trist, a leading member of the TIHR and a major influence on Bowlby. See Bowlby, *op. cit.* (note 13), 7.

35. R. Money-Kryle, *Psychoanalysis and Politics* (London: Duckworth, 1951), 106–22.

36. Quoted in B. Turner and T. Rennell, *When Daddy Came Home* (London: Pimlico, 1996), 41–2.

37. W. R. Bion, 'Psychiatry at a Time of Crisis', *British Journal of Medical Psychology*, 21 (1948), 81–9: 81, 83. See also D. W. Winnicott, 'Some Thoughts on the Meaning of Democracy', *Human Relations*, 3 (1950), 1744-86, and J. C. Flugel, *Man, Morals and Society: A Psychoanalytical Study* (London: Penguin 1962 edn, 1st published, 1945).

38. Dicks, *op. cit.* (note 28), 115–6, 143.

39. Senn Interview, *op. cit.* (note 29), 12.

40. *Ibid.*, and Paddington Group, *The Tavistock Clinic* (note 28), 16; Tavistock Library: IMM. Uk. Acc. No. X1150, 'Description of the

Tavistock Project, March, 1948-1951' (Hereafter 'Tavi Project, 1948-1951'), para 32.

41. When the Ford Foundation began its Mental Health Research Programme in 1955, the official Tavistock application was from Bowlby, who received 225,000 dollars over five years. Trist, *op. cit.* (note 32), 11-12; Frank, *op. cit.* (note 30). Frank became Chair of the Macy Foundation, which gave financial support to Bowlby. The Foundation became the main sponsor of child development studies, advocating a mother-centred approach in pursuit of the stable personality. Graebner, *op. cit.* (note 15), 621; H. Dicks, 'In Search of Our Proper Ethic', *British Journal of Medical Psychology*, 23, 3 (1950), 1-14. See also M. Thomson, 'Mental Hygiene as an International Movement', in P. Weindling (ed.), *International Health Organisations and Movements, 1918-1939* (Cambridge: Cambridge University Press, 1995), 283–304 and his 'Before Anti-Psychiatry: "Mental Health" in Wartime Britain,' in Marijke Gijswijt-Hofstra and Roy Porter (eds), *Cultures of Psychiatry and Mental Health Care in Postwar Britain and the Netherlands* (Amsterdam: Rodopi, 1998), 43–59.

42. CMAC, PP/BOW/F.3/1, Transcript. The lecture also appeared 'Psychology and Democracy', *Political Quarterly*, 17, (1946), 61–76. For similar concerns, see Winnicott, *op. cit.* (note 37).

43. 'Tavi Project, 1948-1951', *op. cit.* (note 40), para 5.

44. Bowlby, *op. cit.* (note 13), 11 and 91.

45. *Ibid.*, 157.

46. John Bowlby, *Child Care and the Growth of Love* (Harmondsworth: Penguin, 1953).

47. Kenneth Shoddy, 'Maternal and Mental Health', *Mental Health*, xi, (1952), 70–5.

48. 'Tavi Project, 1948-1951', *op. cit.* (note 40), paras 30, 37–9. Also Tavistock Library, IMM. UK. Acc. No. X1151, 'Report by the British Team to the International Children's Centre', May, 1952 (Hereafter 'Report by the British Team'.

49. Tavistock Library, IMM. UK. Acc. No. X1153, 'Report on Work Done in Years 1951-55 to the Regional Office for Europe of WHO', (December, 1956), 3.

50. 'Report by the British Team', *op. cit.* (note 48).

51. 'Tavi Project, 1948-1951', *op. cit.* (note 40), para 58.

52. 'Report by the British Team', *op. cit.* (note 48), (B) The Sick Child.

53. 'Tavi Project, 1948-1951', *op. cit.*(note 40), paras 17–18. See also Robertson and Robertson, *op. cit.* (note 2), 10–11. Robertson had been a conscientious objector during the war and had worked in Freud and Burlingham's residential nursery where he had been trained by

Anna Freud.

54. Robertson and Robertson, *op. cit.* (note 2), 10–12.

55. *Ibid.*, 22.

56. *Ibid.*, 23, 45, 12–13.

57. *Ibid.*, 23.

58. *Ibid.* See also James Robertson, *A Two Year Old Goes to Hospital. A Scientific Film Record* (London: Tavistock Publications, 1953).

59. *Ibid.*, 43–7. Interview with Mrs. Joyce Robertson (notes), 1998.

60. Senn Interview, *op. cit.* (note 29), 27–8. CMAC, PP/BOW/J. 6/1-11, Box 57: Film Guides. The film (and a later one made in 1958) was shown in a carefully prepared manner, accompanied by explanatory leaflets.

61. James Robertson, *Young Children in Hospital* (London: Tavistock, 1958), x.

62. *Ibid.*, 12–14.

63. Interview with Sir George Godber, March 1999.

64. Interview with Dr Mary Lindsay (notes), 1998.

65. Having said this, it would be wrong to suggest that Bowlby was the only significant influence. Mention has already been made of Burlingham and Freud and Anna Freud was certainly an important figure in the debate around the impact of maternal separation. See Janet Sayers, *Mothering Psychoanalysis* (Harmondsworth: Penguin, 1992). Aside from Bowlby, the other major figure was Donald Winnicott, child analyst and paediatrician, who was a dominant influence among social workers and whose radio talks on mothers and children were published as 'The Ordinary Devoted Mother and Her Baby', Nine Broadcast Talks (Autumn, 1949. Privately distributed). However, it was suggested that Winnicott missed what he should have seen, namely the suffering of young hospital patients. See CMAC, PP/BOW/A5/27. David Malan, 'Notes for Reminiscences and Reflections – Dr. John Bowlby', 1990. For useful general discussion of the issues and the times, see Rose, *op. cit.* (note 22) and, for a feminist account, Denise Riley, *The War in the Nursery: Theories of the Child and the Mother* (London: Virago, 1983). For excellent studies of Bowlby and his work, see Susan Van Dijken, *John Bowlby: His Early Life* (London: Free Association Books, 1998), and Jeremy Holmes, *John Bowlby and Attachment Theory* (London: Routledge, 1993).

66. T.J. Csordas, *Embodiment and Experience: The Existential Ground of Culture and the Self* (Cambridge: Cambridge University Press, 1994).

67. Ronald McKeith, 'Children in Hospital', *Mother and Child*, 25, 3 (1954), 58–61: 58, 61.

68. Michael Fordham, 'Some Observations on the Self in Childhood',

British Journal of Medical Psychology, 24 (1951), 83–95; Hilda Lewis, 'The Child Without his Parents', *Nursing Mirror*, 9 February 1951, 279-80; Annual Conference of National Baby Welfare Council, 'The Child and His Environment', *Mother and Child* , 21, 5 (1950), 130–47; A.T.M. Wilson, 'The Child and Family Relationships', *Nursing Mirror*, 8 August 1952, 419–20; W.M. Burbury, 'The Development of the Child into the Citizen', *Nursing Times*, 3 April 1948, 240–1; Editorial, 'The Mind of a Young Child', *Nursing Times*, 15 November 1957, 1289; Editorial, 'The Child as a Person in Hospital', *Nursing Times*, 14 November 1953, 1153.

69. The Platt Report, *op. cit.* (note 4), 10, para 3.

70. Interview with Mary Stott (notes), June 1999; *Observer*, 15, 22, 29 January 1961.

71. Robertson and Robertson, *op. cit.* (note 2), 59.

72. Interview with Peg Belson (notes) May 1999; Peg Belson, 'Children in Hospital', *Children and Society*, 7, 2 (1993), 196-210; Constitution of MCCH in ASC Archive.

73. A. R. Hochschild, 'The Sociology of Emotion as a Way of Seeing', in Gillian Bendelow and Simon J.Williams (eds), *Emotions in Social Life* (London: Routledge, 1998), 3–15: 5.

74. Deborah Lupton, *The Emotional Self* (London: Sage Publications, 1998), 5.

75. N. Denzin, *On Understanding Emotion* (San Francisco: Josey-Bass, 1984), x.

76. P. Freund, 'The Expressive Body: A Common Ground for the Sociology of Emotions and Health and Illness', *Sociology of Health and Illness*, 12, 4 (1990), 452–77: 458.

77. A. R. Hochschild, *The Managed Heart: The Commercialization of Human Feeling* (Berkeley, C.A.: University of California Press); A. R. Hochschild, 'Emotion Work, Feeling Rules, and Social Structure', *Amercian Journal of Sociology*, 85, 3 (1979), 551–75.

78. Hochschild, *op. cit.* (note 73), 6.

79. *Ibid.*

80. Quoted in Robertson and Robertson, *op. cit.* (note 2), 57. See also Ronald MacKeith, *op. cit.* (note 67), 61.

81. Freund, *op. cit.* (note 76), 466; Hochschild, *Managed Heart* (note 77), 173.

82. Lupton, *op. cit.* (note 74), 19.

83. Hochschild, *op. cit.* (note 73), 6.

84. Freund, *op. cit.* (note 76), 461 and 466.

85. *Ibid.*, 465.

86. Bendelow and Williams, *op. cit.* (note 73), xvi.

87. J. Finkelstein, 'Considerations for a Sociology of the Emotions', *Studies in Symbolic Interactionism*, 3 (1980), 111–21: 119.

88. For children as historical actors, see Harry Hendrick, 'The Child as a Social Actor in Historical Sources: Problems of Identification and Interpretation', in Pia Christensen and Allison James (eds), *Research with Children: Perspectives and Practices* (London: Falmer Press, 2000), 36–61.

11

The Problem of Sex Education in the Netherlands in the Twentieth Century

Hugo Röling

The sexual behaviour of the young has always been a source of worry to authorities of all kinds. Though first and foremost a moral problem, by the end of the nineteenth century in much of the Western world, religious and moral issues became subordinate to the urgency of threats to national health, as the grave consequences of venereal disease and abortion became manifest. At the same time, concerns about the debilitating consequences of failing sex education developed, just as the new disciplines of psychology and psychiatry were revealing their diagnosis of modern neuroticism. These developments meant that the public debate on sexuality in the twentieth century changed. Sexuality was considered a medical hazard, but it was also seen as the centre of private life. Thus, there was a continuing conflict between, on the one hand, the urge to intervene, and, on the other hand, a reluctance to bring this domain under any kind of external, or worse governmental, control. At the end of the twentieth century, the threat to national health of the consequences of sexual behaviour is still a source of concern, but the circumstances of that concern have fundamentally changed, beyond all recognition.

There are radical changes in the history of human behaviour and morals that seem to have gone undisputed or questioned by historians. Since beginning work on the history of sexuality and sex education I have been surprised by the almost unanimous acceptance of the changes in twentieth-century sexual experiences (in particular of the young) as if they required no explanation. Yet, until very recently, a majority of people endorsed the idea that children and adolescents should know as little as possible about sex. It was almost unthinkable that they should display any sexual activity, the possibility of young people engaging in full intercourse at an average age of 15 would have been considered a serious disruption of society only half a century ago. Today, some people may still be worried, but proposals to change the situation seem to have little chance of success.

In this article,[1] I will try to elucidate the development and problems of sex education in the Netherlands by considering a number of crucial issues. I will first consider the slow and cumbersome introduction of sexology, which resulted from a failure of the majority of experts to face essential facts. Second, I will discuss the role of fashion and convention in the debate on sex education. The third section will discuss both the moral panic and, in very restricted circles, the enthusiasm which accompanied the revelation, in the 1920s and 1930s, of the sexual activities of the young. The fourth section will consider the way sexuality continued to be treated as a non-issue from 1945 until the so-called sexual revolution of the 1960s. The final section will analyse the experiences of young people, according to their reported memories of youth.

In the course of the twentieth century, the desirability and necessity of sex education has become self-evident. It is now hard to imagine that at the end of the nineteenth century a vast majority of experts in educational philosophy and practice favoured an absolute minimum of information on sexual matters for children and adolescents. At that time, there was a solid consensus that what little needed to be told to prevent disasters such as premarital pregnancies and venereal diseases should be left to parents. During the twentieth century, sex education became a subject for public debate. Questions as to how far it could be left to the family were considered urgent, as it became evident that a majority of parents could not summon the courage to offer adequate advice. In the Netherlands, the pressure to prevent sex education in school from confessional political parties (in particular the Catholics) was strong. This dominated the opinions of authorities in health and education, who only changed their opinion slowly as they became convinced that any damage that might occur from untimely information was small, compared to the real risks of secrecy and ignorance. Once convinced, educational policy changed in an astonishingly short time. These changes form part of the sexual revolution or revolutions of the twentieth century.

In interpreting these changes, contemporary commentators have taken a consistently negative approach. Historians writing about the great transformation of sexual behaviour in the twentieth century have generally had a low opinion of the results. This began with Herbert Marcuse's influential *Eros and Civilisation*, first published in 1955.[2] He argued, crudely, that sexual liberation was a trick of the ruling classes to deflect the attention of the workers from the miseries of capitalist societies. Another view was that the scientific study of sex, and the spread of sex education in accordance with the findings of sexology, had established a domination over people more threatening to human autonomy than the traditional suppression of sexual activities had been. This idea became popular as a simplified rendering of Michel Foucault's ambitious history of sexuality.[3] The regulation of sexuality has invariably been represented as a stifling infringement of authentic experience.[4] The commercial exploitation of sex, it is suggested, has resulted in a nauseating over-consumption forced upon people.[5] I hope to argue that whilst a continuing concern about sexuality and its discontents may be characteristic of the way health authorities have to deal with the subject, commentators have neglected the gains of sexual liberation in the twentieth century.

The introduction of sexology in the Netherlands and its effect on sex education

At the end of the nineteenth century, the pioneers of sex education were inspired by the emergence of modern sexology. Havelock Ellis' books were received with detached interest. In 1915, part of his *Psychology of Sex* was translated into Dutch.[6] The comprehensive collection of sexual variations and curiosities had a liberating effect, proving as it did, by sheer force of evidence, the wide range of possible ways of regulating sexuality in different times and cultures. The inventory of expert opinions diverging widely or contradicting each other put the whole subject in a reassuring perspective. The German psychiatrist, Albert Moll, wrote the first large monograph on childhood sexuality; however, in reviewing it, Dutch readers noticed that he considered sex education desirable, not necessary. Moll was sceptical about those enthusiasts who expected so much of it.[7] Freud was little known before the First World War,[8] but when he began to attract attention in the Netherlands, writers who adhered to psychoanalysis joined in with warnings against the overestimation of sex education. The popularisation of psychoanalytic concepts stimulated a fascination with everything that had to do with sexuality. Psychoanalytically influenced pedagogues took sex instruction for granted, but they were sceptical too; they believed one could spoil much, but gain little by doing it right and thus it did not really matter. These contributions to sex education in the first half of the twentieth century show a typical ambivalence. The subject was declared to deserve or even demand attention from all those concerned with the health of Dutch youth, but no one wrote about

245

it without deploring the fact that it was necessary to discuss it in public.

In the debate on education, Freud elicited hostile comments in the Netherlands. Lodewijk van Mierop, a purity crusader, remarked in a review of one of the first translations of Freud in Dutch, that he reduced everything to a 'pansexualism'.[9] Disseminating knowledge of Freud's theories among the lay public was considered undesirable, as it could make girls and boys insecure in the 'affectionate relation' respectively to their fathers and mothers. Things were too much associated with sex.[10] Formulated more forcefully, the exaggeration of the Oedipus complex defiled the relation between mothers and sons, between fathers and daughters.[11] Such were the opinions of Andrew de Graaf, an influential writer on sexuality, actively engaged in the campaign against prostitution. He was given to unrestrained defamation of the idea that the senses, religious sentiments included, were sexual in origin. He wrote, 'I used to think it the diseased exaggeration of the unbelieving sex maniac, which is indeed my opinion on Freud, based on many other statements'.[12] However, by the early 1920s even he had to admit that psychoanalysis contained important insights.

The concept of child sexuality was received in Holland with revulsion. It was taken as a reversal of childhood innocence, which had been the dominant idea in the debate on sex education. Not only Christian inspired authors but also the fiercely atheist pioneer of sexology in the Netherlands Dr J. Rutgers (1850-1924) defended the concept. Rutgers had devoted his life to the practice of Neo-Malthusianism (he taught Margaret Sanger the use of the diaphragm). In 1916, his opinion was that the child is not sexual and that a healthy child does not have sexual daydreams.[13] In the 1920s, psychoanalysis gained ground rapidly, but among writers on education resistance was evident. In 1926, Philip Kohnstamm, by then the most prominent professor of education in the Netherlands, had come to accept that the stimulation of the skin of babies was a source of pleasure as infantile sexuality. This sexual gratification of infants was normal, he decided, but it ought not to be encouraged. The warning on that point was worded in a threatening way that probably brought about the opposite of what psychoanalysts were trying to achieve.[14]

Public denouncements of the 'satanic opinions on infantile sexuality'[15] were frequent, especially in Catholic medical and educational circles. It seemed that the basic assumptions of psychoanalysis were widely accepted in the 1920s and 1930s, but a need to keep warning against excesses prevailed in the debate. Thus, full endorsement of psychoanalysis was scarce in the debate on sex education before 1940. Freud was often twisted to support the call for self-control in the young or, especially by Kohnstamm, as a warning against over-indulgence. The first fully Freudian advice-book for parents of small children appeared in 1940.[16] It broke with the past, for example, by urging a relaxed attitude to toilet training. It also advised that infantile masturbation should be completely ignored. The author tried to make these heresies acceptable by playing down their importance, but she wrote like a true believer.

The hesitant but irresistible rise of psychoanalysis in the Netherlands mirrored events in other countries, especially the United Kingdom. Another phenomenon similar in both countries was the appearance of sex manuals for adults in which an almost ecstatic celebration of marital love was the main point. Mary Stopes' books were a success in Dutch translations, but they were surpassed by Dutch gynaecologist Th.H. van de Velde's *Het volkomen huwelijk* (1926, in English *Ideal marriage* (1928)). The mild atmosphere of scandal surrounding this new type of manual underlined a change in the general attitude towards sex; though it remained restricted to wedlock, the pursuit of pleasure as an end in itself was no longer condemned.

After 1945 psychoanalysis soon became the dominant strain in psychiatry and had a strong influence on pedagogical thinking. Despite the fact that, in the 1950s, psychoanalysts kept warning against too much sexual freedom for the young and against the lack of discipline in sex education, Freud was seen mainly as a prophet of the idea that sexual needs demanded a proper outlet. In confessional circles, this still gave offence. In 1946 the Catholic psychologist A. Chorus wrote, 'The principal cause of Freud's success lies in the fact that he provided people with scientifically impressive motives to unbridle their sexual urges'. Of course, he had a point in warning that 'the "let go" of psychoanalysis is about to erode Christianity in practice, on which our civilisation rests.'[17] However, fewer and fewer people saw this erosion as a threat to civilisation.

Second thoughts about sex education

In progressive circles positive and explicit sex education had been popular since the 1890s. There had always been sceptics, but, after 1910, a distinct reaction set in. In a leading magazine on child-rearing, which had customarily proclaimed the necessity of sex education, a long debate began with a growing number of participants subscribing to the slogan, 'Don't do it'.[18] There was little argument, mainly expressions of disgust. 'We can't bear those haughty wise children who look upon their pregnant mother with a knowing glance, aware that they too were once cherished in mother's womb... If one were able to consult the children, one would probably find that they are not by far as eager to learn about these things as the pamphlet-writing lady pedagogues suppose.'[19]

The champions of sex education liked to present themselves as the ones who cleaned out old prejudices. Though arguing against sex instruction, sceptics took care not to seem insensitive to the needs of the young. This explains the international success of the German pedagogue Friedrich Foerster. He emphasised the importance of sex education, but criticised writers on the subject as confused over ends and means.[20] 'There are a great number of writings nowadays, devoted to the so-called sexual enlightenment, which seem to see it as their assignment to preface their ideas on proper sexual behaviour with such enthusiastic glorification of human procreation that it looks as if a new cult of *Astarte* and *Priapus* is to be prepared.'[21] Foerster reiterated frequently that to trust in the dissemination of knowledge on sexuality was a rationalist error. Instruction, he argued, was a relatively unimportant aspect of sex education. The point should be to train the willpower and the moral sense. This kind of rhetoric was received as the ultimate wisdom for a long time. A feminist freethinker translated his books. Protestant[22] and, in the 1920s, Catholic writers on education[23] accepted his line of reasoning. Especially appealing was Foerster's objection to explicit instruction on the grounds that it aroused too great expectations of sexual life.[24]

Emilie Knappert was a leading personality in Dutch education. She had become the head of the first school for social workers while making her contribution to the debate, which epitomised the predicament. Though she accepted some kind of sex instruction was necessary, the title of her series of articles, warmly received in 1917, was *Speak by Keeping Silent.*[25] While an earlier generation had been worried by the absence of sex instruction, in the 1930s the disadvantageous consequences of this were played down. According to the head of the municipal health department in Amsterdam, L. Heijermans, who also wrote in the Labour Party daily newspaper, even if children got the facts completely wrong, it was not a serious problem. Healthy children solved the riddles of secrets, lies, and dirty talk among themselves.

Among Catholics, keeping silent on sexuality had been practised for a long time. The answer to the primal question was that children were sent by God. Some formulas from moral theology were repeated regularly such as *ignoti nulla cupido* (one does not desire what one does not know) and *ne quid nimis* (never too much).[26] Systematic sex instruction for everybody was condemned. The debate among priests engaged in working with youths was restricted to questions about what cases would make the giving of some kind of information unavoidable. It was the parents' task to give attention to this; the many observations that parents generally failed to do so was not considered a serious problem. The papal bull *Divini illius magistri* (1929) rejected sex instruction. At the same time, however, it is obvious that more Catholic books and pamphlets on sex education were published in the 1930s than ever before. Even if not every young person needed it, the fact that there were boys and girls in the care of Catholic schools and institutions who ran the risk of sinning as a consequence of ignorance was acknowledged more freely.

Moral panic

The ambivalence towards sex education deepened in the increasingly open culture of sexuality during the 'roaring twenties'. Changes in fashions and the behaviour of women were experienced as a sexual revolution. There was no way to avoid the young seeing the seductive images offered by the cinema. Pedagogues who had championed open instruction became less sure. The professor of education, J.H. Gunning, described two conflicting strategies. On the one hand, there was a continuation of the old tradition of screening off children, and, on the other, the practice of exposing children to the facts of life to a degree that seemed intended to make them immune. Both methods were wrong and Gunning could not choose between them.[27] Ph. Kohnstamm, another star of educational thinking, was also insecure. He diagnosed a 'crisis of sexual relations'. He feared a return to primitive promiscuity and thought only self-discipline could save civilisation. However, he asked, how were the young to learn self-control at a time when the older generation was giving the opposite example?[28] Until 1940, sex education was a captive of this dilemma. The more it was discussed in public, the more sexuality was trivialised. The less children were told or knew accurately, the more dangerous the experiments that would occur. The debate continued to run strongly, but did not make any progress as long as there was a rejection of sexual activity amongst the young.

In the economic crisis of the 1930s the moral climate hardened. Powerless against the depression, politicians called for a toughening of the fight against depravity. Contraception had always been considered unacceptable for the masses, but it was practised by increasing numbers of people. The Dutch Neo-Malthusian League (founded in 1881) had been able to promote the knowledge and use of contraceptives relatively freely. In 1927, however, when the legal recognition of the organisation had to be renewed, the Catholic dominated government refused to do so. Dutch Neo-Malthusians anticipated the complete prohibition of their organisation. It did not come to that (and no proof has been found to show that this threat was imminent) but their fear indicated the atmosphere that pertained during this period.[29] It may have been a response to the rising public presence of sex. There was certainly a connection between noting that young people were sexually active and the proposals of some daring writers that this did not forcast a catastrophic decline of civilisation

The observation that most people did not wait for marriage to have sex was not new. However, this behaviour had been interpreted either as associated with the traditional, pre-modern, rural population or with demoralised factory labourers. At the other end of the social spectrum, the aristocracy had been notoriously libertine, but the solid, middle classes were supposed to refrain from irresponsible behaviour of this kind. In the 1920s, it appeared that young white-collar workers, sometimes highly educated, were taking liberties, and were breaking with the traditions of bourgeois convention. A report published in 1921 stirred the imagination. Shop girls in Amsterdam were inspected as they left work and were all found to have contraceptives in their purses.[30] A pessimistic commentator observed that whereas the previous generation had waged an idealistic struggle to free itself from conventions, the young practised this freedom thoughtlessly.[31]

In this climate of opinion, the publication of Ben Lindsey's *The Revolt of Modern Youth* (1925, Dutch translation 1927) created a sensation. Why exactly this publication of an American judge should have triggered a discussion on premarital sex is difficult to establish. Probably, it was the positive aspects of youthful delinquents that Lindsey depicted that took the breath of the Dutch away. Lindsey described them as exceptionally nice and attractive young people and proposed that something should be done about the unwanted consequences of their actions, rather than the actions themselves.[32] Lindsey's facts were indisputable. His approach was that of 'Realpolitik'. According to the dermatologist Van Leeuwen it was wrong to give in to reality on this matter, but, on the other hand, he realised that 'our young come to sexual intercourse on a continually larger scale and a continually younger age'.[33]

In 1932, a scandal was caused by a book in which a well-known Dutch politician and his wife, both active in the Dutch Labour Party, expressed their views. In *Wordend Huwelijk (Marriage Coming into Being)*, F.M. Wibaut, deputy mayor of Amsterdam and his wife, Mathilde Wibaut-Berdenis van Berlekom, wrote on education and the position of women. *Wordend huwelijk* recommended the people should make love before getting married. This, they argued, would make better marriages or at least avoid mismatches.[34] Few people dared to support these heresies (the Wibauts also hinted at not having lived monogamously) and they came under heavy criticism, not only from conservative and confessional sides, but also in their own party.[35] As he was about to speak on radio about the book, Wibaut's announcement that he would touch upon the 'controlled sexual gratification of engaged couples' caused his lecture to be banned.[36]

Though there was general dismissal of the new freedom, discussion of the topic at least made it clear that actual sexual conduct deviated from public morality. A small avant-garde came into being amongst whom ideas on the necessity of sex were defended more openly. They argued that sexual tensions were unhealthy. The old debate on the (im)possibility of sexual continence was reopened this time not in defence of prostitution but as a justification for free love. It was a small group, which soon discovered Wilhelm Reich as a source of inspiration, but some members of this group were to play a prominent role in the movement for sexual reform after 1945. During the 1930s, however, repression remained firm. For example, a doctor, known for his radical views, had a complaint filed against him by the parents of his servant. They claimed he had supplied her with contraceptives and had allowed her to receive her boyfriend in his house. The doctor was suspended by the medical board for half a year.

After 1945

After 1945, adhering to unfeasible rules of moral conduct became more difficult. The war had been experienced as a *demasqué* of the established values. The explosive increase of births out of wedlock and of venereal diseases made proper instruction appear less objectionable than it had been before. Empirical knowledge on sexual behaviour became more precise. Kinsey's publications drew a large response, though quite a few experts could not believe what they read. A new phenomenon in writing on sex education was the tone of insecurity. Educators doubted their ability in this area. Having been brought up in an atmosphere hostile to sexuality, they felt unable to keep an open mind.[37]

The old neo-Malthusian movement had been disbanded by the German occupiers. With great idealism, plans were made to revive it on a broader basis. The *Nederlandse Vereniging voor Seksuele Hervorming* (NVSH, Dutch Association for Sexual Reform) wanted to do more than distribute contraception. It aspired to become a 'people's movement for happiness', teaching people to enjoy their sexuality in full and preparing the young for a better life without frustration. In the first years of its existence the organisation was managed by some enthusiasts from the Reich circle, as is evident from the wording of the lofty aims they produced for the organisation. In the tradition of the great sexual reformers, they expected a better quality of sexual life to contribute to a more peaceful world, the abolition of prostitution, and an end to inequality between the sexes. The self-appointed vanguard had great expectations. However, the leaders overlooked the fact that it was the refusal of Dutch medical authorities to further adequate contraception that directed people to the NVSH, not a desire to reform their sexual lives, let alone to make a better world. Still, members flocked in and made the NVSH a tremendous success for at least two decades although, dominance of the Catholics in Dutch politics meant that legal recognition of the NVSH was denied up until 1957.[38]

The impression that the war and occupation had had a devastating effect on Dutch morality in general, and of youth in particular, prevailed in the years after 1945. 'Mass youth' was the catch phrase for all manner of problems which seemed to be caused by open unruliness and impatience in sexual matters. In what was meant to be an example of large-scale modern social scientific research, 'mass youth' was described in downright alarmist fashion. A majority of the researchers saw the young as a problem threatening the stability of Dutch society. It was the old moral panic of the 1920s all over again. However, a new element that would later have great influence, emerged at this time. A group of progressive Catholic psychologists and pedagogues drew attention to the lack of sexual knowledge and instruction. This subtle but stubborn struggle of a loose group of Catholic intellectuals for the 'spiritual liberation' of the faithful was to last for decades.[39] Their message was that the demands of the church in sexual matters were too harsh for ordinary people.

An almost masochistic invocation of sexual incompetence is characteristic of the debate in the 1950s. Psychiatrists suggested to parents that they were authoritarian and harmful to the development of their children. They said that the goal of education had been too much about making children obedient and that parents and educators were making children feel insecure and guilty.[40]

It was small wonder that so many people believed all this. 'Revolutionary' young people in the sixties simply repeated the same message. Sex education writers were attracted by the idea that the obtaining of knowledge necessarily brought about anxiety. Sex instruction was too much a presentation of facts without meaning.[41] The irreligious activities of the NVSH were criticised. They showed no understanding of the emotional consequences of telling people in general that their sex-lives were inadequate. The young worried too much when told they were responsible for the sexual happiness of future partners. The deep ambivalence towards sex instruction went deep into the avant-garde of the mental health movement. Psychiatrists active in the NVSH went on record with warnings that education in these matters could be too free, for example, parents should not appear naked in front of their children. In the opinion of psychoanalyst H. Musaph, 'It is wrong to leave the child alone with its sexual drives'. He argued that infant sexuality should be recognised, but it should also be controlled.[42] It was typical that, at this time, a book by the German sociologist H. Schelsky, deeply sceptical of the attention given to sexuality in general and of the young in particular, was translated by the chairman of the NVSH. Schelsky had warned that the young had their emotions prescribed to them too much by all the instruction booklets.[43]

The 60s and after:
Sexual revolution

Looking back on the debate surrounding sex education in the post-war decades it is obvious that the experts had given up the possibility of making the young live in sexual continence until marriage. At last, though unhappily, they recognised the facts. Behaviour in public became more free, encouraged by cinema, literature, popular music and mass-culture in general. However, established conventions were tenacious and in the atmosphere of economic recovery, the rhetoric of self-control and responsibility was important to the older generation. The guardians of morality had lost touch with reality, but during the 1950s the image had been maintained.

The release of this tension took on a spectacular character during the 'sexual revolution' of the 1960s. It was primarily a revolution in mass media. There was endless talk about sexual freedom and the need to do away with the old restraints. All the publicity reinforced the impression that sexual conduct was changing very rapidly, but there are many indications that this was far more of a long drawn out process than recognised by contemporaries. In the Netherlands, there was a surprising discovery when large-scale surveys were carried out in 1969 and 1981. Opinions and conduct turned out to be far more conservative in 1969 than expected, while in the 1970s, at the time generally experienced as a period of conformism, a majority proved to have adopted permissive views on premarital sex, the use of contraceptives by the young, homosexuality, etc.[44] Information on contraception had become widely available after 1945, but the awkwardness of the methods available restricted their mass use. The introduction of the pill after 1964 changed that, but even then, it took years for practice to catch up with the new possibilities.

The reputation of the 1960s was built up by unlimited talk, discussions on TV that lasted whole nights and a persistent searching for taboos ready for demolition. 'Everything' was possible and up to a certain point obligatory. The tone in the 1970s changed. The debate was dominated by feminists, who saw little gain in the proclamation of sexual freedom. The emergence of the gay liberation movement fitted in more smoothly with ideas of sexual liberation, advocating as it did alternative views of sexuality and an extrovert cultivation of free sexual gratification. This movement, however, turned in on itself and was therefore of limited interest to the general public.

The ideals of innocence, sexual continence, and silence had been unrealistic for many years, but they became completely untenable with the explosion of publicity about sex in the twentieth century. Based on these, now obsolete, ideals, sex education had been considered to belong to the domain of the family. The revelation that in the vast majority of families the subject was totally neglected had not been enough to change this. However, during the 1960s and 1970s the role of schools was gradually recognised. Sex instruction became part of the curriculum from nursery school to secondary education, something confessional politicians had resisted successfully for years.

When surveys made clear that the young ran considerable risks in their first sexual encounters, the call for more instruction grew louder, even though unwanted pregnancies had less drastic consequences after the introduction of the morning-after-pill and the liberalisation of abortion (around 1980). The illusion that venereal diseases were no longer a serious threat was destroyed by the advent of AIDS at the beginning of the 1980s. At this point, another limit was passed when sex instruction was permitted during prime time television. Government information campaigns were initiated on a broad scale. A landmark in Dutch television history was the appearance of the popular hostess of a TV news programme for children, witnessing a condom demonstration on a stout model of an erect penis on 14 April 1987. It is ironic that public sex education became acceptable in the Netherlands at the same time as large groups of Muslim immigrants, with ideals of modesty and obligatory innocence, became resident in the country. This group was criticised as backward looking because they forbade their daughters to attend sex instruction classes, even though this had only recently been accepted by the large majority in Holland. Even orthodox Catholics and Protestants seemed to have forgotten just how recently they had considered sex education outside the home an infringement of morality.

The experiences of young people
according to autobiographical evidence

What was the result of this highly ambivalent but sustained effort to let children know as little as possible? In recent surveys, young people have talked freely about their problems with sexuality. They appear to have no lack of sources of information and a majority have positive expectations about what sex will mean for them.[45] One suspects, however, a considerable amount of wishful answering. For the period up to the 1960s one can consult memories of youth that tell a different story. The secrecy of parents regarding sexuality was recorded as inevitable, but in retrospect, quite a few children resented this. Parents could have spared some painful insecurities, for instance, when in religious instruction children were told how sinful it could all be.

> That's how it went, suddenly one came across the seventh commandment in confirmation class, that appeared to mean a lot more than breaking a marriage. You were not even allowed to think of things linked to these feelings, and the catechism contained the terrible and untranslatable word 'impurity' for it. Acts, gestures, words, thoughts and anything bringing one onto that subject was cursed by God. How miserable and rejected I felt after each fall. How despair and remorse consumed me with every sensation of

255

pleasure or spontaneous erection. I could not talk this over with the boys, I think they would have laughed at me. Neither with father and mother, because they lived in the tacit assumption that such things did not exist or ought not to exist. One cannot break such a code.

A feeling of agonising loneliness was the result.[46]

Almost all Dutch and Flemish autobiographers when bringing up the subject of sexuality mention the lack of sex education and instruction. The birth of brothers and sisters was often the occasion for youngsters to realise something had been kept from them. 'I understood the meaning of the "terrible toothache", my mother was literally moaning about the night before. It all left me with a confused feeling of pity and contempt because of the deceit.'[47] Pretending to know nothing was such an obvious posture that quite a few memoirists cannot remember whether they were curious at all. Thinking about the mystery, in retrospect, seemed an unreal activity for some children. 'Girls raised like myself thought much about love without knowledge of the natural facts. Love was the big secret that would change our existence. It was as if I were a caterpillar thinking about the butterfly it would meet, after becoming a butterfly itself.'[48] Some witnesses recall the clumsy stammering of their father; at the time, the sons did not want to hear from fathers about these things any more.

> My good father failed to do more than produce an incomprehensible formula [on masturbation] he brought up with a blush, adding, 'Something like that is very wrong. You must never do it.' His generation never understood what long years of self-torment such categorical statements cause in a young and ignorant mind.[49]

It was the great historian Johan Huizinga who is here exposed by his son as an impossible prude.

Looking back, autobiographers appear to have experienced sexuality as the source of a wide gap between adults and children. This gap had functioned at a time when the distinction between old and young was clear and was considered desirable. In modern pedagogical doctrine, such an absence of trust and intimacy was increasingly unwanted. Testimony cited so far proves that, by and large, children did not appreciate the breaking of the silence around sex in well-meant attempts to maintain confidence between the generations. Many autobiographies mentioned the necessity of hiding sexual exploration. A classic response to a sudden breakthrough into consciousness of the sexual act was the idea, 'Do my parents do such a dirty thing?'

> Birth was still more mysterious than death. As becomes decent people my parents had kept me ignorant. Sexual enlightenment was unknown at home... Stork and cabbage had never had a chance with me. But what was it then! How had I come into the world? I was not particularly interested in the others. But me...! ... At best, they said, 'You'll hear that as a matter of course and now leave off quickly this funny talk'. I had to gather my knowledge from the gutter and the gutter did not disappoint me. I can still see the illuminated confectioner's shop window before my eyes, where a precocious friend explained the whole business to me in subtle detail. At first, I laughed at him, but when someone else confirmed his exposition, I was deeply shocked. I do not recall anything making such a devastating impression on me as the delicate secret of birth. Stained with the mud from the gutter the mystery came to me. I hardly dared to look my father and mother in the face any more. I had to think all the time of that... Shame! Bah! - Like dogs! Other parents might do it, but mine too! It took a long time before I was able to behave normally with them again. What misery one confidential conversation with my father could have spared me.[50]

Disbelief was frequently the answer to enlightenment in these stories by boys (girls are less well represented). The fact that the sturdy bringers of the shocking news hardly knew half themselves did not enhance their credibility.

> It was the same P. who as a small boy of about eight informed me on human procreation. He did this in such a preposterous way, that I shook with laughter and believed nothing. He did know something about the genital organs, but told me moreover about a drop of urine, from which man arises.[51]

On the other hand, there were children who were not disturbed, even as friends tried to keep them in suspense. However, not all were as sensible as the daughter of a physician, Louise Kaiser.

> The girls next door offered to tell me how children come into the world. During the walk we took for this purpose, they were overcome with all kinds of scruples. When I asked whether it was like dogs and cats, they answered vaguely in the affirmative. But what had to happen first was such a vile thing, so vile, they lamented. I answered that something applying to all people could

never be vile. In the end, they told their story, which did not affect me much.[52]

Contrary to the stories of bewilderment and frustration there are only a few reports of careful attention to sex education in the family. Even these do not seem to have been an unmixed blessing. 'I caused a sensation in the neighbourhood when my brother was born. A neighbour asked whether the stork had paid a visit and I answered pedantically: "Small children are not brought by the stork, they come out of their mothers belly."'[53] This seems to be a triumph of modern education, but careful sex instruction at a time when it was not common practice threatened to isolate children. 'I did not realise I lived through an enlightened education. I did not know that some of my many friends and girlfriends were not allowed to play with me any more, after I had said there was a brother or sister in their mothers' belly.'[54]

At a time when sexuality began to attract more and more attention in public life, people contemplating their youth were surprised that they had allowed convention to divert their attention. The sudden breakthrough of something vaguely classified as forbidden had been a shock. What else had they suppressed? It was not necessarily the revelation of sexual facts that was most shocking, but confronting proof that one had been able to ignore something so important, so omnipresent. Sex education was, apparently, an embarrassing experience, irrespective of whether parents expressly engaged in it, or left it to the confused information of contemporaries. It is likely to remain that way. However, the more relaxed attitude of recent times shows that it can be less frightening and agonising than it used to be.

Conclusion:
Gains and losses, or progress too?

It seems very old-fashioned to describe developments in society in terms of gains and losses,[55] but radical changes in the experience of such an important part of human life calls for a weighing up of the pros and cons. It is absurd to deny that the opportunities to cultivate and enjoy sexuality have increased enormously. However, this has been taken for granted and one seldom finds a recognition of this, as something that could have happened differently. The obsession with the negative aspects of sexual liberation in the last quarter of the century (for example, sexual violence, child abuse and AIDS) indicate in my view a classic case of blinding by abundance. Anyone discovering the doleful bungling of the sexual needs of even the most talented young people a century ago will feel some kind of relief as they review the changes that have taken place. Only a few enlightened doctors would give reassurance on the harmlessness of masturbation and even they would discourage any yearning for sexual gratification. For girls it was unthinkable that they would try to find out about their sexual capacities. Boys could move on the path of prostitution if they could put aside their revulsion. Well-to-do boys, similarly overwhelmed with feelings of guilt, could try to abuse a servant or other lower-class girl. In the labouring classes, inhibitions were less stifling, but early marriages were burdened with too many babies. Secretiveness allowed outsiders (mainly women) to become victims of the sexual misconduct of others but clear instruction on venereal diseases was considered immoral. For young homosexuals there was no explanation of their inclination available, if one was to find something it was the description of a creepy deviation.

In the last century, all this has changed. The catchwords are secularisation, individualisation, and emancipation: the most important factor probably being a rise in the standard of living resulting in better health; more living space; and more leisure time. Inevitably, people have become more active sexually. The slow, sexual emancipation of women, homosexuals and the young raised protest, but it has been irrepressible and apparently irreversible. The sexual autonomy of unmarried people was long disputed but has ceased to be so. Changes in the actual conduct of people ultimately resulted in a reversal of attitude. Experts and politicians lagged behind and claimed to be doing their best to stop it. However, the spectacular change in the way sex was talked about in public seems best explained as a reluctant facing of the facts that could no longer be ignored. Those facts were the consequences of failing instruction; the obvious sexual unhappiness as a result of insecurity; and conflicts between the rules and actual conduct becoming too acute. Moralists, who upheld a code of conduct nobody observed, became implausible. The gains in freedom of action, which have finally been accepted, have since been treated as if it could never have been any different. This kind of amnesia in the discussion of sexuality seems to me short-sighted. The concentration on a 'culture of complaint' in which feminists and gay liberators hold on to the position of victims is confusing the issues. The scandals around child-pornography could easily be turned against the freedom of the young. To dismiss the idea that some kind of progress was achieved with sexual liberation carries a risk.

Overabundance of freedom does bring about problems. The old saying 'set a beggar on horseback and he'll ride to the devil' may apply. Indeed, as a concerned pedagogue shortly after 1945 observed, 'The greater number of difficulties we experience are always the outcome of greater possibilities'.[56] For one thing, greater freedom of choice implies an obligation to achieve. Those who lived in sexual continence used to be regarded as virtuous and admirable, but nowadays will tend to feel as if they are losing out. The individual's needs may have become more afflicting and consequently sexual envy may have become more bitter. The expectations of sexual life have been stirred up in an unprecedented way, which possibly makes the young feel more insecure. Their helplessness may have been exacerbated by the accurate knowledge of the facts of life preceding any opportunity to put them into action.

Notes

1. Based on H.Q. Röling, *Gevreesde vragen. Geschiedenis van de seksuele opvoeding in Nederland* (Amsterdam: Amsterdam University Press, 1994).
2. Herbert Marcuse, *Eros and Civilization. A Philosophical Enquiry into Freud* (Boston: Beacon Press, 1955).
3. Michel Foucault, *La volonté de savoir* (Paris: Gallimard, 1976).
4. Jeffrey Weeks, *Sex, Politics and Society: The Regulation of Sexuality since 1800* (Harlow: Longman, 1989).
5. Lawrence Birken, *Consuming Desire. Sexual Science and the Emergence of a Culture of Abundance* (Ithaca: Cornell University Press, 1988). For a recent summing up of the negative interpretation of sexual liberation, see R. Commers, *De val van Eros. Over seksuele armoede vandaag* (Antwerpen: Houtekiet, 2000).
6. Havelock Ellis, *Psychologie der sexen*, with an introduction by A. van Renterghem (Baarn: Hollandia, 1915).
7. A. Moll, *Das Sexualleben des Kindes* (Leipzig: Vogel, 1909), 278-9.
8. I.N. Bulhof, *Freud en Nederland. De interpretatie en invloed van zijn ideeën* (Baarn: Ambo, 1983).
9. *Levenskracht* 8, 5 (May 1914), 104.
10. F. van Beeck Calkoen, N. van Leeuwen-Vos and A.F.S. Schepel-Kerdijk, 'Indrukken van een cursus voor vrouwen en meisjes over sexueele hygiëne', *Sexueele hygiëne*, 1 (1921-22), 72–5.
11. A. de Graaf, 'Sexueele Paedagogiek', in Ph. Kohnstamm, H.Y. Groenewegen and A. de Graaf (eds), *Paedagogische en ethische vragen op het gebied van het sexueele leven* (Zeist: Ploegsma, 1925), 149–205: 117.

12. A. de Graaf, *Over gezinsregeling* (Putten: Terwee, n.d.[1938]), 25.
13. J. Rutgers, *Het geslachtsleven van den man* (Almelo: Hilarius, 1916), 351, 356.
14. Ph. Kohnstamm, *Sexueele opvoeding* (Zeist: Ruys, 1926), 8–9.
15. R. ter Meulen, *Ziel en zaligheid De receptie van de psychologie en van de psychoanalyse onder de katholieken in Nederland 1900-1965* (Baarn: Ambo, 1988), 75.
16. Ada Citroen, *Kinderpsyche en opvoeding volgens psycho-analytische opvattingen* (Amsterdam: Kosmos, 1940).
17. A. Chorus, *Ontstaan en ontwikkeling der psycho-analyse* (Nijmegen: Dekker en Van de Vegt, 1946), 54. Quote from R. ter Meulen, *op. cit.* (note 15), 109.
18. The discussion in *Het Kind* lasted from July 1914 to February 1915.
19. C.A.F. Zernike (ed.), *Paedagogisch Woordenboek* (Groningen: Wolters, 1905), 998, 995.
20. Cf. P. Selten, 'Het volle leven tegemoet. Katholieke opvattingen over de psyche van de rijpere jeugd', in J.J.H. Dekker *et al.* (eds), *Pedagogisch werk in de samenleving* (Leuven: Acco, 1987), 181–94.
21. F. Foerster, *Levenswandel. Een boek voor jonge menschen* (Zwolle: Ploegsma, 1910), 76.
22. H. Bavinck, *Opvoeding der rijpere jeugd* (Kampen: Kok, 1916), 163.
23. G. Lamers [review article] *DUX*, 1 (1927-28), 133–5.
24. G. Kapteyn-Muysken, 'Sexueele paedagogiek', *Belang en Recht*, 8. (1903-04), 157–8, 165–6.
25. E.C. Knappert, 'Spreken door zwijgen', *Leven en werken. Maandblad* (June 1917), 507–14.
26. Heathens had their stock of Latin slogans too: *ab assuetis non fit passio* (what you are used to, does not arouse the passions) and foremost: *naturalia non sunt turpia* (what is natural is not disgraceful).
27. J.H. Gunning, *Problemen der rijpere jeugd* (Utrecht: Ruys, 1924), 49.
28. Ph. Kohnstamm, *Persoonlijkheid in wording* (Haarlem: Tjeenk Willink, 1929), 450–1.
29. G. Nabrink, *Seksuele hervorming in Nederland* (Nijmegen: SUN, 1978), 115.
30. The story was launched in *Levenskracht* in 1921 and repeated until after 1945.
31. P.H. Ritter, Jr., *De drang der zinnen in onzen tijd* (Amsterdam: Scheltens & Giltay, n.d. [1933]), 217.
32. A solidly argued review: A. Hijmans, *Ben Lindsey's nieuwe sexueele ethiek* (Zeist: Ruys, 1929).
33. Th.M. van Leeuwen, 'Sexueele voorlichting', *Sexueele Hygiëne*, 7, 1

(November 1930), 1–31: 7.

34. M. Wibaut-Berdenis van Berlekom and F.M. Wibaut, *Wordend huwelijk* (Haarlem: Tjeenk Willink, 1932).

35. Cf. C. Pothuis-Smit and S.J. Pothuis, *Zoo kan het huwelijk worden* (1932). In a new introduction in the second edition the Wibauts answered the critics, *Wordend huwelijk* (Haarlem: Tjeenk Willink, 1932), 7–50.

36. F.M. Wibaut, *Verboden rede over Wordend Huwelijk* (n.p., 1932), 9.

37. S.M. Rubens, 'Verslag', *Verstandig Ouderschap*, 27, 9 (October 1947), 8.

38. The Neo-Malthusian League had had 30,000 members in 1939. The newly-refounded NVSH had 40,000 in 1948, passed the 100,000 mark in 1955 and in 1965 reached its peak of 205,000 members. In 1966 the law of 1911 restricting the availability of contraception was withdrawn and soon membership of the NVSH had dwindled to some tens of thousands. Nabrink, *op. cit.* (note 29), 100, 388.

39. Hanneke Westhoff, *Geestelijke bevrijders. Nederlandse katholieken en hun beweging voor geestelijke volksgezondheid in de twintigste eeuw* (Baarn: Ambo, 1996).

40. *De gevoelsmatige ontwikkeling van het kind* (Rotterdam: De Koepel, 1957), 18–20.

41. N. Beets, *Lichaamsbeleving en sexualiteit in de puberteit* (Utrecht: Bijleveld, 1964), 157.

42. H. Musaph, 'Voordracht Kaderconferentie 10.1.1954', *Ledencontact*, 50 (February 1956), 1–13.

43. H. Schelsky, *Sociologie der sexualiteit* (Assen: Born, 1957), 123–33.

44. *Sex in Nederland* (Utrecht: Prisma, 1969); *Sex in Nederland. Het meest recente onderzoek naar mening en houding van de Nederlandse bevolking* (Utrecht: Prisma, 1983).

45. Janita Ravesloot, *Seksualiteit in de jeugdfasen vroeger en nu. Ouders en jongeren aan het woord* (Amsterdam: Het Spinhuis, 1997).

46. Fedde Schurer, *De beslagen spiegel* (Amsterdam: Moussault, 1969), 26–7.

47. A. Romein-Verschoor, *Omzien in verwondering* (Amsterdam: Arbeiderspers, 1970), 35, 38–9.

48. Jeanne van Schaik-Willing, *Ondanks alles* (Amsterdam: Querido, 1955), 74–6.

49. Leonhard Huizinga, *Mijn hartje wat wil je nog meer* (Den Haag: Leopold, 1968), 37.

50. Piet Bakker, *Jeugd in de Pijp* (Amsterdam: Elsevier, 1946), 122.

51. S. van Praag, *Een lange jeugd in Joods Amsterdam* ('s-Gravenhage: Nijgh & Van Ditmar, 1985), 69.

52. Louise Kaiser, *Een persoonlijk witboek* (Amsterdam: Polak & Van Gennep 1968), 41–2.

53. Hilda Verwey-Jonker, *Er moet een vrouw in* (Amsterdam: Arbeiderspers, 1988), 44.

54. Louka Wolf Catz, *Kind in de schaduw* ('s-Gravenhage: Nijgh & Van Ditmar 1985), 18–19.

55. In spite of the example of L. Stone, *The Family, Sex and Marriage in England 1500-1800* (New York: Harper & Row, 1977), 683–7.

56. J.C. van Andel and O.van Andel-Ripke, *Moeilijkheden en mogelijkheden der rijpere jeugd* (Utrecht: Bijleveld, 1949), 17.

12

'Tall, Spanking People':
The Idealisation of Adolescents in a
Dutch Therapeutic Community

Gemma Blok

One day at Amstelland - a Dutch therapeutic community for adolescents, founded in 1969 - a psychotic boy flew into a tantrum and smashed a window, and another, and another. In the end, he smashed about thirty windows. None of the psychotherapists present interfered. On the contrary, they were almost cheering him on. It was considered healthy to show your emotions.[1]

This anecdote symbolises a change in attitudes towards adolescence and psychological crisis, which occurred during the 1960s and 1970s. Whereas during the fifties much concern was expressed about the supposed licentiousness of modern youth, in the course of the sixties a growing chorus of scientists, politicians and journalists started to applaud rebellious adolescents. These young people, they argued, were bringing to light a crisis in Western society.

According to these cultural critics, modern society was filled with conformists, whose existence was like 'death in life'. They went about their jobs mechanically, as cogs in a mass, capitalist society. Living a 'respectable' life, they stuck with the person they married and lived 'happily ever after'. Or so it seemed. In fact, it was argued, they had forgotten how to be spontaneous or to think or feel independently. Internally, they felt anxious and insecure, out of touch with their 'true selves'. They tried to dull this unpleasant feeling with consumer goods. It was considered that World War II was the ultimate consequence of such a passive attitude to life. Obviously, Western society needed some kind of 'shock therapy'. Perhaps adolescents could administer it.

As this article attempts to show, events in the therapeutic community of Amstelland reflected the cultural developments hinted at above. They serve to demonstrate that there was a close relationship between trends in mental health care and the more general climate of the 1960s, which was as much psychological as political in nature.

Magic mountain

The founder of Amstelland was psychiatrist and psychoanalyst Jan van de Lande, 32 years old at the time of Amstelland's foundation. His therapeutic community was part of Santpoort, a large psychiatric hospital near Amsterdam. Amstelland catered for about 60 people aged from 15 to 25 years of age. The main pillars of treatment were to be the writings of Maxwell Jones and the principles of psychoanalytic group therapy.

Especially during its early years, a revolutionary spirit and a feeling of superiority were dominant in the young community, which liked to present itself as critical of both 'bourgeois' society and 'traditional' psychiatry. As Van de Lande stated in 1971, 'Supposing we call all deviant individuals "weeds", then, as long as we continue to remove these weeds from society and lock them behind plates saying "Dune and Field", "Light and Water", "Bogland and Valley", a mono-culture will come into being in which possible changes without compulsion will have to be waited for for a long time'.[2]

According to sociotherapist John Bassant, 'at the time we felt nobody was as good as us'. Social worker Leo Folgering compared Amstelland with the tuberculosis-sanatorium in Thomas Mann's *Magic Mountain*: 'We looked down with disdain on the world below. They just didn't know, they just lived on... We, on the contrary, possessed the wisdom.' Many members of the Amstelland personnel identified with their patients and projected their own desires, feelings, or self-image onto them. For example, Van de Lande, who presents himself as a true rebel in his writings and interviews, was sympathetic to the playful anarchy of adolescents. He recounts how he was himself once expelled from high school, 'My parents were Catholic, so I went to a Jesuit School. I hated it, and in the fifth grade I was forced to leave after I delivered an anti-Catholic speech from the roof of the bicycle shed!'

The young people who, likewise, climbed onto the barricades in the late sixties filled him with enthusiastic optimism. As he put it in 1980, 'In 1968, adolescents displayed revolutionary powers... The revolt in Paris, the Maagdenhuis affair [an Amsterdam student revolt], pop music and soft drugs showed that the instinctive life still had chances to offer. "Freedom" and "Love" became key words, which inevitably had to enter psychiatry... This led to an extra emphasis on the adolescent as, on the one hand, the victim who had to be liberated, and on the other hand, the hero, who would bring salvation.'[3]

Bassant describes similar feelings. 'Like most people at Amstelland, I found young people attractive because of their seeming freedom to live life to the full. In those days, adolescents were almost identification figures for older people; they were truly glorified. At the time we never talked about it in those terms, but I think this was the implicit feeling of many of us.' Social worker Folgering regarded Amstelland as a therapeutic community for the personnel as well as the patients, 'Many people working there, including myself, felt their education had been too restrictive. In offering young people at Amstelland a more tolerant environment, the kind you would have wanted to have yourself, it was possible to do some "*Wiedergutmachung*", to repair some of the damage that was done to yourself when you were younger.'

War on the family

As youthful non-conformists were idealised during the 1960s, criticism of the family grew. In the eyes of its critics, the family represented, on a micro-level, exactly the kind of society they wanted to change. The warm womb of the family, it was argued, was actually a hotbed of horrible psychodramas. All the general evils of Western society were present. In families, the 'alienation' and lack of 'authentic' communication were especially abrading. The need to achieve and to be 'normal' was forcefully instilled into little children, while weak or deviant family-members were cruelly victimised. Revolutionary movements often attack the family as the ultimate bulwark of a 'wrong' kind of society and, in similar fashion, it fell under attack during the 'cultural revolution' of the sixties.

In Amstelland, these trends were translated into therapeutic practice. A positive approach to adolescent identity crisis was combined with a strong devaluation of parental authority. Van de Lande was convinced that psychoses and deviant forms of behaviour should be considered as 'rites of passage' which were to be understood, not repressed. He argued that not only the individual but also society at large could benefit from the new values expressed by young people. As he once put it,

> Young people today seem more impressive, not only because of their growth in length, width, and number, but also, and mostly, because of their significance in a psychological sense. [But] they hardly get a chance to show their own face. Their portrait is already drawn, based on prejudice and the jealous ideas or unfulfilled wishes of oldsters... Recently, a number of rebellious American students were submitted

to a psychological investigation, because they were thought to suffer from some mental disorder. To the astonishment of many, they turned out to be decidedly intelligent, well informed, critical, good observers, open to their fellow human beings, averse to inauthentic routine, distrustful of unclear traditions and not particularly interested in material gain. Thus, prejudices were unmasked and a portrait arose of the youth of today: tall, spanking people, who are not easily frightened![4]

Consciousness III

In his fascination for adolescents, Van de Lande was perfectly in tune with his time. During the post-war decades, young people had become a popular subject of attention in the Western world.[5] Of course, interest in adolescents was not a new phenomenon[6] but after 1945, it reached a new height. This was partly the result of new perceptions, and partly of concrete phenomena such as the post-war baby-boom, the growth of affluence, the longer duration of education and the earlier onset of puberty thanks to improved nutritional and health standards. Teenagers had more time and money to spend which led to a separate, internationally oriented youth culture coming into existence, with its own magazines, music and clothes. Non-conformist subcultures were born, such as the 'beat generation' in America, 'existentialists' in France and the English 'angry young men'.

Commercial entrepreneurs quickly discovered the rapidly expanding teenage market. At the same time, social scientists, psychologists, and psychiatrists started to pay more attention to adolescence. The writings of psychologist Erik Erikson were especially influential. They were certainly an important source of inspiration for Jan van de Lande. Erikson was a Freudian, but his views differed from Freud's in several important ways. In classical psychoanalysis, the crucial developmental stages of the individual occur only in the first years of life. Erikson, however, believed that the development of personality was a continuing process, divided into stages stretching into old age. Like Anna Freud, who had analysed him, he did not think the 'ego' was just a mediator between the 'id' and the 'super-ego'. Erikson considered the ego to be a source of strength in its own. He argued that Man was an individual with his own identity. Adolescence was the crucial stage in the formation of this identity and was often a period of conflict and experiment. During this stage, according to Erikson, 'delinquent and "borderline"

268

psychotic episodes are not uncommon'.[7]

The tone of those commenting on youth culture was mixed. Many critics expressed concern about the nihilism, hedonism, and delinquent tendencies among the 'youth of today'. Others welcomed their non-conformism, 'classlessness', and exciting energy. Influential American social scientists like Paul Goodman in *Growing up Absurd* (1960) and Kenneth Keniston in *The Uncommitted: Alienated Youth in American Society*, (1965) portrayed modern youth as the main victims of the 'alienation', loneliness, and disintegration in Western society. Slowly, a shift of focus came about, 'from teenagers as real or potential delinquents to teenagers as young adults in the making'.[8] Young adults, moreover, who could pay an important contribution to the evolution of society.

Some put forward a decidedly romantic image of young people as the embodiment of a natural spontaneity, freedom of mind, energy, happiness, and sexuality that many people felt they themselves had lost. For example, Charles Reich, a law teacher at Yale University, argued in his best-seller *The Greening of America* (1970) that in the wake of the 'hippies', mankind was entering a new and better stage of consciousness. He propounded that after Consciousness I, of religious man in rural society, and Consciousness II, the abysmal state of mind of modern man in the technological state, some people were now evolving into Consciousness III. These people were spiritually more awake, more tolerant, willing to think for themselves in a critical way and unwilling to renounce personal responsibility. Reich wrote, 'There is less guilt, less anxiety, less self-hatred. Consciousness III says, "I'm glad I'm me"... Perhaps there was always a bit of Consciousness III in every teenager, but normally it quickly vanished.'[9]

In the Netherlands, views on adolescents were also changing. As historian James Kennedy argues, during the sixties 'for many older people, youth became the embodiment of their inability to control the future'.[10] As the Dutch minister of social welfare, Marga Klompé expressed it in 1967, 'At the moment, so many changes are taking place in society that the whole of mankind has become a bit insecure. Young people as well. If adolescents revolt against society, which in fact operates with obsolete structures, it is a healthy phenomenon.'[11]

In his dissertation, *In Praise of Maladjustment* (1969), sociologist H. Milikowski argued that innovative and creative people, like Socrates, Jesus or Luther, had always been considered 'weird' and maladjusted in their own times, whereas today they are presented as heroes. Why then, he asked, are Ho Chi Min, Fidel Castro or the young people who seem to 'go against the grain' today not given the same credit? In his book, which sold well in Holland during the 1970s, Milikowski further elaborated on his objections to the 'industrial world, where people become more and more like each other in looks, behaviour and ideals'.[12]

Psychological breakdown: a necessary ordeal

The young Van de Lande was an admirer of 'anti-psychiatrists' Laing and Cooper. He sometimes compared Amstelland with Cooper's 'Villa 21', and a large portrait of Laing adorned one of Amstelland's walls. Anti-psychiatrists firmly held to a concept of personal growth through crisis. This was an important theme within the whole of mental health care during the sixties and seventies. However, anti-psychiatrists took this to an extreme, they stated that 'psychiatric patients' were perhaps more 'aware' and healthy than supposedly normal people. Van de Lande reflected, 'I especially liked Laing's notion of the psychotic breakdown in adolescence as a phase in life they had to go through, a necessary ordeal that would bring them to a higher level of psychological integration'.[13] If adolescents were psychotic, then this had to be regarded as a searching for new ways, an attempt at reintegration, 'possibly at a new and higher level: "*réculer pour mieux sauter*"'. [14]

'Schizoid' young adults were central to Laing's first and most famous book *The Divided Self* (1960). He presented them as 'ontologically insecure' individuals with a poor sense of 'integral selfhood and personal identity'. Their insecurity, Laing thought, was due to a gap between the 'true' and the 'false' self. The true self had become estranged from the 'surface persona' or the mask presented to the outside world. Laing attempted to trace this estrangement back to profound interpersonal disjunctures in the first years of personal development.[15]

In his later work he elaborated on this theme, becoming progressively more radical. The psychotic individual, Laing argued, had fled into madness as an escape from an undesirable situation.[16] However, a breakdown could be a breakthrough. In 1965, Laing established an experimental community, Kingsley Hall in London, where people could live through their breakdown without medical or therapeutic interference.

A few years earlier Cooper had founded Villa 21, 'an experiment in anti-psychiatry'. The Villa was a therapeutic community within a large psychiatric hospital near London, and catered for about 20 young 'schizophrenics'.[17] It was closed down in 1966. It had become too experimental for the hospital management to tolerate. The staff at 'the Villa' had started to doubt the divisions between sanity and insanity and one day had simply decided to renounce all their traditional tasks. They withdrew from household matters and stopped activating the 'patients'.

Although Villa 21 did not survive, Amstelland did. Partly this was due to differences between them. Despite Van de Lande's sympathy for anti-psychiatric theories, his therapeutic community was much less experimental, anarchistic, or 'anti-therapeutic' than Kingsley Hall or Villa 21 had been. Amstelland was no anti-psychiatric stronghold. Traditional psychoanalytic principles and theories about how a therapeutic community should function were always upheld and there was no abandonment of rules or daily structure.

Despite the feeling of being special and revolutionary at Amstelland, as Bassant put it, 'looking back I realise Amstelland was just as psychiatric as any other institution for mental health care. We admitted individuals who were ill and tried to make them better. A medical model, in spite of everything we built around it. We just had different ideas about how psychiatry should be practised. We just thought there should be more attention for the social context of illness and for the patient as an individual.'

From traditional hospital to therapeutic community

All in all, the 'revolution' of Amstelland was a comfortable one. The rebellious community was offered a great deal of money and space for their experiment due to developments in Dutch hospital psychiatry. On the one hand, during the sixties, dissatisfaction prevailed about the growing number of chronic, elderly patients and the precarious phenomenon of 'hospitalisation'. The status of psychiatric hospitals was diminishing and they were in danger of silting up, whereas facilities for ambulatory mental health care started to increase.

On the other hand, hopes were raised by modern social and psychological methods of treatment, made possible by the introduction of the new psycho-pharmaceuticals.[18] Half-way houses were founded and both individual and group psychotherapy gained ground. A few therapeutic communities were founded in Holland during the 1950s and early 1960s, and experiments with group therapy and sociotherapy were conducted in some university clinics and psychiatric hospitals. However, it was not until the 1970s, that psychotherapeutic communities and group psychotherapy truly began to flourish.[19]

Things were slowly changing in Santpoort, too. For a long time, Santpoort had remained a 'traditional' hospital. Patients spent their days either working or in bed. They were differentiated according to their behaviour (quiet or restless) and sex. In 1967, 62 percent of the patients had lived in Santpoort for ten years or more. Eighty-one percent of the population was more than 40 years old.[20] Psychotherapy was hardly used and most therapeutic energy was directed at psycho-pharmaceutical research.

In 1964, however, a wind of change began to blow. A new director was appointed, who had studied in Switzerland with Carl Jung. He wanted to transform Santpoort into a therapeutic community, where sociotherapy and group psychotherapy would be the leading principles of treatment. P. Bierenbroodspot, a psychiatrist already working in Santpoort, was given the chance to write a dissertation on the idea and practice of a therapeutic community and its implementation within a 'traditional hospital'. The resulting book, published in 1969, became a psychiatric best-seller in the Netherlands.[21] By the end of the 1960s, some Santpoort wards had started experimenting with 'patient-staff meetings' and group therapy. In 1971, Bierenbroodspot established his own therapeutic community in the hospital, called Rijnland. The biggest symbol of this change, however, was to be Amstelland, the most experimental off-shoot of the Santpoort tree.

The directors of Santpoort allotted Amstelland one of the finest parts of the hospital building, a ward that had recently been completely refurbished. Originally, the ward was intended for a group of chronic patients who had been living in Santpoort for years and were finally to be given more privacy and a better living environment. At the last moment, however, youth was given precedence.

'To the directors, the concept of the therapeutic community seemed interesting', Van de Lande recounts. There were no special facilities for young patients in Santpoort, they simply wandered around on the wards amid the chronic patients. 'Of course, I had to play the management a little', Van de Lande claims. 'For instance, I put Bierenbroodspot and Maxwell Jones in the foreground and didn't mention Laing, although I doubt if they would have known him anyway. And when I told them I wanted to handle disturbed behaviour in a permissive fashion, I didn't let on that I actually wanted to leave all doors unlocked.'[22] Thus, negotiations passed off smoothly and the deal was satisfactory to both sides. Santpoort offered Van de Lande an opportunity to do challenging, innovative

272

work based on modern ideas, and Van de Lande offered Santpoort the prospect of presenting itself as a progressive hospital, in tune with modern times.

An ideal state

At Amstelland, psychotic and neurotic patients (or 'residents', as they were to be called) were mixed during therapy as well as in the sociotherapeutic 'living-groups'. In this way they could help and support each other. The neurotic person could see that things could be worse, whereas the psychotic one could benefit from being among people who were less ill than himself. After all, it was assumed, their underlying problems were, basically, the same. 'We didn't use traditional diagnoses in those days', Van de Lande recalls. 'We were very much against that. Instead, we labelled almost everything an identity crisis: an identity crisis with depressive symptoms, an identity crisis with psychotic symptoms, and so on.'

The basic tenet of treatment was that psychological problems should be muffled as little as possible. Therapists aimed to use as little medication or force as possible, although isolation cells did exist and psycho-pharmaceuticals were administered. However, the therapeutic culture was against it, as the memories of ex-Amstelland personnel show. 'Sometimes we let a person walk around psychotic for months on end', Van de Lande claims. 'We really admired them sometimes. How they turned their flight from distress into psychotic behaviour: we used to call that creative.' This creativity had to be acknowledged and listened to, though it was difficult at times not to intervene. Van de Lande commented, 'Sometimes we really had to say to each other: "Hold on, hold on!"'

Bassant remembers an episode in which a psychotic resident stood near the exit door for days,

> jumping up and down, moaning and screaming 'Oh god, no, oh god no'. Well, in those days a situation like that could last for days, weeks maybe. So I went up to this boy and tried to chat with him. The idea was that if you could find the right words, the right attitude, the right therapeutic intervention, then you could make this person take a turn for the better. So the well-being of a person depended on your actions, really. That's how it felt. It was a bit like magical thinking.

To pursue such a form of treatment a loyal team was essential. Van de Lande was given the chance to attract personnel who shared his points of view.[23] He wanted colleagues who 'worked from the heart' instead of the mind, and who focussed on the healthy aspects of individuals, instead of regarding them as walking diagnoses. Proper training was less important. Like Cooper, Van de Lande believed that unschooled people could have more healing power than trained personnel could.

In this way, a young and progressive group of people came to work in the new therapeutic community. The building had been painted in bright colours and contained three huge attics: one for creative therapy; one was for play and contained a ping-pong table, a billiard table and a pin-ball machine; and the third was a 'beat'-attic to throw parties in. According to Bassant, 'To me, Amstelland was a bit like an ideal state… At the time, I was sympathetic to anarchist ideas. I thought that as long as everyone at Amstelland would be allowed to take responsibility for themselves, things would turn out all right. An extraordinarily optimistic view of man, as I look back on it now.'

Life in Amstelland was organised in a liberal way. There were some basic rules, such as the daily patient-staff meetings and regular group therapy or psychodrama sessions. Aside from these obligations, however, there was a lot of free time to enjoy. Many hours were spent talking and listening or singing to guitar music. There was room for all kinds of spontaneous activities. Van de Lande recalled, 'Everyone invented something new. Putting the tables in the corridors and cooking a meal for the whole group. Taking a long walk to the beach. We played football all the time.'[24] The psychiatrists' reasoning was, 'Let's act like normal people, that will help the residents most'[25] which demonstrated an important adjustment to psychoanalytic thought. The therapist was not to be a 'distant mirror', but an open, honest person, not afraid to show himself in his true colours.

The enemy: the super-ego

While spontaneity and the primary forces of the 'id' were valued, all that was felt to represent the 'superego' was resisted, such as the main Santpoort hospital itself. Santpoort looked upon the beautiful new ward (nicknamed the 'Hilton-hotel') with mixed feelings. Amstelland was strikingly more liberal than the rest of the hospital. Whereas in Santpoort, nurses and doctors were still in uniform and many patients still wore 'asylum clothes', everyone at Amstelland wore their own clothes. Moreover, in Santpoort most doors were locked whilst at Amstelland all the doors were open and there were no restrictions on the freedom to move about. This meant that residents walked on the grass, swam in the pond, demolished trees, rang the hospital chapel's bell, played loud music, and used drugs.

Officially, drugs were forbidden at Amstelland and indeed the use of hard drugs such as speed was heavily combated, but the smoking of marihuana was often tolerated.

Most shocking of all, boys and girls were allowed to do all kinds of things together, even engage in sexual activities. In Santpoort, not only the patients but also the nurses were kept strictly apart while sexual relationships between Amstelland residents were freely tolerated. 'In those early days', Van de Lande recalls, 'experimenting with sex had a central meaning. Considering the whole "family-atmosphere" it is surprising that pregnancies were an exception.'[26] According to Bassant, however, there was hardly any sex at Amstelland.

> Sure, the atmosphere was such that much would have been allowed, but only few took the opportunity. Much to our surprise, by the way. We thought that those young, physically healthy people would raise the roof. But they didn't! Most of them were too insecure and scared of intimacy. I think there was more sex among members of the personnel.

Although Amstelland was not the Valhalla of sex, drugs and rock 'n roll some believed it to be, it was still much more tolerant than the other Santpoort wards. This excited a feeling of injustice. For years, the people at Santpoort had had to obey strict rules and now these impertinent newcomers broke them one by one, without being punished. The 'Amstellanders' seemed to enjoy and cultivate a special status and provocative attitude. Van de Lande himself grew his hair, started to wear trendy clothes, and walked on the lawns in the park, which was forbidden.

In the meantime, he offered his fellow psychiatrists a clinical analysis of his 'over-identification' with adolescents.[27] He manoeuvred cleverly between the roles of rebel, charismatic community leader, and ambitious, talented newcomer in the world of psychiatry, but always showed himself enthusiastic about his creation. As he proudly and frequently pointed out, since 1969 there had not been any suicides at Amstelland.[28] In the treatment of suicidal patients, 'the shared responsibility of every worker or resident at Amstelland has taken the place of an isolating architecture or a magic electroshock'.

Family afternoons

From the beginning of Amstelland's foundation, the ultimate representatives of the super-ego, and thus the ultimate enemies, were the parents. Van de Lande wrote in 1976, 'many members of staff experienced the parents as "the cause" of a failed development, or as "guilty" of the identity crisis of their child'.[29] Similar hostility towards parents was present in England, where anti-psychiatrists were among the leaders of an all-round attack on the 'bourgeois' family. 'The bourgeois nuclear family unit', wrote David Cooper in *The Death of the Family* (1971), 'has become the ultimately perfected form of "non-meeting"'. It was the main location for a 'chronic murder of selves' and of the socialisation of children towards 'normality' and 'conformism'. 'Bringing up a child in practice is more like bringing down a person', Cooper fulminated.[30] Laing was no friend of families either. He worked hard to show that they bred madness, as parents damaged their children with 'double binds' (conflicting messages) and by 'scapegoating' vulnerable family-members.[31]

This 'war' against parents was part of the broader spirit of cultural revolution.[32] Central to this revolution was the conviction that the individual no longer had to adjust to society; it had to be the other way around. What historian Roy Porter called a 'shift of culpabilisation' occurred within psychiatry as well.[33] For a long time, any family-member who did not 'fit in' was considered to be the main problem, and was therefore given psychiatric treatment. Freud dealt the first blow to the idyll of the happy family. In 1949, neo-Freudian Frieda Fromm-Reichman coined the infamous term 'schizophrenogenic mother'. In the 1950s, 'parent-blaming' had become popular in American psychiatry.[34] During the next two decades, family therapy blossomed and the concept of the family as a pathogenic unit reached a peak.

Of course, this concept did not always take on the radical forms of the anti-psychiatrists. Not all who theorised about the role of the family as a cause of mental distress were critics of culture and suspicious of parents, but some were. Amstelland was not alone in this respect. Zandwijk was one such example. This was a Dutch institution for the psychiatric treatment of adolescent boys, many of whom were referred through the police or the juvenile court. Around 1970, the theoretical basis of treatment was that much of the deviant behaviour of adolescent boys was due to their social background, in particular the closedness and isolation of families, the false 'idyll of the harmonious family' and the moral of achievement in Western society.[35] Van de Lande often visited Zandwijk and adopted many ideas from their example.

Joost Mathijsen, a psychiatrist working at Amstelland around 1970, remembered,

At Amstelland I constantly encountered situations that made me think, 'Ah, that's so typically Laing'. For example, a dialogue between a father and his daughter, 'Father, you must think I'm the loser of the family'. 'Oh no my dear, on the contrary, we really pity you.' So he denies what his daughter says, while at the same time confirming it by using the word 'pity'. It's all so subtle.[36]

'Amstelland fully participated in blaming the parents', said Joke Meillo, who worked at Amstelland as a psychodrama therapist from the mid-seventies. 'I did, too. It was just the spirit of the times.'[37]

Ideas about the negative influence of parents made the Amstelland staff adopt a distant attitude towards families. Until 1973, parents were kept away as much as possible. The residents were encouraged to leave home and live independently. Social worker Folgering claimed nobody went back home after Amstelland. However, slowly, parents became more involved in the treatment. From 1973 onwards, they were invited to come to Amstelland for 'family afternoons'. These meetings had a theme. 'For example, "Who is actually ill here?"', as one ex-resident remembered.[38]

Officially, these family afternoons were organised to explain to parents about the treatment at Amstelland and improve communication between parents and children. However, according to Van de Lande, he and many other members of staff, still had a bone or two to pick with their own parents.[39] Emotions could get heated. Van de Lande recounts how,

> I once treated a 19-year-old boy. He was autistic and had lost all contact with his surroundings. Medication hadn't helped. The symbiotic relationship with his mother seemed to be a typical example of all the descriptions of schizophrenic processes within the family. But the parents were determined to remove the boy from the pernicious influence of Amstelland. When they took their boy away, I experienced it as theft; me and a social worker reacted to this event by taking a long walk in the park, both of us moved to tears.[40]

Sociotherapist John Bassant recalls similar scenes,

> Those family-afternoons were organised like regular therapy sessions. Just wait and see which emotions start to surface, and then work with that. The more emotional the better. The idea was to confront parents with their children's feelings. It could get very heavy. Some children became really emotional and then were ashamed of it afterwards. They had lost it in front of the 'troops', so to speak.

Folgering vividly remembers those family afternoons. The residents sitting with the staff, the parents all sat together. According to Folgering

> Jan could be very theatrical. Once, he walked up to the parents of a psychotic boy and, in front of all those other patients and their parents, he started to shout at the father, 'You! You, sir, you have poisoned your son!' Everyone almost applauded. Embarrassing, that's what I think of it now. But, it was our hero who did it, and it seemed an act of liberation, a brave deed. And of course, I too felt that my father had failed… Well, at some unconscious level it worked as a liberation for yourself, as well.

Sera Anstadt, a Dutch writer whose son was admitted to Amstelland in the early-seventies, went to one of the first family afternoons at Amstelland. She returned shocked and saddened. She wrote,

> Most parents looked frightened, helpless, and shy. They knew little about the illness of their child, who in the meantime had adopted the language of the staff. Obviously, they had been taught how to behave towards their parents. Without reserve, one accusation after the other was expressed through the microphone. The parents had little chance to respond. Few of the children went to sit by their side. I was under the impression that some of them wanted to do so, but they also wanted to keep their countenance in the presence of their fellow patients… Many of the parents left with tears in their eyes.[41]

Anstadt claimed that one psychiatrist accused her of being happy to be rid of her son saying 'You think he is well put away here, I notice'. Andstadt protested. The psychiatrist had judged her too easily, she said. She disagreed with her son finding a place of his own in Amsterdam, as the staff of Amstelland had suggested. She desperately told the psychiatrist, 'He can't live alone, but he can't live with people either. Whole families are destroyed because they have to live with someone who is impossible to live with.' However, the psychiatrist told Anstadt in a lecturing manner 'No madam, that's not how it works. It's the families who destroy their weaker members.'

This same attitude towards parents was represented in two films, *Family Life* by Ken Loach (1972) and its Dutch counterpart, *Kind van de zon* ('Child of the sun', 1975), which was based on the situation at Amstelland. Van de Lande gave psychiatric advice to the director of the film and had a big hand in the editing. *Kind van de zon*, which was released nationally, concerns Anna, a young girl who lived with her parents in a small village.[42] She leaves for Amsterdam, much against the will of her parents. However, things do not go as planned. She finds that she is sexually inhibited and tends to withdraw from people.

Returning home, she pours out her heart to her mother, who is portrayed as cold and demanding. Anna cries and calls herself a failure. Her mother neither touches nor comforts her but says, 'Do you think it makes me happy to see you like this? You know all I want is for you to be happy!' Anna cries out, 'Leave me alone mummy! I am not a little plaything that you can push and then it starts to play, because it doesn't play! It just doesn't work with me! Oh, why don't you just hug me, I know you can't, but I'm so sad about that…'. After this failed attempt at communication, Anna is committed to Amstelland.

After being there for a period, Anna's mother talks with a psychiatrist. She asks whether Anna is well again, and when she can come back home. In a drawling, passive-aggressive manner, the psychiatrist answers, 'Well, you do notice that I do not give you a clear answer to that question, don't you? Like yes or no, ill or well.' Anna's mother is confused and filled with indignation, 'But who else can I ask? Should I see the director of the hospital? Please, tell me, is Anna well or not?' 'Well, I don't think you'll be getting any certainty on that point, do you?', the psychiatrist continues. 'I believe it's quite a disappointment to you, isn't it, that Anna can't come home with you, and that I don't sit down and scribble something official on a piece of paper.'

Together the sources show clearly that during the pioneering decade of Amstelland, parents were treated as if they were children, even naughty children, who had to be taught a lesson. Children, however, were supported, given a great deal of freedom and were even put on a pedestal. I would argue that the Amstelland staff practised something like 'resistance-therapy', a popular term in the 1970s. It meant that treatment consisted of making patients aware of the external forces that repressed them, so that they would start to rebel against them. As the Dutch sociologist, Milikowski described it: 'Resistance therapy occupies itself with fighting the social causes of mental illnesses. Doctors and patients take part in it together.'[43] In an extreme form, this kind of therapy was used by the radical German 'Socialist Patients Collective', who wanted to stimulate the protest of 'patients' against the capitalist 'system'. The Collective believed that psychological problems were actually frustrated attempts at becoming aware of the external powers that repressed them. Focussing on the pathogenic family and trying to get adolescents in crisis to break away from their parents was a milder form of the same concept.

Paradise lost

Tragically, in 1974 four suicides in a row occurred at Amstelland.[44] The dismay was intense; they were the first suicides to take place within five years. In the case of one 19-year-old boy, the staff thought, suicide might have been prevented. The boy had been described as 'rigid, intellectualising, with a strong defence against emotions, a superior attitude towards the staff and his fellow patients'. According to his closest friend, who helped him to his fatal dose of pills, the boy had cultivated a 'romantic death cult', involving astrology, magic and occultism. He had organised secret ritual meetings in his bedroom.[45] Several residents knew about this and joined a secret club under the leadership of the boy. One Saturday night, music by Vivaldi was heard playing loudly in the boy's room. The staff decided to let him be. The next morning he was found lying dead on his bed, his hand on a book by Plato, which lay open at the scene of Socrates' death.

The last of the four suicides was especially traumatic for the Amstelland personnel. A patient hanged himself in his room while at the very same moment staff and group-leaders were sitting in the living room discussing how to handle his continuing suicidal tendencies.[46] The series of suicides led to very emotional staff-meetings. The collective 'hubris' had been dealt a severe blow. In Bassant's view, this 'hubris' was not just arrogance but also a necessity, in keeping up the often chaotic and difficult psychiatric experiment at Amstelland. Furthermore, the ideal of 'openness', so important in a therapeutic community, had been betrayed.

These events were not the only reason for the gradual change of climate in Amstelland after 1975. However, they did strengthen pre-existing doubts. There had already been conflict over the situation at Amstelland after one group had been on a holiday. During this vacation, a group leader had had sex with a resident. On top of this, a psychotic boy had deteriorated to a catatonic state and nothing had been done about it. Apparently, it was thought that this was something he wanted or needed to do. The boy had stood immobile in the corner of the room for days. When the holiday was over, these events led to heated discussions within the team.[47]

Slowly, from the mid-seventies onwards a new course was set.[48]

First, closer attendance and more structure in the daily activities were thought to be necessary. Adolescents were to be trained in social skills, assertiveness, and bodily hygiene. Second, the conclusion was reached that it was impossible to treat the patients without involving the family more. Social worker Folgering played an important part in the resulting expansion of family therapy. He commented,

> To be honest, I did not want to be a traditional social worker anymore, I wanted to play with the 'big guys', be a psychotherapist. And so I did. First, we focussed on eliminating pathological patterns, following the ideas of Watzlawick and Palazzoli, for example. Later on, we also started to aim at repairing the affectionate and pedagogical bonds between the family-members. Healing the whole family, restoring parents in their authority. Well, that led to a lot of protest. It went against the whole traditional idea of parents being 'poison' for the patients, the notion that you had to liberate them and that in the meantime, Amstelland was to be their home. I started to fight that model, calling it 'pedagogical kidnapping'.

Third, a closed unit was installed, for patients with strong psychotic symptoms, suicidal tendencies, or a tendency to keep running away. The unwillingness to use medication or force diminished. Moreover, the concept of psychosis as a possible breakthrough and attempt at solving conflicts, which had to be given time, slowly changed into the notion of psychosis as a dangerous phase in life, which could lead to total disintegration of the personality and a phase which had to be mended as soon as possible.[49] Thus, the reality of treating disturbed adolescents ultimately forced the Amstelland staff to adjust their original ideals and practice.

Negotiation between autonomous individuals

The kind of hostility towards parents and idealisation of adolescents present at Amstelland during the first period of its inception, was probably to be found only within a relatively small social vanguard. However, in many people's lives less revolutionary but nevertheless important developments were taking place. Divorce was becoming common and thanks to 'the pill' people could experiment more sexually. At the beginning of the twenty-first century, there are more one parent and one person households than during the 1950s and 1960s. Although the nuclear family as an institution has far from disappeared, relationships within it have changed. Women have more chances to develop themselves. The interaction between parents and children seems less formalised and authoritarian. To put it in very simplified terms, the model of men commanding their wives and parents commanding their children is now strongly combated by a model of negotiation between a group of autonomous individuals. This model has become the basis for many families.[50] Of course, similar changes in power structures and an informalisation of manners are perceptible throughout society.[51] The situation at Amstelland was an extreme expression of such structural changes.

At the turn of the millennium, there is again much anxiety about the status of the family, though it has a different content. The alleged demise of the family is now thought to cause social disintegration, psychological problems, and criminality.[52] The family has always been a prime candidate for use as a metaphor for cultural discomfort – just as psychiatric illnesses are.

Notes

1. Interview G. Blok with J. Bassant, 13 October 1999 and with L. Folgering, 28 October 1999. All quotes in this article from mr. Bassant and mr. Folgering are from these interviews. For this anecdote, see also S. van 't Hof, 'De geschiedenis van Amstelland, voormalige jeugdafdeling van het Provinciaal Ziekenhuis te Santpoort, 1968-1994', in *idem*, J. Broerse and L. de Goei, *Tulpenburg en Amstelland 1951-1994. Bladzijden uit de geschiedenis van de Nederlandse kinder- en jeugdpsychiatrie* (Utrecht: Trimbos-instituut, 1997), 101-81: 127. In writing this article, this book on Tulpenburg and Amstelland has been a great help and inspiration. I would also like to thank mrs. Van 't Hof for kindly allowing me to use the transcripts of her interviews with psychiatrist Jan van de Lande.

2. J. van de Lande, 'Verandering zonder macht', *Maandblad voor Geestelijke Volksgezondheid*, 27: 7/8 (1972), 360-71: 370.

3. J. van de Lande, 'Borderline-adolescenten; relatie tussen concept, behandeling en tijdsbeeld', in M. Eijer (ed.), *Adolescenten en psychiatrie. Enkele specifieke stoornissen in de adolescentie en haar behandeling* (Deventer: Van Loghum Slaterus, 1982), 89-99: 93.

4. J. van de Lande, *Kind van de zon. Naar aanleiding van de Nederlandse speelfilm van René van Nie* (Haarlem: J.H. Gottmer, 1976), 26-7.

5. A. Marwick, *The Sixties: Cultural Revolution in Britain, France, Italy and the United States, c.1958-1974* (Oxford: Oxford University Press, 1998), 41-112; R. Abma, *Jeugd en tegencultuur. Een theoretische*

verkenning (Nijmegen: SUN, 1990); C. In 't Velt, *Jong in de jaren '50. Tijdsbeeld van een generatie* (Utrecht: Kosmos, 1994); J. Janssen, *Jeugdcultuur. Een actuele geschiedenis* (Utrecht: De Tijdstroom, 1994); G. Tillekens, *Nuchterheid en nozems. De opkomst van de jeugdcultuur in de jaren vijftig* (Muiderberg: Coutinho, 1990).

6. See, for example, J. Neubauer, *The fin-de-siècle Culture of Adolescence* (New Haven: Yale University Press, 1992).

7. E. Erikson, *Identity: Youth and Crisis* (New York: Norton & Company, 1968), 131-2.

8. Marwick, *op. cit.* (note 5), 46.

9. C. Reich, *The Greening of America* (New York: Random House, 1970).

10. J. Kennedy, *Nieuw Babylon in aanbouw. Nederland in de jaren zestig* (Amsterdam: Boom, 1995), 45.

11. *Ibid.*, 161.

12. H. Milikowski, *Lof der onaangepastheid* (Meppel: Boom, 1977).

13. Van 't Hof, *op. cit.* (note 1), 109.

14. Van de Lande, *op. cit.* (note 3), 93.

15. R.D. Laing, *The Divided Self. Existential Studies in Sanity and Madness* (London: Tavistock Publications, 1960).

16. D. Burston, *The Wing of Madness. The Life and Work of R.D. Laing* (Cambridge, Mass./London: Harvard University Press, 1996), 58.

17. D. Cooper, *Psychiatrie en anti-psychiatrie* (Meppel: Boom 1973; original title *Psychiatry and Anti-Psychiatry*, 1967), 94-117.

18. G. Blok, 'Wetenschap en wederopbouw', in G. Blok and J. Vijselaar, *Terug naar Endegeest. Patiënten en hun behandeling in het psychiatrisch ziekenhuis Endegeest 1897-1997* (Nijmegen: SUN, 1998), 147-86; P. Schnabel, 'Dutch Psychiatry after World War II', in M. Gijswijt-Hofstra and R. Porter (eds), *Cultures of Psychiatry and Mental Health Care in Post-War Britain and the Netherlands* (Amsterdam and Atlanta: Rodopi, 1998), 29-43.

19. J. van de Lande (ed.), *Opgenomen in de groep. Psychotherapeutische gemeenschappen in Nederland* (Deventer: Van Loghum Straterus, 1982).

20. Van 't Hof, *op. cit.* (note 1), 101.

21. P. Bierenbroodspot, *De therapeutische gemeenschap en het traditionele ziekenhuis* (Meppel: Boom, 1969); see also J. Vijselaar, 'Vrijheid, gelijkheid en broederschap', in *idem* (ed.), *Gesticht in de duinen. De geschiedenis van de provinciale psychiatrische ziekenhuizen van Noord-Holland van 1849 tot 1994* (Haarlem: Verloren, 1997),192-238: 201.

22. Interview G. Blok with J. van de Lande, 7th June 1999. Unless

mentioned differently, all quotes from Van de Lande stem from this interview.

23. Van 't Hof, *op. cit.* (note 1), 110.

24. *Ibid.*, 116.

25. J. van de Lande, 'Adolescenten roepen gevoelens op', *Tijdschrift voor Psychiatrie*, 15 (1973), 89-98: 92.

26. Van de Lande, *op. cit.* (note 3), 96.

27. Van de Lande, *op. cit.* (note 25).

28. Van de Lande, *op. cit.* (note 2), 367; G. Dijkhuis, '"Daar ligt een galblaas, die huilt zo". Interview met Jan van de Lande', *Avenue* (February 1974), 27-9.

29. J. van de Lande, 'Gezinsmiddagen op Amstelland', *Maandblad voor Geestelijke Volksgezondheid*, 31:1 (1976), 3-14: 3.

30. D. Cooper, *The Death of the Family* (Harmondsworth: Penguin, 1971), 5–6.

31. R.D. Laing and A. Esterson, *Sanity, Madness and the Family* (London: Tavistock Publications, 1964); R.D. Laing, *The Politics of the Family* (London: Tavistock Publications, 1969).

32. K. van Meel, 'Begeestering en ontnuchtering', in G. Hutschemaekers and M. de Winter (eds), *De veranderlijke moraal. Over moraliteit en psychologie* (Nijmegen: SUN, 1996), 35-49.

33. R. Porter, 'Anti-Psychiatry and the Family', in Gijswijt-Hofstra and Porter (eds), *op. cit.* (note 18), 257-83.

34. E. Dolnick, *Madness on the Couch: Blaming the Victim in the Hey-Day of Psychoanalysis* (New York: Simon & Schuster, 1998), 83-169; C.E. Hartwell, 'The Schizophrenogenic Mother Concept in American Psychiatry', *Psychiatry: Journal of the Biology and the Pathology of Interpersonal Relationships*, 59 (1996), 274-97.

35. J. Schouten, S. Hirsch and H. Blankenstein, *Laat je niet kennen. Over residentiële behandeling van adolescenten* (Deventer: Van Loghum Staterus, 1974).

36. B. Bruins, Interview with Joost Mathijsen, in K. Trimbos (ed.), *Dat wordt me te gek. De psychiatrie kritisch bekeken* (Amsterdam: Contact, 1972), 155-65.

37. Meillo quoted in Van 't Hof, *op. cit.* (note 1), 148.

38. Van 't Hof, *op. cit.* (note 1), 122.

39. Van de Lande, *op. cit.* (note 29), 3-14.

40. Van de Lande, *op. cit.* (note 25), 94-5.

41. S. Anstadt, *Al mijn vrienden zijn gek. De dagen van een schizofrene jongen* (Den Haag: BZZTôH, 1983), 50-68.

42. R. van Nie, *Kind van de zon* (Pandora-movie 1975).

43. H. Milikowski, 'Daarom wil ik pleiten voor verzetstherapie', in

Trimbos (ed.), *op. cit.* (note 36), 202-6.

44. L. van Eck, W. Knol-Schoonhoven and J. van de Lande, 'Suïcide en psychiatrische behandeling', *Tijdschrift voor Psychiatrie*, 18 (1976), 761-808.

45. *Ibid.*, 'Suïcide', 790-1.

46. Interview G. Blok with J. Bassant.

47. Van 't Hof, *op. cit.* (note 1), 129; Interview G. Blok with J. Bassant.

48. Van 't Hof, *op. cit.* (note 1), 141-56.

49. Van de Lande, *op. cit.* (note 3), 98.

50. G. van Schoonhoven, 'Een heel nieuw leven', in *idem* (ed.), *De nieuwe kaaskop. Nederland en de Nederlanders in de jaren negentig* (Amsterdam: Prometheus, 1999), 240-9: 245.

51. A. de Swaan, 'Uitgaansbeperking en uitgaansangst: over de verschuiving van bevelshuishouding naar onderhandelingshuishouding', in *idem*, *De mens is de mens een zorg* (Amsterdam: Meulenhof, 1982), 81-116.

52. M. Neve, 'Nuclear Fallout: Anxiety and the Family', in S. Dunant and R. Porter (eds), *The Age of Anxiety* (London: Virago Press, 1996), 107-23.

13

In the Name of the Child Beyond

Roger Cooter

Ten years ago *In the Name of the Child* was conceived as a means to bridge a gap between the history of childhood and the history of medical and welfare provision for children. Unlike the social and cultural history of childhood, which was rich and flourishing in the wake of the debate initiated by Ariès in the early-1960s, the historical literature on the medical welfare of children was meager and dull. Where not immersed in narratives of progress, it was dominated by the anachronistic triumphalism of mid-twentieth-century welfareism. *In the Name of the Child* claimed new perspectives. It aimed to locate child welfare initiatives in their full and appropriate socio-economic, intellectual and cultural contexts. More crucially, it sought to reveal how those initiatives were constitutive of the political and ideological interests that they often served to mask. For the period from the 1880s to the 1940s, it revealed how child-centered medico-humanitarian concerns expressed by moralists, pedagogues, philanthropists, politicians, doctors and the state served to mediate political and social self-interests and idealisations. Children did not gain a voice over the period; rather, 'in their name' they became an effective mouthpiece for legitimating the power agendas of adults. *In the Name of the Child* illuminated why the child, relative to other available rhetorical resources (such as animals, prostitutes, or the elderly) became so favoured from the late nineteenth century in the articulation of interests. To expose the construction of that focus and the way it was sustained was central to the book's purpose.

So where are we now? How have we shifted ground? First, it has to be said that there have been no significant developments in the literature on child health and welfare over the past decade or, for that matter, on the history of childhood. No inspirational study has emerged to drive the field forward, as was partly the case for *In the Name of the Child* through Vivian Zelsizer's *Pricing the Priceless Child* (1985). A glance at the references in the present collection confirms the recent observation of Harry Hendrick, that children and childhood have yet to become a major focus of historical research, 'either in terms of prestige or of popularity'.[2] To the extent that they have gained some purchase, it has been in relation either to wider, more general historical agendas, or in connection with specific foci, such as the history of sports, masculinity, and 'mental defectives'.

Secondly, it is evident that many of the chapters in this volume could easily have been incorporated into *In the Name of the Child*. To some extent, Deborah Thom's chapter continues a discussion actually begun in that volume, while Nelleke Bakker's closely parallels the chapter by Cathy Urwin and Elaine Sharland on childcare advice in inter-war Britain. Several of the chapters cover the same territories: schools, custodial institutions, the family, political parties, child guidance clinics, and parental advice literature. They elaborate some of the same processes and issues: professionalisation, medicalisation, psychologisation, experimentation, legislation, pedagogy, social policy and, not least, the difficulty of defining 'the child'. At root they are animated by a similar curiosity about how the material, educational, legal, psychological and other circumstances of children in the West today have come to differ so substantially from those of a hundred years ago when the 'Century of Childhood' was proclaimed. And similar is their unstated suspicion that, whatever the changes and modulations in the comprehension of childhood over the century, it was around the century's beginning that the modern idealisation was constructed.

Yet, differences between these two books are no less apparent, and they extend beyond merely the introduction of new historical material such as that on law, rights, delinquency, and children's emotions. Most apparent is the explicit comparison with the Netherlands, which highlights the common and peculiar features that molded the investment in babies and children in both countries. Inherent to this comparative exercise is questioning the boundaries of the social and the cultural in the construction of childhood. What are we to make of the fact that welfare efforts on behalf of children in urban-industrial, secular, class-ridden, and reformist Britain appear more alike than different from those in the less-industrialised, sectarian, conservatively 'pillarized' society of the Netherlands? How much does immediate context matter? And how much, or how little, the role of contingencies? Some of the essays here address these questions directly; others do so simply by virtue of the different national perspectives they bring together between a single set of covers. The exercise is welcome, for transnational comparisons have been conspicuously absent from the history of child health and welfare. (Absent, too, have been regional comparisons within single states, or regional/ethno-religious comparisons such as those conveniently provided by the case of the Netherlands, or by England relative to Scotland.) Historians have long been aware of parallel developments in child health and welfare c.1900 in Western states, and that many international forums and agencies were involved.[3] It is striking, however, how national, Protestant, and Anglo-American dominated the research has remained.[4]

There are also significant differences in emphasis and nuance between these essays and those in *In the Name of the Child*. Although some of the subject matters may be the same, the graining is often finer. Predictably, perhaps, more weight is attached to the analysis of discourse, gender, and concepts of citizenship, rights, and identity – the latter three having mushroomed in historical writing during the 1990s. There is also greater attention to difference, temporal as well as spatial, as in John Welshman's reflections on the thinking around physical education in the 1930s, as opposed to the 1920s, or in Bakker's sensitivity to the discontinuities in the advice literature issued in the Netherlands between the 1890s and 1950s. Spatial differences (beyond those opened up by the UK/Netherlands comparison) are further exposed in the chapter on the reformer, Mulock Hower, which demonstrates how American Republicanism - a political space - instrumentally affected pedagogical techniques. Mark Jackson's analysis of the 'arrested' evolutionary conceptualisation of feeble-minded children, and the 'borderlands' of insanity that they were held to occupy, reminds us how metaphors of time and space were themselves central to discussions of children's minds and bodies. Overall, these essays broaden the themes of child health and welfare. They further remove us from the narrow corridors of hospitals and clinics, and the micro-politics of medical professionalisation and specialisation. Hence they also further distance us from the sociologically vulgar forms of 'medicalisation' lamented in *In the Name of the Child*. In many ways this broadening is captured by Bernard Harris' regard of the development of the School Medical Service in the UK as a branch of a public education service rather than 'a medical service which happened to be located in schools'.

Two essays in particular serve to illustrate how we have moved beyond the theoretical anchoring of *In the Name of the Child,* insofar as that rested on interests theory. The first is that by Lyubov Gurjeva on the middle-class nursery. While there have been many studies of late-nineteenth century professional inroads into the nursery and baby-care, Gurjeva's casting in terms of material culture is novel and revealing. The nursery emerges not only as an ideal, but also as a work sphere, a unit of production (as well as consumption), and a source of class distinction, division and identity. Clearly, one can locate specific interests here - middle-class families, manufacturers and salesmen of nursery products, doctors, scientific experts, and the state - but the model is more dynamic and interactively creative or 'performative' than reference to interests only would allow, or, indeed, reference merely to human agency. Although Gurjeva does not consider the feeder-bottle as an 'actant' in the Latourian sense, she comes near to it in her disclosure of how scientific and commercial artifacts and agents were enrolled in the middle-class nursery (and beyond). As such, she provides a perspective that was largely absent from *In the Name of the Child*. As other chapters in this collection also remind us, it was often neither crudely nor subtly 'in the name of the child' that action around children's minds and bodies was performed; frequently it was in the name of commerce, crime and punishment, scientific prowess, and theory itself. Above all, Gurjeva's chapter makes manifest that the history of child health and welfare turns on more than merely the aggrandisements of the medical profession, or on the machinations of politicians, charity workers, and ideologues. Religion, sexuality, concepts of minds, rights, citizenship, law, family, and identity (as well as the spaces within and between these discursive formations) might almost be juxtaposed historiographically to crude versions of interests theory. The competing agendas revealed through the latter exercise can often serve even to obscure the *creation* of interests forged through the relations between knowledge and politics, and the mobilisation of the forces around them.

The other essay that beckons significant theoretical departure from *In the Name of the Child* is that by Harry Hendrick. Whereas Gurjeva's essay reflects recent trends in the social history and sociology of science, Hendrick's study of the debate over the visiting of children in hospital - a subject hitherto largely neglected by historians - takes its cue from the pioneering work of Peter Stearns and his colleagues in the history and sociology of emotions. Again, like the late nineteenth-century nursery, the hospital in relation to the children within it can easily be historicised in terms of a site exploited by different kinds of professional interests. And Hendrick reveals those interests in the course of his mission to explain the cultural shift whereby professionals came to conceive of, and popularise, the emotional needs of children. But his essay hints at more: a history of children's own experience of illness and medicine.

Capturing children's own experience of reality is of course notoriously difficult. Beyond the obvious problem of a lack of sources for the historical study of children's interiority, there is the almost insurmountable burden of finding an adequate language to reveal the subjectivity of pain and sickness. Some of the parameters (and difficulties) of this pursuit have recently been addressed by Russell Viner and Janet Golden, but the promise they raise, of gaining 'a richer understanding of the historical experience and meaning of medicine' through the capture of children's experience of it, remains far from fulfilled. [5] Alternative ways of understanding 'reality', and of theorising childhood seem required; at the very least, as Hendrick appreciates, there is a need to link the history of childhood to the history of subjectivities, identity, and the emotional links between parents and children. Historians have dealt with children's minds and bodies in relation to health, disease and poverty, in connection with natalism, nationalism and maternity, and with regard to the professionalising manoeuvres of child psychologists and others, but they have hardly begun to consider the emotional world of children in relation to the historically shifting affections and roles of fathers, mothers, other siblings and families (not to mention guardians, orphanages and adoption agencies).[6]

A part of the problem here, as Hendrick has remarked elsewhere, lies in the preoccupation in recent years with the concept of *childhood* as a social construction, to the neglect of the historical study of *children* as social actors with their own strategies.[7] Insufficiently appreciated have been the differences between these two enterprises, the study of the latter being largely precluded by treating as unquestionably 'natural', rather than political, the distinction made (by adults) between children and adults. In equating personhood only with adulthood, we have been implicitly ageist or 'adultist' in our approach to the historical study of children and childhood, denying children even the possibility of an authentic voice or, in their own way, exercise of power. Although none of the contributors to this volume, including Hendrick, confronts this problem head-on, they nevertheless suggest some of the borderlands where it might fruitfully be pursued - in relation to the history of children's rights, around juvenile delinquency, the 'discovery' of adolescence, and over the efforts of various children's institutions to draw age limits for entry.

The call to re-enfranchise the child in history by confronting and de-naturalising agism in the writing on children is a sign of how the imperatives to the historical pursuit of child health and welfare have shifted over the decade since *In the Name of the Child*. Although it may still be too soon to reflect deeply on the wider cultural context in which we were impelled to our task, the essays in the present volume highlight at least some of our biases, assumptions, and silences. Two such features now stand out. The first is the overemphasis on Britain in *In the Name of the Child*, or rather, the book's Anglo-centricism, despite its inclusion of chapters on America, parts of the European Continent, and Africa. The emphasis is understandable insofar as the 'big picture' of child health and welfare *c.*1900 — the preoccupation with 'fit' populations for industrial and imperial advantage - is best characterised in relation to what was then the world's dominant nation state. But the 'little picture' can be considerably different and historically revealing. To be reminded of the 'pillarized' denominational organisation of Dutch society is to be made aware of national contexts where divisions other than class, and concerns additional to those of economic efficiency, have had significant bearing on interventions in child health. The American 'melting pot' and the Canadian 'vertical mosaic' may not have been experienced with the same daily intensity as the 'pillars' of Dutch society, but they alert us to societal configurations (as well as issues of race and ethnicity) which were unlike the British and which, in turn, nuanced differently the rhetoric around the child. In these other places, as in the Netherlands, the idea of 'national fitness' (if it existed at all), was seldom so strident or so mobilising a force for child health as in militaristic and imperialistic Britain. 'Fitness' might well have been pursued in the interest of social accommodation to, or the strengthening of, religio-ethnic groupings. In some places, at certain times, it may have been pursued in the interest of creating 'good citizens', but the meaning and rhetorical exploitation of 'citizens' is hardly neutral. Indeed, the lesser reliance on citizenship rhetoric in Britain reflects the fact that in the USA and France, for instance, 'citizenship' was (and is) predicated upon and serves to celebrate a notion of belonging to an independent republic. In monarchical Britain, as Jordanova has noted with respect to the contemporary practice of history, 'notions of citizenship are not particularly strongly promoted'; here political identity rotates more around the idea of a strong and efficient nation state.[8] Among other things, escaping the 'big picture' usefully provides a perspective on past historical practice in the area of child health.

The other 'bias' of *In the Name of the Child* highlighted by the present collection is its chronological focus. Although a few of its chapters strayed into the 1950s, the concentration was on the heroic period of interest in the child, between 1880 and 1940. Several essays in this volume move the discussion forward in time, beyond the Second World War into a world bearing very differently on the realities and representations of the child. John Pickstone has recently characterised as 'communitarian' the medicine of the period c.1945-1970, in contrast both to the earlier 'productionist' medicine (preoccupied with the supply and health of populations for productive purposes), and the later 'consumerist' type with which we currently wrestle.[9] The values promoted in the age of communitarian medicine, he notes, were those of social inclusion and professional progress – a fairly good approximation in fact to the democratic concerns that Hendrick illuminates as emerging in the field of child psychology in the late-1930s.

What, practically, this new ideological and political-economic context meant for child health and welfare is something yet to be fully sorted out — country by country, pillar by pillar, class by class, and profession by profession. The *pace* of change and its *extent* in different locations also requires attention. (As Deborah Thom's chapter reminds us in relation to the use of corporal punishment in post-war Britain, shifts from body to mind could be far later and much less sudden than certain writings of Foucault might lead us to believe.) Some straightforward questions also need asking about the role of iatrogenic medicine in the post-war period, as opposed to the effects simply of greater welfare provision and family income; indeed, for the earlier period, too, more has been *assumed* about the impact of modern medicine on child mortality and morbidity than has actually been demonstrated. More problematic, though, are the implications of the post-1945 context for the figure of the child in socio-political rhetoric and discourse. Insofar as the welfare state was that which the political Left had struggled for partly 'in the name of the child' since the late nineteenth century, the child as ideological midwife could disappear. It is clear, especially from the contributions here by Gemma Blok and Hugo Röling, that in the post-war years socio-political concerns with (and psychologically mediated constructions of) 'adolescents', 'juveniles' and 'youths' overtook an earlier focus on 'the child'. To a degree, the beauty and rhetorical value of the icon of the innocent child was tarnished by the psychological leveling of all humans. Long before the unfolding of the Bolger tragedy in Britain in the 1990s, children had lost innocence; they could even be demonised.[10] A different set of cultural parameters than those existing c.1900 must prevail for the study of the mid-century figure of the 'troubled adolescent', the 'juvenile delinquent' and the 'reckless youth'. The historiography of child health and welfare needs to develop accordingly - the perils of metaphors of growth notwithstanding.

Where exactly the child fits in the post-welfare society of individual consumers remains an even greater unknown. The child as an object of 'medicalisation' has certainly not disappeared, and it may be fair to say from the point of view of surveillance (and perhaps in other ways too) that we have all been rendered child-like. But in culture generally and in body politics, the figure of the child has been superseded by the moral and commercial focus on the foetus, and, increasingly, on the gene. Consequently, the child no longer seems an intelligible category, even if, in the academy, 'childhood studies' has acquired its own momentum. (Interestingly, the latest textbook on the subject, while offering a variety of perspectives on childhood, contains no reference to medicine.)[11] In some ways, then, the plot of *In the Name of the Child* has run dry. Still, the transformation of the child into a non-intelligible category only begs questions about the nature of that process - not least, about the relations between medicine, capital and consumerism in different national contexts and within shifting global cultures.

The title of this volume, 'Cultures of Child Health' is itself an indication of how we have shifted ground since *In the Name of the Child*. In the singular, 'culture' is of course notoriously difficult to define, but within its use there is at least the recognition of mediums less fixed, less structural, and less causal than those invoked by 'the social'. As 'health' is broader than some definitions of 'medicine', so 'culture' seems more flexible and inclusive than 'society'. Inherent to 'the cultural' is a plurality of spaces for the medical, pedagogical and psychological mediation of the child. In that awareness, moreover, lies the further realisation that child health and welfare concerns ought never be reduced simply to competing social and ideological interests, or in any easy way reduced merely to social structures and ideologies. We have moved on then, not because the interest theory that informed *In the Name of the Child* has been rendered untenable, but rather, because we have gained a wider and deeper understanding of the contextual construction of interests both over time and place. And we have moved on because it is no longer necessary to insist on the social construction of 'the child' and the concept of 'childhood'; by now the point has been made. We accept that it cannot be otherwise, just as we accept that 'social history' is a tautology if all history is 'social.'[12]

'Cultures' in the plural, is all the more apposite, invoking not only different social contexts, but a multiplicity of forms (human and material) as well as sites (physical, social, intellectual, political, economic, financial, medical and educational) in which concerns and conceptualisations of child health and welfare have been taken up and negotiated. Appropriately, too, 'cultures' suggests the crossing of boundaries, national as well as conceptual. In that sense these essays beckon us on, not to the 'stale and tasteless' repetition of case studies (as Margaret Mead cautioned against as early as the 1950s when children and childhood were newcomers in the social sciences),[13] but to new untrammeled problems and forms of material for analysis. In sum, they open a door on inquiries beyond *In the Name of the Child.*

Notes

1. Roger Cooter (ed.), *In the Name of the Child: Health and Welfare, 1880-1940* (London: Routledge, 1992).

2. Harry Hendrick, *Children, Childhood and English Society 1880-1990* (Cambridge: Cambridge University Press, 1997), 1.

3. See John Hutchinson, 'Promoting Child Health in the 1920s: International Politics and the Limits of Humanitarianism', paper presented to the conference on 'The Healthy Life', Almunecar, Granada, September 1999.

4. Work in progress by Claudia Casaneda takes the transnational history of children considerably further, by revealing how the national child study literatures of c.1900 were decontextualised as they were brought into the international arena and simultaneously re-contextualised as they were read and incorporated in regionally and nationally organised Child Study programmes. See also Claudia Casaneda, *Worlds in the Making: Child, Body, Globe* (Durham: Duke University Press, forthcoming).

5. Russell Viner and Janet Golden, 'Children's Experiences of Illness', in Roger Cooter and John Pickstone (eds), *Medicine in the Twentieth Century* (Amsterdam: Harwood Academic, 2000), 537-87.

6. The tide is changing, however; see Anthony Fletcher and Stephen Hussey, *Childhood in Question: Children, Parents and the State* (Manchester: Manchester University Press, 1999), which considers the formation of identity and the emotional world of children since the seventeenth century.

7. Harry Hendrick, 'The Child as a Social Actor in Historical Sources: Problems of Identification and Interpretation', in Pia Christensen and Allison James (eds), *Research with Children: Perspectives and*

Practices (London/New York: Falmer Press, 2000), 36-59.

8. Ludmilla Jordanova, *History in Practice* (London: Arnold, 2000), 8.
9. John Pickstone, 'Production, Community, and Consumption: The. Political Economy of Twentieth-Century Medicine', in Cooter and Pickstone (eds), *op. cit.* (note 5), 1-19: 14.
10. See Blake Morrison's novel *As If* (London: Grant, 1997), based on the juvenile kidnap and murder of James Bulger in 1993.
11. Jean Mills and Richard Mills (eds), *Childhood Studies: A Reader in Perspectives of Childhood* (London: Routledge, 2000).
12. Charles Rosenberg, 'Framing Disease: Illness, Society, and History', introduction to his and Janet Golden (eds), *Framing Disease: Studies in Cultural History* (New Brunswick, N.J.: Rutgers, 1992), xiv.
13. Margaret Mead, 'Theoretical Setting – 1954', in Margaret Mead and Martha Wolfenstein (eds), *Childhood in Contemporary Cultures* (Chicago: University of Chicago Press, 1955), 5.

Index

A

Addams, Jane 176
Adler, Alfred (and Adlerian psychology) 135, 139, 143
 delinquency and 196
adolescence (and adolescents) *see* delinquency; puberty; youth
Adolescence 191
adulthood, feeble-minded occupying space between childhood and 151
advertisements, child/infant products (incl. food) 103, 104, 105, 108, 109–11, 114
Advice to a Mother... (1839) 109–10
Advisory Committee on Nutrition 71
Aggressive Youth and Wayward Girls 192
Aichhorn, August 175, 177–8, 181
 delinquency and 193
Aldrich, Anderson and Mary 218
Allbutt, Henry A 109
Allebé, GAN 37, 38
Allenbury's advertisements 109, 110
Allers, Rudolf 139
America 292
 hospital visiting and psycho-medical research 218–19

youth culture and social scientists in 269
Amersfoort, *Zandbergen* in 169, 173, 177, 178
Amstelland 23, 265–85
 early years 266–7
 family afternoons at 275–80
 family criticised at 267–8, 275–80
 paradise lost (1970s) 280–1
 Santpoort and 272
  comparisons between 274–5
Amsterdam
 children's hospital (1865) 34
 Observatiehuis (boy's assessment centre) 169, 171
Anson, Sir William 96
Anstadt, Sera 278
anthropometric measurement 114–20
anti-psychiatric views and adolescence 23, 270
anti-social behaviour
 children, as symptom of emotional disturbance 206
 in families, Netherlands 48–9
Arbeiders Jeugd Centrale (AJC) 43–4, 45
 disbandment (late 1950s) 47
Arbeidswet (1889) 10
artificial feeding 113–14
'assertiveness', extreme and frustrated 136, 137, 140, 142

297